Gene Delivery Systems

DRUGS AND THE PHARMACEUTICAL SCIENCES

A Series of Textbooks and Monographs

Series Editor

Anthony J. Hickey

RTI International, Research Triangle Park, USA

The Drugs and Pharmaceutical Sciences series is designed to enable the pharmaceutical scientist to stay abreast of the changing trends, advances and innovations associated with therapeutic drugs and that area of expertise and interest that has come to be known as the pharmaceutical sciences. The body of knowledge that those working in the pharmaceutical environment have to work with, and master, has been, and continues, to expand at a rapid pace as new scientific approaches, technologies, instrumentations, clinical advances, economic factors and social needs arise and influence the discovery, development, manufacture, commercialization and clinical use of new agents and devices.

Recent Titles in Series

Gene Delivery Systems
Yashwant V. Pathak

Percutaneous Absorption: Drugs, Cosmetics, Mechanisms, Methods
Nina Dragićević and Howard Maibach

Handbook of Pharmaceutical Granulation Technology
Dilip M. Parikh

Biotechnology: the Science, the Products, the Government, the Business
Ronald P. Evens

Filtration and Purification in the Biopharmaceutical Industry, Third Edition
Maik W. Jornitz

Handbook of Drug Metabolism, Third Edition
Paul G. Pearson and Larry Wienkers

The Art and Science of Dermal Formulation Development
Marc Brown and Adrian C. Williams

Pharmaceutical Inhalation Aerosol Technology, Third Edition
Anthony J. Hickey and Sandro R. da Rocha

Good Manufacturing Practices for Pharmaceuticals, Seventh Edition
Graham P. Bunn

Pharmaceutical Extrusion Technology, Second Edition
Isaac Ghebre-Sellassie, Charles E. Martin, Feng Zhang, and James Dinunzio

For more information about this series, please visit: www.crcpress.com/Drugs-and-the-Pharmaceutical-Sciences/book-series/IHCDRUPHASCI

Gene Delivery Systems

Development and Applications

Edited by
Yashwant V. Pathak

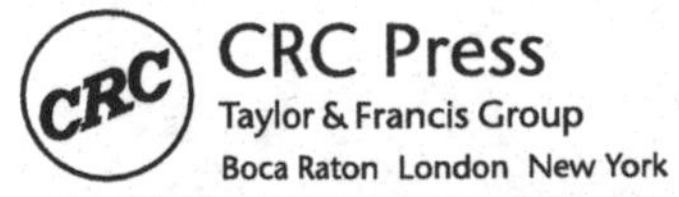

CRC Press is an imprint of the
Taylor & Francis Group, an **informa** business

First edition published 2022
by CRC Press
6000 Broken Sound Parkway NW, Suite 300, Boca Raton, FL 33487–2742

and by CRC Press
2 Park Square, Milton Park, Abingdon, Oxon, OX14 4RN

CRC Press is an imprint of Taylor & Francis Group, LLC

Library of Congress Cataloging-in-Publication Data
[Insert LoC Data here when available]

ISBN: 978-1-032-02550-6 (hbk)
ISBN: 978-1-032-02972-6 (pbk)
ISBN: 978-1-003-18606-9 (ebk)

DOI: 10.1201/9781003186069

Typeset in Times LT Std
by Apex CoVantage, LLC

To the loving memories of my parents and Dr. Keshav Baliram Hedgewar, who gave proper direction to my life; to my beloved wife Seema, who gave positive meaning; and to my son Sarvadaman, who gave a golden lining to my life.

I would like to dedicate this book to the loving memories of Ma Chamanlaljee, Ma Lakshmanraojee Bhide and Ma Madhujee Limaye, who mentored me selflessly and helped me to become a good and socially useful human being.

Yashwant V. Pathak

Contents

Preface

Human gene therapy was in a conceptual stage in the 20th century, but come the 21st century, it has become a reality. The recombinant adeno-associated virus (rAAV) has become a major gene therapy vector and spawned a multibillion dollar industry. With the advent of the COVID-19 pandemic in the last two years, gene therapy has become a great tool to treat new virus infections. Most of the COVID-19 virus vaccines are using messenger RNA (mRNA) technology as a treatment tool.

The possibilities of rAAV gene therapy are continuing to grow. In addition, advances in structural biology provide easier access to the molecular details responsible for cell entry and escape from neutralizing antibodies. This is helping investigators design increasingly sophisticated capsid modification schemes to improve rAAV vector properties. Newer challenges are forthcoming in developing drug delivery systems to deliver various gene-based treatment, including mRNA, small interfering RNA (siRNA) and other gene therapies for treatment of various diseases. These treatments are providing incredible solutions, especially for the treatment of chronic diseases, including cancers and infectious diseases.

There is a lot to be understood about the key molecular interactions of capsids with host factors, and one would anticipate continuing feedback into vector design over the coming years. There are also areas in which the salient molecular interactions remain largely uncharacterized, such as cellular immune responses, and so progress in vector delivery now involves empirical mitigation strategies. It is important to emphasize that identification of the most critical host factors for entry is recent, their characterization is ongoing and exploitation of the emerging understanding for improved vector delivery is only just starting.

In the recent pandemic, two companies used gene-based mRNA technology to develop a vaccine for COVID-19 and successfully administered millions of doses around the world. Using mRNA as a medicine is a fundamentally different approach than treating diseases with other drug classes. mRNA plays a fundamental role in human biology. It is the set of instructions by which cells make proteins and send them to various parts of the body. mRNA medicines take advantage of normal biological processes to express proteins and create a desired therapeutic effect. This enables the potential treatment of a broad spectrum of diseases, many of which cannot be addressed with current technologies.

Seven scientists in the United States and Britain who have come up with a revolutionary gene therapy cure for a rare genetic form of childhood blindness won a 1 million euro ($1.15 million) prize in 2018 from Portugal's Champalimaud Foundation. Their gene augmentation therapy involved the delivery of healthy genes using engineered harmless viruses, described by the foundation as "an elegant solution."

A significant boost to gene therapy research was given in 2020 with the Nobel Prize in Chemistry given to Emmanuelle Charpentier of the Max Planck Unit for the Science of Pathogens and Jennifer Doudna of the University of California, Berkeley, for their discovery of the CRISPR/Cas9 genetic scissors that have revolutionized genome editing.

It is believed that mRNA has the potential to transform how medicines are discovered, developed and manufactured—at a breadth, speed and scale not common in our industry.

This book, titled *Gene Delivery Systems: Development and Applications*, is a collection of 15 chapters written by some of the best scientific minds working in this field. The topics that are covered in this book include an overview of the development of gene therapy, technology involved in gene therapy, clinical applications of siRNA, non-viral vector–based mRNA delivery using nanotechnology, RNA-based vaccines for treating the infectious diseases, CRISPR technology for gene editing and so on.

I am extremely indebted to all the authors who took lot of effort to complete the chapters on time and made sure that all aspects related to gene delivery development and applications are covered. I am aware that gene delivery is a vast area, and it will be hard to cover everything related to this area of research, but the authors of the chapters have done phenomenal work and definitely deserve kudos from readers.

I am extremely thankful to Ms. Hillary Lafoe and Tony Hickey of Taylor & Francis for encouraging me to edit this book. Several people from Taylor & Francis have helped me to bring this to the market. To mention a few, Ms. Danielle Zarfati, Ms. Laura Piedrahita and many others from the press have helped a lot.

I would like to express my sincere thanks to my university authorities and administration of Taneja College of Pharmacy, who have always supported my endeavors in editing books.

I will be failing in my duties if I do not mention my sincere thanks to my family, who always have to compromise their time for such efforts.

Thanks to our readers—they are the ultimate judge of our efforts and provide feedback to improve the book. I am sure it will be a very useful reference book for people who are working in this field. If there are any suggestions to improve the book, please do not hesitate to e-mail me the corrections and they will be implemented in the second edition.

Yashwant V. Pathak, M Pharm, Executive MBA, MSCM, PhD
Professor and Associate Dean for Faculty Affairs
Health Taneja College of Pharmacy, University of South Florida
Adjunct Professor, Faculty of Pharmacy
University of Airlangga, Surabaya Indonesia
E mail: ypathak1@usf.edu

About the Editor

Dr. Yashwant V. Pathak completed a PhD in pharmaceutical technology at Nagpur University, India, and an EMBA and MS in conflict management from Sullivan University. He is professor and associate dean for Faculty Affairs at the College of Pharmacy, University of South Florida, Tampa, Florida. With extensive experience in academia as well as industry, he has more than 100 publications, two patents and two patent applications, and has had 20 edited books published, including 7 books in nanotechnology and 6 in nutraceuticals and drug delivery systems. Dr. Pathak is also a professor of global health with the College of Public Health at USF, and recently his student completed a PhD in global health on homeopathy medicine and its efficacy, based on a survey of 1274 patients in Pune, India.

Contributors

Ismaila Adams
Department of Medical Pharmacology
University of Ghana Medical School
Accra, Ghana

Ofosua Adi-Dako
Department of Pharmaceutics and Microbiology
School of Pharmacy
University of Ghana
Accra, Ghana

Ashish Kumar Agrawal
Department of Pharmaceutical Engineering and Technology
Indian Institute of Technology (BHU)
Varanasi, India

Seth Kwabena Amponsah
Department of Medical Pharmacology
University of Ghana Medical School
Accra, Ghana

Mansi N. Athalye
NLM College of Pharmacy, Ahmadabad
Gujrat, India

Sonia Barua
Chung Ang University
Republic of Korea

Kwasi Agyei Bugyei
Department of Medical Pharmacology
University of Ghana Medical School
Accra, Ghana

Aiswarya Chaudhuri
Department of Pharmaceutical Engineering and Technology
Indian Institute of Technology (BHU)
Varanasi, India

Preetam Dasika
Judy Genshaft Honors College
University of South Florida
Tampa, Florida

Deepa Dehari
Department of Pharmaceutical Engineering and Technology
Indian Institute of Technology (BHU)
Varanasi, India

Khushboo Faldu
Department of Pharmacology
Institute of Pharmacy Nirma University
Ahmedabad, Gujarat, India

Nana Kwame Gyamerah
Department of Pharmaceutics and Microbiology
School of Pharmacy
University of Ghana
Accra, Ghana

Kalpana Joshi
Department of Biotechnology
Sinhgad College of Engineering
Savitribai Phule Pune University
Vadgaon Budruk, Pune
Maharashtra, India

Doris Kumadoh
Department of Pharmaceutics
Centre for Plant Medicine Research
Mampong-Akwapim, Ghana

Robert Moffatt
Florida State University Research Foundation
Tallahassee, Florida

Yuvraj Singh Negi
Indian Institute of Technology Roorkee, Saharanpur Campus
Saharanpur (UP), India

Disha Patel
Postgraduate Research Scholar
Department of Pharmacology, Institute of Pharmacy
Nirma University, Sarkhej
Gujarat, India

Jayvadan K. Patel
Nootan Pharmacy College
Faculty of Pharmacy
Sankalchand Patel University
Visnagar, India

Kshama Patel
Judy Genshaft Honors College
University of South Florida
Tampa, Florida

Manish P. Patel
LM College of Pharmacy
Ahmedabad, India

Mukesh Patel
Experis Engineering
Edina, Minnesota

Yashwant V. Pathak
Taneja College of Pharmacy
University of South Florida
Tampa, Florida
Adjunct Professor at Faculty of Pharmacy
Airlangga University
Surabaya, Indonesia

Sagar A. Popat
LM College of Pharmacy
Ahmedabad, India

Jigna Shah
Department of Pharmacology
Institute of Pharmacy
Nirma University
Ahmedabad, Gujarat, India

Mansi S. Shah
LM College of Pharmacy
Ahmadabad, Gujrat, India

Vandit Shah
Department of Pharmacology
Institute of Pharmacy
Nirma University
Ahmedabad, Gujarat, India

Rakesh Sharma
Florida State University Research Foundation
Tallahassee, Florida
Government Medical College
Saharanpur (UP), India

Sanjay Singh
Department of Pharmaceutical Engineering and Technology
Indian Institute of Technology (BHU)
Varanasi, India

Shashi Prabha Singh
Biochemistry Department
Government Medical College
Saharanpur (UP), India

Sakshi Thassu
Department of Neuroscience
University of Pittsburgh
Pittsburgh, Pennsylvania

Kavita Trimal
Department of Technology
Savitribai Phule Pune University
Pune, Maharashtra, India

Arvind Trivedi
Government Medical College
Saharanpur (UP), India

Govind Vyas
Invahealth, Inc.
Cranbury, New Jersey

1 Overview of Development of Gene Therapy

Ofosua Adi-Dako, Doris Kumadoh, Yashwant V. Pathak and Nana Kwame Gyamerah

CONTENTS

DOI: 10.1201/9781003186069-1

1.1 INTRODUCTION TO GENE THERAPY

The awareness of the genetic basis of disease brought about the concept of "gene therapy." This kind of therapy involved the replacement of abnormal genes with healthy exogenous DNA for the treatment of genetic, neuronal and immune disorders; cancer; blindness; and other diseases with no effective pharmacological and surgical intervention (Maeder & Gersbach, 2016).

The pharmaceutical industry is entering a new era where the underlying cause of a disease is targeted rather than the symptoms in the treatment and management of such diseases (Lee et al., 2017). Many of these diseases are a result of a mutation or deletion of a particular gene (Patil et al., 2018). Gene therapy has the potential to transform medicine by using guided gene transfer to treat human disease, in part because this strategy can treat the disease's fundamental cause rather than just its symptoms, where an exogenic nucleic acid sequence is made to target mutated or affected cells in the body (Lee et al., 2017). Despite repeated setbacks over the years, gene therapy continues to expand and improve as scientists search for new ways to cure some of the world's most severe health problems (Lee et al., 2017).

Gene therapy involves the transfer of genetic material in order to modify a particular phenotype. The application of gene transfer to tissue engineering results in the transient or permanent genetic modification of the engineered tissue to produce proteins for internal, local or systemic use; helping to protect the engineered tissue; and providing stimuli for the engineered tissue to grow and/or differentiate (Keeler, ElMallah, & Flotte, 2017).

Gene therapy has encountered fundamental challenges with respect to its safety, efficacy and precision over the control of the transfer of genetic material. Nevertheless, the technologies for the addition of exogenous healthy genes for treatment have made steady and remarkable progress during this time and a now showing promising clinical results across a range of gene therapy strategies and interventions (Maeder & Gersbach, 2016).

1.2 THE HUMAN GENOME

All living organisms, including humans, have a genome containing all essential biological information required for existence. Human genomes consist of deoxyribonucleic acid (DNA), whereas some viruses have ribonucleic acid (RNA). Aside from the polymeric nature of DNA and RNA, they also contain chains of nucleotides which are monomers or subunits. The nuclear and mitochondrial genomes make up the human genome. Well over 3 million nucleotides of DNA are found in the nuclear genome, which are subsequently divided into 24 chromosomes. The 24 chromosomes comprise 22 autosomes and the two sex hormones, X and Y. However, the mitochondrial genome consists of circular DNA, containing over 16,000 nucleotides, which are found in the mitochondria. The cells in the human body have a unique copy or copies of the genome with the exception of a few cells (e.g., red blood cells).

Moreover, the human genome comprises approximately 20,000 protein-encoding genes that influence biological processes in the body (Brown, 2002; Gibbs, 2020; Hanna, Rémuzat, Auquier, & Toumi, 2017).

1.3 OVERVIEW OF GENE THERAPY

Gene therapy presents a revolutionary approach to the prevention and treatment of previously untreated diseases. This innovative strategy involves the inactivation of a dysfunctional mutated gene, replacement of a disease-causing gene with a healthy gene or the introduction of new genes for the prevention of disease.

Dysfunctional genes cause several rare diseases, often associated with poor prospects of an effective treatment outcome, but this offers the opportunity for gene modifications or correction of abnormal mutated genes for therapeutic treatment. Gene therapy is a promising intervention in the treatment of disorders that are usually unresponsive to conventional drug treatment. In addition, it involves the use of gene designs and suitable delivery mechanisms to ensure expression in the cells of interest or target cells and holds great promise in treating genetic disorders (Hanna et al., 2017; Kumar, Markusic, Biswas, High, & Herzog, 2016).

Disorders that are alleviated with the use of gene therapy include inherited disorders; recessive gene disorders such as sickle cell anemia; hemophilia; cystic fibrosis; and acquired genetic diseases such as cancer, viral infections, ocular, hematological and neurodegenerative diseases. In this case, genes are introduced into a patient's cells to induce the expression of healthy genes or for the production of therapeutic proteins to modulate genetic disorders (Gonçalves & Paiva, 2017; Sung & Kim, 2019).

Techniques such as recombinant DNA technology are applicable in this regard, whereby the healthy gene or normal gene is inserted into the genome to replace an abnormal or disease-causing gene with the help of a carrier or a vector, which could be viral or non-viral (Gonçalves & Paiva, 2017).

1.4 STRATEGIES IN GENE THERAPY AND GENE DELIVERY SYSTEMS

Gene therapy entails either delivering fully active genes (gene transfer) or blocking native gene expression by transfecting cells with short nucleic acid chains (oligonucleotides). These single-stranded DNA molecules are utilized in medicine to prevent mRNA- or DNA-binding proteins from becoming inactive (Xiang, Oo, Lee, Li, & Loh, 2017). The vector may be transferred ex vivo, where the modified gene is transferred into the particular cell of interest and then the modified cell is then restored into the patient, or in vivo, where the modified gene is directly administered into the patient (Gowing, Svendsen, & Svendsen, 2017). Gene therapy is a simple concept but difficult to implement. The design of the vector, how the vector is delivered to the cell population of interest, translocating the vector/expression cassette from outside the cell to the nucleus and the expression of the gene to achieve the desired therapeutic effect are all major issues relating to successful gene therapy (Sinclair, Islam, & Jones, 2019). Independent of the gene transfer vector's choice and design, successful gene therapy necessitates decisions about the amount of vector needed to change the number of target cells required to achieve the desired therapeutic effect, as well as consideration of whether the vector will elicit a host immune response and/or cause unacceptable toxicity. The gene therapist must also consider how to get the vector to the target cells, as well as the vector's targeting specificity and affinity for the relevant receptor (Sinclair et al., 2019). The gene cargo within the vector must be translocated from outside the cell to within the nucleus once it reaches the cells of interest. It is critical to decide whether the gene will be inserted into the target cells' chromosomal DNA when designing the gene transfer strategy. Finally, the transferred gene must be expressed, which raises issues such as the amount and control of expression, as well as host immunity and toxicity that may be triggered by the gene's expression (Lundstrom, 2018).

1.5 EX VIVO AND IN VIVO GENE THERAPY

Ex vivo transfer of genetic material with later transfer of the transformed cells or tissue to the host and in vivo transfer with direct injection of the gene therapy vectors to the patient are the two most common procedures for genetic engineering using gene therapy technology (Sharma, Arora, Singh, & Layek, 2021).

1.6 EX VIVO GENE THERAPY

Cells are obtained from the patient's own body (autologous) or from other healthy people in an ex vivo delivery system (allogeneic or donor), which are then purified, enhanced and/or activated outside the body using genetic engineering tools before being transplanted back into the patient, which then proliferate and spread throughout the body (Gowing et al., 2017). The ex vivo technique permits a gene or genes to be transferred to a specific cell subpopulation without impacting other cells or organs; however, the vectors utilized must be able to integrate the genetic material into the genome for long-term therapeutic effect (Sinclair et al., 2019).

1.7 IN VIVO GENE THERAPY

Direct injection of the gene therapy agent into the body is known as in vivo gene therapy. In vivo gene therapy can be given intravenously, injected into muscles, infused or injected into an organ or physiological structure or injected directly into a tumor, depending on the vector and the target (Sinclair et al., 2019).

1.8 VECTORS IN GENE THERAPY

Modified forms of natural viruses and plasmids are among the vectors used in gene therapy (Hardee, Arévalo-Soliz, Hornstein, & Zechiedrich, 2017). Viruses have been changed to replace disease-causing genes with the gene(s) to be transmitted and the sequences that control its expression, while preserving the viral envelope or coat, which promotes transfer (Sauderson, Castro, & Lowenstein, 2013). Plasmids are DNA segments with no natural coat or envelope that can be enclosed in a manufactured lipid membrane or polymer to promote transmission. Commonly used DNA viruses are adeno-associated viruses (AAVs) (a non-pathogenic but abundant tiny virus); adenoviruses (responsible for upper respiratory infections); and herpesviruses. Retroviral vectors produced from lentiviruses (such as human immunodeficiency virus 1 [HIV-1]) and gamma-retroviruses are examples of RNA viruses, which can all integrate a DNA copy of their genetic material into the host genome (Yazdani, Alirezaie, Motamedi, & Amani, 2018).

The choice of vectors depends on the size of the gene or genes it can carry, the target cells (dividing or non-dividing and cell type), whether the virus will insert into the target cells' genome or remain separate and the antibody status of potential patients (Lundstrom, 2018). Because the gene is kept after cell division, insertion into the genome provides the most long-lasting expression (Gowing et al., 2017). Controlling the insertion site is crucial, because putting the gene in the wrong place can result in the inserted gene not being expressed (if it inserts into a silenced section of the genome) or tumors emerging from the disruption or activation of nearby genes implicated in cancer development (Sauderson et al., 2013).

1.9 RETROVIRUSES

Retroviruses such as HIV are viruses that can transform RNA genomes into double-stranded DNA and integrate into the chromosomes of their host cells (Keeler et al., 2017). One issue with retrovirus-based gene therapy is that the integrase enzyme can insert the virus's genome into any position in the host genome (Sauderson et al., 2013). If the genetic material is put in the middle of one of the host cell's main genes, the gene's function will be harmed (insertional mutation) (Yazdani et al., 2018). If a gene is inserted during the cell division process, the result is uncontrolled cell division (cancer) (Yazdani et al., 2018). The use of zinc finger nucleases and particular sequences such as the beta globin control region has helped to alleviate this challenge in part by directing the insertion of the gene into specific chromosomal locations (Lundstrom, 2018).

1.10 ADENOVIRUSES

This group of viruses has a double-stranded DNA genome and infects people in the respiratory, digestive and ophthalmic systems (Oliveira, da Costa, & Silva, 2017). When these viruses infect a cell, they insert their DNA molecules into the host, yet the adenovirus's genetic material does not integrate with the host cell's genetic material. Instead, the DNA molecule remains inside the nucleus of the host cell, where it is transcribed like any other gene (Lundstrom, 2018). The sole difference with adenoviruses is that the foreign genes are not reproduced when the host cell divides; as a result, cells produced during division will lack extra genes. As a result, treating a growing cell population with adenoviruses necessitates reinjecting them (Yazdani et al., 2018).

1.11 ADENO-ASSOCIATED VIRUSES

AAVs are a small group of viruses that have single-stranded, uncoated DNA. They can infect both dividing and non-dividing cells and produce constitutive expression in both (Naso, Tomkowicz, Perry, & Strohl, 2017). These viruses are a good possibility for gene therapy since they can be found in cells in both lysogenic and lytic forms (Naso et al., 2017). Another notable aspect of these viruses is their lack of pathogenicity for humans in the absence of auxiliary viruses such as adenoviruses and herpes viruses, and these viruses can insert their genetic material into a specific place on chromosome 19 in the absence of auxiliary viruses (Naso et al., 2017).

1.12 HERPES SIMPLEX VIRUS

Viruses in this class infect a specific type of brain cell with double-stranded DNA. Cold sores and fever blisters are caused by type 1 herpesvirus infection, which is a common human pathogen. Herpes simplex virus (HSV) is a human neurotropic virus that is mostly used in the neurological system for gene transfer (Sauderson et al., 2013). Although the wild HSV-1 virus can infect neurons and evade the host's immune response, it can also be inactivated, resulting in a lytic cycle of viral reproduction, and as a result, a mutant HSV-1 strain that cannot replicate is commonly employed (Lundstrom, 2018).

1.13 NON-VIRAL METHODS

Non-viral approaches are now more advantageous than viral ways (Keeler et al., 2017). The advantages are ease of manufacture on a large scale and fewer immune responses by the host (host immune system reactions) (Xiang et al., 2017). Previously, the method's shortcomings were thought to be the high degree of transfection and low gene expression (Helal et al., 2017). However, recent advancements in vector technology have resulted in the development of compounds and techniques that are as effective as viral techniques (Helal et al., 2017).

1.14 ORMASIL

Another non-viral way is to employ ormasil (silica or modified organic silicate), and because of its relative ease of use, silica has become a popular choice for gene delivery (Rejeeth & Vivek, 2017). Due to its toxicity, the most frequent approach of employing silica in gene therapy is to combine nanoparticles with amino silicones (Rejeeth & Vivek, 2017). However, because of the reaction between serum proteins as a limiting factor, administration in the presence of serum lowers the efficacy of this approach (Yazdani et al., 2018).

1.15 INJECTION OF NAKED DNA

The simplest non-viral transmission approach is to inject naked DNA. Despite the fact that clinical studies of this technology were successful, gene expression is significantly lower than with other methods (Yazdani et al., 2018). Experiments with naked polymerase chain reaction (PCR) products have been carried out in addition to those with plasmids, and the absorption of bare DNA by cells is often ineffective (Keeler et al., 2017). As a result, researchers have worked on enhancing DNA absorption efficiency, leading to the invention of new methods such as electroporation, sonoporation and the use of the "gene gun," which introduces DNA coated with gold particles into a cell with helium gas at high pressure (Oliveira et al., 2017).

1.16 DEVELOPMENTS IN GENE THERAPY AND GENE DELIVERY SYSTEMS

Genetic material such as anti-sense oligonucleotides, DNA and mRNA are introduced into dysfunctional cell or tissues for the restoration of appropriate genetic function or to eliminate a defective gene causing a disorder (Goswami et al., 2019).

Genetic material is usually delivered to the nucleus of the cell. The transfection process involves the use of two kinds of vectors: viral and non-viral vectors. The vector is the vehicle for the delivery of genetic material. Ideally, delivery of the genetic material to the target cell should subsequently result in the expression of the gene product without toxicity to the cell. Viral vectors are rendered safe by making them unable to replicate and are able to infect cells via the transfer of DNA without triggering an immune response.

Transduction involves the transfer of genes via viral vectors, while the use of non-viral vectors is transfection. Oral delivery of genes through the introduction of DNA by calcium phosphate, liposomes, lipid or protein complexes is referred to as chemical transfection.

Formulation of a liposome or lipid vector is the combination of plasmid DNA and a lipid solution. These lipid vectors introduce plasmid DNA into the nucleus, after merging with the cell membrane, for the expression of the gene of interest. Physical transfection is achieved through microinjection; parenteral injections; aerosols; and electroporation, where high-voltage electrical current is delivered to the cells, pores are formed and the gene of interest is introduced into the cell (Mali, 2013).

Recent reports indicate the use of viral vectors or viral gene delivery systems based on RNA, DNA and oncolytic vectors. The non-viral gene delivery systems employ physicochemical techniques involving polysaccharides, cationic polymers and poly-L-lysine. Challenges with gene delivery are constantly being investigated and evaluated for improvement (Sung & Kim, 2019)

1.17 PHYSICAL METHODS FOR IMPROVING DNA TRANSFER

1.17.1 Electroporation

Electroporation is a technique for transferring DNA from cell membranes that involves a high-voltage brief pulse, where small pores are produced on the membrane's surface temporarily as a result of the electrical shock, making it permeable to nucleic acid (Oliveira et al., 2017). Although electroporation can be used on a wide range of cell types, high rates of cell death have limited its usage in clinical settings (Yazdani et al., 2018).

1.17.2 Gene Gun

Another physical approach for DNA transfer is particle bombardment, sometimes known as a gene gun, where the DNA is coated with gold particles and then placed into a device that provides the necessary force to enter the cell in this procedure (Sharma et al., 2021). However, if the DNA is in the wrong place in the genome, such as in a tumor suppressor gene, it can cause a tumor to form (Oliveira et al., 2017). This approach was tested in clinical studies on patients with X-linked severe immunodeficiency (X-SCID), where hematopoietic stem cells (HSCs) were infected with a retrovirus harboring the modifying gene, and T-cell leukemia was successfully treated in 3 out of 20 patients (Yazdani et al., 2018).

1.17.3 Magnetofection

DNA is complexed with magnetic particles in magnetofection, and a magnet is put beneath the cellular tissue culture container to expose the DNA-containing compound to only one cell layer. The therapeutic gene is linked to magnetic nanoparticles in this technology, which is based on the notion of targeted medication delivery. The complex deposition and transfection rate are additionally accelerated by the electromagnetic field gradient produced by the ground beneath the cell culture medium (Oliveira et al., 2017). In vivo, the gene-magnetic complex is given intravenously, and it is absorbed and approaches the target with the help of strong external magnets and finally, intermolecular restriction enzymes, charge interaction or matrix degradation are used to isolate the gene from the magnetic particles (Yazdani et al., 2018). This method is frequently used in laboratory investigations to transfer a gene to primary cells and other cells to which previous methods are ineffective (Sharma et al., 2021).

1.17.4 Sonoporation

Ultrasonic frequency is used to introduce DNA to a cell in sonoporation, which results in DNA movement in the cell and is referred to as ultrasound cavitation in the cell membrane (Sharma et al., 2021).

1.18 CHEMICAL METHODS FOR IMPROVING DNA TRANSFER

1.18.1 Oligonucleotides

Gene therapy employs synthetic oligonucleotides to deactivate and inactivate genes implicated in the disease process (Yazdani et al., 2018). The use of specific antisense for the target gene prevents defective genes from being transcribed. Another option is to employ small interfering RNA (siRNA), which causes a specific sequence of the faulty gene's messenger RNA (mRNA) to break down, halting translation and, consequently, expression (Xiang et al., 2017).

1.19 DENDRIMERS

The dendrimer is a branching spherical macromolecule in which the particle surface can be charged in a variety of ways, and it determines many features of the particle's final structure (Sharma et al., 2021). The extra charge causes a brief nucleic acid connection with the cationic dendrimer in the presence of genetic material such as DNA or RNA. Endocytosis allows the nucleic acid–dendrimer complex to enter the cell (Oliveira et al., 2017).

1.20 LIPOPLEXES AND POLYPLEXES

A polyplex is a mixture of DNA and cationic polymers, which are formed by particle buildup caused by polyplex interactions. DNA should be safeguarded from damage and a positive charge to facilitate fresh DNA transport to the cell. As a result, anionic and neutral liposomes are used as synthetic vectors for the creation of lipoplexes (Rasoulianboroujeni et al., 2017).

1.21 HYBRID METHODS

Each method of gene transfer has its own drawbacks; as a result, hybrid methods, which combine numerous procedures, are being developed. A hybrid method is a virosome, which is made up of a liposome and an inactive HIV or influenza virus. In pulmonary epithelial cells, this hybrid technique of gene delivery is more efficient than the viral or liposome method alone. This strategy entails combining several viral vectors with cationic liposomes or hybrid viruses in general (Yazdani et al., 2018).

1.22 CHALLENGES WITH GENE THERAPY AND GENE DELIVERY

One challenge encountered in gene therapy is associated with the release of the healthy gene into the cell. The carrier or vector used should have the required characteristics. It should:

i. Have high specificity
ii. Exhibit efficiency when releasing the appropriate size of gene
iii. Not be seen as a foreign body by the host's system

iv. Show capability of being purified in high concentrations on an industrial scale
v. Should not induce allergic reactions in the host
vi. Should be non-inflammatory to the host's system
vii. Enhance normal functions with the delivery of the gene
viii. Correct the abnormality or deficiency
ix. Be safe for the patient and the health professionals handling it and the environment
x. Have the ability to express the gene of interest for the entire lifespan of the host

Findings from studies have confirmed the benefits and efficacy of viral vectors. However, there are some limitations to be addressed. For example, the presence of viral genetic material in the plasmid could trigger an acute immune response, coupled with probable oncogenic and epigenic alterations. Some of the limitations associated with the transfer of genes to the desired target sites are poor efficacy of gene transfer and safety issues such as immunogenicity and toxicity (Gonçalves & Paiva, 2017).

1.23 GENE EDITING TECHNOLOGIES

1.23.1 Genome Editing for Gene Therapy

The addition of genes to human cells is essential for gene therapy; however, the development of genome editing technologies, where the human genome could be manipulated, presents various strategies to obtain a therapeutic effect. Hence, the correction of mutations that cause genetic disease, or the addition of genes to certain sites in the human genome or the elimination of harmful genome sequences is made possible with the adoption of these technologies (Maeder & Gersbach, 2016).

1.24 THE GENE EDITING APPROACH

The basis of gene editing is the realization that targeted DNA double-strand breaks could be used to stimulate endogenous cellular repair pathways. Homology directed repair or non-homologous end joining pathways are key in the repair of DNA breaks. After the strand invasion of the broken end into a homologous sequence, mechanisms of varied genome editing strategies demonstrate the available common nuclease-based platforms such as the CRISPR/Cas9 system and transcription activator–like effector nucleases zinc finger nucleases (TALENs) and meganucleases (Maeder & Gersbach, 2016).

1.24.1 Basic Gene Therapy Approaches

Some genetic approaches in gene therapy are (1) gene addition, (2) gene correction, (3) gene silencing and (4) cell elimination techniques. With gene addition, a new gene such as plasmid DNA is added into the desired target cells for the formation of new proteins. This kind of gene therapy is being investigated to treat hemophilia or congenital blindness.

Gene correction makes use of gene editing to remove defective aspects of the gene or a dysfunctional DNA portion is replaced. In effect, gene repair aims at producing a functional protein and inhibits the expression of defective and dysfunctional proteins. Recent developments indicate that gene correction could be employed in removing HIV from infected mice and in correcting genes in Huntington's disease.

Gene silencing involves the use of certain sequences of RNA to bind to the target mRNA. Consequently, the double-strand DNA that is produced is degraded. This is an effective strategy in treating disease caused by the overexpression of a protein.

Cell elimination techniques are effective in destroying cancer cells and benign tumors. Oncotropic viruses are carriers for genes that cause cancer cell death (Alhakamy, Curiel, & Berkland, 2021; Hanna et al., 2017).

1.25 CELLULAR GENE THERAPY

Cellular gene therapy involves the transfer of genetic material into the target cells, where the altered cells are expected to provide the much-needed therapeutic effect. For instance, genetically engineered stem cells are effective in improving conditions such as the need for continuous administration of enzymes or transfusion. Cellular gene therapy is being used to treat not only hereditary or genetic diseases but also acquired disorders. For instance T cells are useful in cancer immunotherapy (Alhakamy et al., 2021).

1.26 SOMATIC AND GERMLINE THERAPY

Gene therapy can be done directly in body cells (somatic) or in the egg or sperm cells (germline) to pass on the change to future generations. The genome is altered by targeting somatic cells, but the change is not handed down to progeny. Because the alterations to the genome of a patient's egg or sperm are created in germline gene therapy, they will be passed down to the offspring, preventing hereditary disease in future generations. While somatic cell gene therapy is being actively pursued, germline gene therapy is not being actively pursued, in part due to ethical concerns about permanently altering an unborn child's genome (Patil et al., 2018).

1.27 ADVANTAGES AND DISADVANTAGES OF GENE THERAPY

1.27.1 Advantages of Gene Therapy

- Gene therapy may offer a cure to terminal illnesses and not just palliative treatment.
- Gene therapy has the potential to remove and prevent inherited disorders like cystic fibrosis, as well as to treat heart disease, acquired immunodeficiency syndrome (AIDS), and cancer (Patil et al., 2018).

1.27.2 Disadvantages of Gene Therapy

- Gene therapy is very expensive to undertake, which may be a hindering factor preventing people from partaking in it.
- It involves too much uncertainty and scientific risks, and the long-term effects are also unknown (Patil et al., 2018).

1.28 ETHICAL ISSUES CONCERNING GENE THERAPY

Some plaguing questions raised with respect to gene therapy and which have to be addressed are:

- Who will decide which characteristics are normal and which are abnormal?
- Will gene therapy be restricted to wealth creation (economic issues)?
- Is it possible that the spread of gene therapy will reduce the social acceptance of people who are different?
- Should humans be allowed to use gene therapy to enhance important characteristics like height, intelligence or athletic ability? (Riva & Petrini, 2019)

1.29 APPLICATIONS OF GENE THERAPY

Pharmaceutical companies and healthcare agencies are actively involved in current developments in gene therapy. The number of clinical trials investigating gene therapies has increased dramatically, and numerous products have been approved for use (Alhakamy et al., 2021; Hanna et al., 2017).

1.30 DISEASES TARGETED BY GENE THERAPIES

1.30.1 Parkinson's Disease

The effectiveness of gene therapy in Parkinson's disease (PD) has been proved, according to independent research. One of the proposed approaches, for example, raises the level of gamma-aminobutyric acid (GABA) in the brain, a neurotransmitter whose absence causes PD (Kirik, Cederfjäll, Halliday, & Petersén, 2017). Tubes were implanted in the parts of the brain linked with movement in 45 participants with severe PD. Half of the individuals received viruses containing a gene that boosts GABA synthesis, while the other half received a harmless saline solution (as the control group) (Yazdani et al., 2018).

1.30.2 Diabetic Neuropathy

Researchers discovered that gene therapy is promising in the treatment of diabetic polyneuropathy, a prevalent condition caused by persistent diabetes. The intramuscular injection of a vascular endothelial growth factor (VEGF) gene by Boston researchers may assist diabetic neuropathy patients. In this study, 39 patients received three VEGF injections in one leg and 11 patients received placebo injections. Diabetic neuropathy causes leg and foot discomfort, weakness and balance issues. A decrease in touch sensitivity makes it more likely that a foot ulcer may go undetected, leading to amputation. The majority of the patients in the study had severe neuropathy with little possibility of rehabilitation (Yazdani et al., 2018).

1.30.3 Cancer Treatment

Over the last two decades, advances in human genomes have revealed that cancer is caused by abnormalities in the host genome's somatic cells. As a result of these accomplishments, many cancer researchers are turning to medicines based on genetic manipulation and modification to treat cancer and find a potential cure. Gene therapy employing viral (or bacterial) vectors or non-viral vectors, rousing the immune system against tumor cells (immunomodulation), manipulating the tumor cell to diminish tumor tissue and boosting antigens for improved tumor detection by the host's immune system are all examples. The number of treatments with few side effects has increased in general. New-generation viral or non-viral vectors considerably reduce the hazards associated with prior cancer therapy approaches, such as retrovirus integration with the danger of mutagenicity or malignancy, immune reaction against viruses, tumor formation, medication resistance or disease relapse (Yazdani et al., 2018).

Different types of cancer have been the prime focus in clinical trial investigations. Research in skin, blood, breast, prostate, thyroid and gastrointestinal cancers has been conducted for the development of new therapies for gene delivery. A reported 62.5% of gene therapy clinical trials were in the field of cancer research. Applications in genetic diseases such as hemophilia, ocular diseases, cystic fibrosis, sickle cell diseases and thalassemia have also been witnessed, making up 20.6% of gene therapies for inherited diseases. Gene therapy trials for cardiovascular diseases consisted of 5%, infectious diseases 3.9% and other diseases 5.3% (Alhakamy et al., 2021).

1.31 GENE THERAPY CLINICAL TRIALS

In the early stages of gene therapy, there were setbacks such as undesirable immune responses, developmental hurdles, off-target effects, mutagenesis and obsolete regulatory practice applicability, which slowed down progress. However, recently there has been a rebound in momentum due to advancements in gene therapy and editing techniques, leading to a steady rise in research output and gene therapy clinical trials. The successes marked in this area have created a heightened interest in the pharmaceutical and biotechnological fields (Aiuti & Roncarolo, 2009; Baruteau, Waddington, Alexander, & Gissen, 2017; Clément & Grieger, 2016).

More than 2,600 gene therapy clinical trials had been completed, are in progress or have been approved globally. In 2017, for instance, there was an increased percentage of trials about to begin the final phases, but most trials were in phase I and II. These early phase trials demonstrated the proof of concept of gene therapy. Strategies in immunotherapy were also evaluated and had promising potential. Autologous T cells were modified for tumor recognition by using gamma retroviral vectors and were targeted at tumor-associated antigens (Ginn, Amaya, Alexander, Edelstein, & Abedi, 2018; Rakoczy et al., 2015).

The use of chimeric antigen receptor (CAR) T cells in cancer immunotherapy was used to target tumor-associated cell surface antigens. This approach highlights the long-term effects of cytotoxic T cells specific for monoclonal antibodies to help in combating tumors where other cancer therapies had been deemed unsuccessful (Ginn et al., 2018).

Since 2017 to now, 11.1% of clinical trials were aimed at monogenic disease conditions. Clinical trials focused on cystic fibrosis confirmed the use of non-viral gene therapy in improving lung function in a randomized, double-blind, placebo controlled trial. In the study, 78 patients were administered plasmid DNA encoding the *CFTR* complementary DNA (cDNA) complexed with a cationic liposome via lung delivery, after which modest results were obtained. The findings laid a good foundation for further trials (Alton et al., 2015). Clinical trials involving primary immune deficiencies have been showing progress. More than 150 patients have been treated for these disorders with the help of gamma-retroviral and lentiviral gene transfer (Thrasher & Williams, 2017). With regard to adenosine deaminase deficiency (ADA-SCID), over 40 patients have received treatment. More than 70% of these patients experienced a disease-free survival rate (Aiuti, Roncarolo, & Naldini, 2017; Ginn, Alexander, Edelstein, Abedi, & Wixon, 2013; Ginn et al., 2018; Ylä-Herttuala, 2016).

1.32 APPROVED PRODUCTS FOR GENE THERAPY

Gene therapy, as stated by the U.S. Food and Drug Administration (FDA), is the "transcription and/or translation of transferred genetic material and/or integration [of such material] into the host genome and that are administered as nucleic acids, viruses, or genetically engineered microorganisms."

The European Medicines Agency (EMA) also explains a gene therapy medicinal product (GTMP) to be a

> biological medicinal product that contains an active substance which contains or consists of a recombinant nucleic acid used in or introduced into humans to regulate, repair, replace, add, or delete genetic sequences, and its therapeutic, prophylactic, or diagnostic effect relates directly to the recombinant nucleic acid sequence it contains or to the product of gene expression of this sequence.
>
> (Alhakamy et al., 2021)

The improvement of gene vectors and the growth in CAR T-cell immunotherapy strategies, coupled with advances in genome editing technology, have enabled gene therapy to make steady progress. Because of this, more options for clinical therapy of genetic diseases and tumors have become prominent

As of August 2019, 22 gene medicines had been approved by the drug regulatory agencies from different countries. After 2015, with the eminent progress in gene therapy, a dramatic rise in the number of approved gene therapy drugs was observed (Goswami et al., 2019; Naldini, 2015; Wang, Tai, & Gao, 2019). For instance, with Zalmoxis, allogeneic T cells modified with a retroviral vector are beneficial in strengthening the immune system after stem cell transplantation. This therapy was approved by the EMA (Farkas et al., 2017).

Strimvelis is the first corrective ex vivo gene therapy approved for human use by the EMA. It consists of autologous CD34 cells modified to express human adenosine deaminase (ADA), and is useful for the treatment of SCID resulting from ADA deficiency (Hoggatt, 2016; Schimmer & Breazzano, 2016; Stirnadel-Farrant et al., 2018).

The FDA approved both Exondys 51 (eteplirsen) and Spinraza (nusinersen) as antisense oligodeoxynucleotide drugs. Spinraza is useful for the treatment of spinal muscular atrophy and Exondys 51 for Duchenne muscular dystrophy (Aartsma-Rus & Goemans, 2019; Glascock, Lenz, Hobby, & Jarecki, 2017; Korinthenberg, 2019; Ottesen, 2017).

In 2017 the FDA authorized three gene therapy drugs and the Korea Ministry of Food and Drug Safety (MFDS) authorized a gene therapy drug (Morrison, 2019).

Kymriah (tisagenlecleucel) and Yescarta (axicabtagene ciloleucel) were the first CD-19–targeted CAR T-cell immunotherapies approved by the FDA in 2017. Gene therapy with Yescarta involved a CD-19 gene being transferred into recently harvested T cells from a patient (Chow, Shadman, & Gopal, 2018; Yip & Webster, 2018). Kymriah was effective as a CAR T-cell and gene therapy product for the treatment of relapsed B-cell acute lymphoblastic leukemia and is useful for patients under the age of 25 years (Bach, Giralt, & Saltz, 2017; Dolgin, 2017; Maude et al., 2018; Prasad, 2018; Schuster et al., 2019); it is also indicated for adult patients with relapsed or refractory large B-cell lymphoma (Bouchkouj et al., 2019; Locke et al., 2019; Neelapu et al., 2017; Quintás-Cardama, 2018).

Luxturna (voretigene neparvovec-rzyl) was also authorized as an rAAV-based gene therapy drug for the treatment of confirmed biallelic RPE65 mutation–associated retinal dystrophy (Dias et al., 2018; Russell et al., 2017).

The first gene therapy product in Korea, Invossa, consisting of human allogeneic chondrocytes modified with a transforming growth factor-beta 1 (TGF-β1) gene, was authorized by MFSD for therapy in knee osteoarthritis (Evans, Ghivizzani, & Robbins, 2018a, 2018b).

In 2018 one RNA interference (RNAi) drug and one antisense RNA drug were approved by drug regulatory agencies. Both Onpattro and Tegsedi were approved for the treatment of hereditary transthyretin amyloidosis. Onpattro (Patisiran) an RNAi drug, was approved by the FDA and EMA. Tegsedi (inotersen), which is an antisense RNA drug, was also approved by the EMA in July 2018 and the FDA and Health Canada in October 2018 (Chakradhar, 2018).

Subsequently by August 2019, four new gene therapy drugs were approved by the Japan Ministry of Health, Labour and Welfare (MHLW); FDA; and EMA, respectively:

- Collategene, a naked plasmid encoding human HGF gene, was developed for the treatment of critical limb ischemia (CLI) (Suda, Murakami, Kaga, Tomioka, & Morishita, 2014).
- Zolgensma (onasemnogene abeparvovec-xioi) is an a rAAV-based gene therapy drug indicated in pediatric patients with SMA and biallelic mutation in the survival motor neuron (SMN) 1 gene (Hoy, 2019).
- Waylivra (volanesorsen), an antisense oligonucleotide inhibitor of apolipoprotein CIII (apoCIII) mRNA, was used for the treatment of adult patients with familial chylomicronemia syndrome (Paik & Duggan, 2019).
- Zynteglo, a genetically modified autologous $CD34^+$ cell-enriched population that contained HSCs modified with lentiviral vector encoding the $\beta^{A\text{-}T87Q}$-globin gene, has been used for patients 12 years and older with transfusion-dependent β-thalassemia (Cavero, Seimetz, Koziel, Zimmermann, & Holzgrefe, 2020; Ma, Wang, Xu, He, & Wei, 2020).

1.33 THE WAY FORWARD AND THE FUTURE OF GENE THERAPY

The viability of gene therapy has shown great promise, even though there have been constructive debates over the associated moral and ethical issues. There have been positive prospects for the treatment of congenital disease, monogenic disease and cancer, where pharmacological and surgical interventions have not provided the optimal therapeutic outcome (Gonçalves & Paiva, 2017).

Significant strides made in addressing the challenges of conventional gene therapy include the development of new technologies for the precise modification of the human genome. This has helped to unravel solutions for challenges that have plagued the field of gene therapy for years (Maeder & Gersbach, 2016).

Moreover, the field of gene therapy has gained momentum due to advances in gene delivery systems and breakthroughs in genome editing. CRISPR/Cas and other editing technologies have demonstrated unprecedented precision and control. It appears that, for now, approved gene therapies have attracted a high price tag. It is expected that as more products are successfully approved for treatment, the price would also be reduced accordingly.

Regulators have considered precise ways to accelerate access to these new therapies, thereby improving the regulatory process for manufacturers and healthcare professionals (Alhakamy et al., 2021). Challenges due to safety concerns and delivery are being considered to experience the full potential of genome editing for gene and cell therapy. Advances made in this area address these issues by increasing the specificity of genome editing tools and improving the sensitivity of methods required in this regard. Other ways to enhance the safety and efficiency of gene transfer vectors through vector design have been explored and investigated. The design of new vectors for improved efficiency, targeting and specificity and the safety of drug delivery systems are being investigated continually, as these are essential for vector accuracy in targeting T tissues and cell types, with the elimination of off-target effects. Improving vectors would prevent the undesirable stimulation of both the innate and adaptive immune system and provide reproducibility and durable transgene expression (Alhakamy et al., 2021; Gonçalves & Paiva, 2017; Maeder & Gersbach, 2016).

Gene therapy has demonstrated its applications in providing hope for the unmet needs in inherited, degenerative, infectious and other diseases. Several clinical trial models are still being evaluated for the rapid transition of in vivo and ex vivo gene therapy to patients. Since the first approval of gene therapy trials by the National Institutes of Health (NIH) more than 30 years ago, there is still cutting-edge research in gene therapy, which has resulted in various products for the treatment of disorders such as neuronal and immune disorders and blindness.

Originally gene therapies were based on transgene delivery. Gene editing technologies are now based on the precise alteration of human genome sequences. In effect, innovation has led to the next-generation editing technologies with improvement in the accuracy, precision, efficacy and applicability to different disorders.

Currently gene therapy clinical trials, approved products and growing expertise in this exciting field of therapy have experienced significant momentum There are evident possibilities, capabilities with remarkable control over the delivery of nucleic acids and precise modification of human genome technologies.

With such emerging prospects, gene therapy continues to dominate research solutions for previously untreated diseases, leading to new technologies and expanding the scope of genome editing to address the unmet needs in the treatment of disease (Alhakamy et al., 2021; Maeder & Gersbach, 2016).

REFERENCES

Aartsma-Rus, A., & Goemans, N. (2019). A sequel to the eteplirsen saga: Eteplirsen is approved in the United States but was not approved in Europe. *Nucleic Acid Therapeutics, 29*(1), 13–15.

Aiuti, A., & Roncarolo, M. G. (2009). Ten years of gene therapy for primary immune deficiencies. *ASH Education Program Book, 2009*(1), 682–689.

Aiuti, A., Roncarolo, M. G., & Naldini, L. (2017). Gene therapy for ADA-SCID, the first marketing approval of an ex vivo gene therapy in Europe: Paving the road for the next generation of advanced therapy medicinal products. *EMBO Molecular Medicine, 9*(6), 737–740.

Alhakamy, N. A., Curiel, D. T., & Berkland, C. J. (2021). The era of gene therapy: From preclinical development to clinical application. *Drug Discovery Today*. https://doi.org/10.1016/j.drudis.2021.03.021

Alton, E. W., Armstrong, D. K., Ashby, D., Bayfield, K. J., Bilton, D., Bloomfield, E. V., . . . Calcedo, R. (2015). Repeated nebulisation of non-viral CFTR gene therapy in patients with cystic fibrosis: A randomised, double-blind, placebo-controlled, phase 2b trial. *The Lancet Respiratory Medicine, 3*(9), 684–691.

Bach, P. B., Giralt, S. A., & Saltz, L. B. (2017). FDA approval of tisagenlecleucel: Promise and complexities of a $475 000 cancer drug. *JAMA, 318*(19), 1861–1862.

Baruteau, J., Waddington, S. N., Alexander, I. E., & Gissen, P. (2017). Gene therapy for monogenic liver diseases: Clinical successes, current challenges and future prospects. *Journal of Inherited Metabolic Disease, 40*(4), 497–517.

Bouchkouj, N., Kasamon, Y. L., de Claro, R. A., George, B., Lin, X., Lee, S., . . . Pazdur, R. (2019). FDA approval summary: Axicabtagene ciloleucel for relapsed or refractory large B-cell lymphoma. *Clinical Cancer Research, 25*(6), 1702–1708.

Brown, T. A. (2002). The human genome. In *Genomes* (2nd ed.). Wiley-Liss.

Cavero, I., Seimetz, D., Koziel, D., Zimmermann, W.-H., & Holzgrefe, H. H. (2020). 19th Annual Meeting of the Safety Pharmacology Society: Regulatory and safety perspectives for advanced therapy medicinal products (cellular and gene therapy products). *Expert Opinion on Drug Safety, 19*(5), 553–558.

Chakradhar, S. (2018). Treatments that made headlines in 2018. *Nature Medicine, 24*(12), 1785–1787.

Chow, V. A., Shadman, M., & Gopal, A. K. (2018). Translating anti-CD19 CAR T-cell therapy into clinical practice for relapsed/refractory diffuse large B-cell lymphoma. *Blood, The Journal of the American Society of Hematology, 132*(8), 777–781.

Clément, N., & Grieger, J. C. (2016). Manufacturing of recombinant adeno-associated viral vectors for clinical trials. *Molecular Therapy-Methods & Clinical Development, 3*, 16002.

Dias, M. F., Joo, K., Kemp, J. A., Fialho, S. L., da Silva Cunha Jr, A., Woo, S. J., & Kwon, Y. J. (2018). Molecular genetics and emerging therapies for retinitis pigmentosa: Basic research and clinical perspectives. *Progress in Retinal and Eye Research, 63*, 107–131.

Dolgin, E. (2017). Epic $12 billion deal and FDA's approval raise CAR-T to new heights. *Nature Biotechnology, 35*(10), 891–893.

Evans, C. H., Ghivizzani, S. C., & Robbins, P. D. (2018a). Arthritis gene therapy approved in Korea. *JAAOS-Journal of the American Academy of Orthopaedic Surgeons, 26*(2), e36–e38.

Evans, C. H., Ghivizzani, S. C., & Robbins, P. D. (2018b). Arthritis gene therapy is becoming a reality. *Nature Reviews Rheumatology, 14*(7), 381–382.

Farkas, A. M., Mariz, S., Stoyanova-Beninska, V., Celis, P., Vamvakas, S., Larsson, K., & Sepodes, B. (2017). Advanced therapy medicinal products for rare diseases: State of play of incentives supporting development in Europe. *Frontiers in Medicine, 4*, 53.

Gibbs, R. A. (2020). The Human Genome Project changed everything. *Nature Reviews Genetics, 21*(10), 575–576. https://doi.org/10.1038/s41576-020-0275-3

Ginn, S. L., Alexander, I. E., Edelstein, M. L., Abedi, M. R., & Wixon, J. (2013). Gene therapy clinical trials worldwide to 2012—an update. *The Journal of Gene Medicine, 15*(2), 65–77.

Ginn, S. L., Amaya, A. K., Alexander, I. E., Edelstein, M., & Abedi, M. R. (2018). Gene therapy clinical trials worldwide to 2017: An update. *The Journal of Gene Medicine, 20*(5), e3015.

Glascock, J., Lenz, M., Hobby, K., & Jarecki, J. (2017). Cure SMA and our patient community celebrate the first approved drug for SMA. *Gene Therapy, 24*(9), 498–500.

Gonçalves, G. A. R., & Paiva, R. d. M. A. (2017). Gene therapy: Advances, challenges and perspectives. *Einstein (Sao Paulo, Brazil), 15*(3), 369–375. https://doi.org/10.1590/S1679-45082017RB4024

Goswami, R., Subramanian, G., Silayeva, L., Newkirk, I., Doctor, D., Chawla, K., . . . Betapudi, V. (2019). Gene therapy leaves a vicious cycle. *Frontiers in Oncology, 9*, 297.

Gowing, G., Svendsen, S., & Svendsen, C. N. (2017). Chapter 4 - Ex vivo gene therapy for the treatment of neurological disorders. In S. B. Dunnett & A. Björklund (Eds.), *Progress in Brain Research* (Vol. 230, pp. 99–132). Elsevier.

Hanna, E., Rémuzat, C., Auquier, P., & Toumi, M. (2017). Gene therapies development: Slow progress and promising prospect. *Journal of Market Access & Health Policy, 5*(1), 1265293.

Hardee, C. L., Arévalo-Soliz, L. M., Hornstein, B. D., & Zechiedrich, L. (2017). Advances in non-viral DNA vectors for gene therapy. *Genes, 8*(2), 65.

Helal, N., Osami, A., Helmy, A., McDonald, T., Shaaban, L., & Nounou, M. (2017). Non-viral gene delivery systems: Hurdles for bench-to-bedside transformation. *Die Pharmazie-An International Journal of Pharmaceutical Sciences, 72*(11), 627–693.

Hoggatt, J. (2016). Gene therapy for "bubble boy" disease. *Cell, 166*(2), 263.

Hoy, S. M. (2019). Onasemnogene abeparvovec: First global approval. *Drugs, 79*(11), 1255–1262.

Keeler, A. M., Elmallah, M. K., & Flotte, T. R. (2017). Gene therapy 2017: Progress and future directions. *Clinical and Translational Science, 10*(4), 242–248.

Kirik, D., Cederfjäll, E., Halliday, G., & Petersén, Å. (2017). Gene therapy for Parkinson's disease: Disease modification by GDNF family of ligands. *Neurobiology of Disease, 97*, 179–188.

Korinthenberg, R. (2019). A new era in the management of Duchenne muscular dystrophy. *Developmental Medicine & Child Neurology, 61*(3), 292–297.

Kumar, S. R. P., Markusic, D. M., Biswas, M., High, K. A., & Herzog, R. W. (2016). Clinical development of gene therapy: Results and lessons from recent successes. *Molecular Therapy—Methods & Clinical Development, 3*, 16034. https://doi.org/10.1038/mtm.2016.34

Lee, C. S., Bishop, E. S., Zhang, R., Yu, X., Farina, E. M., Yan, S., . . . Wu, X. (2017). Adenovirus-mediated gene delivery: Potential applications for gene and cell-based therapies in the new era of personalized medicine. *Genes & Diseases, 4*(2), 43–63.

Locke, F. L., Ghobadi, A., Jacobson, C. A., Miklos, D. B., Lekakis, L. J., Oluwole, O. O., . . . Timmerman, J. M. (2019). Long-term safety and activity of axicabtagene ciloleucel in refractory large B-cell lymphoma (ZUMA-1): A single-arm, multicentre, phase 1–2 trial. *The Lancet Oncology, 20*(1), 31–42.

Lundstrom, K. (2018). Viral vectors in gene therapy. *Diseases, 6*(2), 42. Retrieved from https://www.mdpi.com/2079-9721/6/2/42

Ma, C.-C., Wang, Z.-L., Xu, T., He, Z.-Y., & Wei, Y.-Q. (2020). The approved gene therapy drugs worldwide: From 1998 to 2019. *Biotechnology Advances, 40*, 107502. https://doi.org/10.1016/j.biotechadv.2019.107502

Maeder, M. L., & Gersbach, C. A. (2016). Genome-editing technologies for gene and cell therapy. *Molecular Therapy, 24*(3), 430–446.

Mali, S. (2013). Delivery systems for gene therapy. *Indian Journal of Human Genetics, 19*(1), 3.

Maude, S. L., Laetsch, T. W., Buechner, J., Rives, S., Boyer, M., Bittencourt, H., . . . Myers, G. D. (2018). Tisagenlecleucel in children and young adults with B-cell lymphoblastic leukemia. *New England Journal of Medicine, 378*(5), 439–448.

Morrison, C. (2019). Fresh from the biotech pipeline—2018. *Nat Biotechnol, 37*(2), 118–123.

Naldini, L. (2015). Gene therapy returns to centre stage. *Nature, 526*(7573), 351–360.

Naso, M. F., Tomkowicz, B., Perry, W. L., & Strohl, W. R. (2017). Adeno-associated virus (AAV) as a vector for gene therapy. *BioDrugs, 31*(4), 317–334.

Neelapu, S. S., Locke, F. L., Bartlett, N. L., Lekakis, L. J., Miklos, D. B., Jacobson, C. A., . . . Lin, Y. (2017). Axicabtagene ciloleucel CAR T-cell therapy in refractory large B-cell lymphoma. *New England Journal of Medicine, 377*(26), 2531–2544.

Oliveira, A. V., da Costa, A. M. R., & Silva, G. A. (2017). Non-viral strategies for ocular gene delivery. *Materials Science and Engineering: C, 77*, 1275–1289.

Ottesen, E. W. (2017). ISS-N1 makes the first FDA-approved drug for spinal muscular atrophy. *Translational Neuroscience, 8*(1), 1–6.

Paik, J., & Duggan, S. (2019). Volanesorsen: First global approval. *Drugs, 79*(12), 1349–1354.

Patil, S. R., Al-Zoubi, I. A., Raghuram, P., Misra, N., Yadav, N., & Alam, M. (2018). Gene therapy: A comprehensive review. *International Medical Journal, 25*(6), 361–364.

Prasad, V. (2018). Tisagenlecleucel—the first approved CAR-T-cell therapy: Implications for payers and policy makers. *Nature Reviews Clinical Oncology, 15*(1), 11–12.

Quintás-Cardama, A. (2018). CAR T-cell therapy in large B-cell lymphoma. *The New England Journal of Medicine, 378*(11), 1065–1065.

Rakoczy, E. P., Lai, C.-M., Magno, A. L., Wikstrom, M. E., French, M. A., Pierce, C. M., . . . Degli-Esposti, M. A. (2015). Gene therapy with recombinant adeno-associated vectors for neovascular age-related macular degeneration: 1 year follow-up of a phase 1 randomised clinical trial. *The Lancet, 386*(10011), 2395–2403.

Rasoulianboroujeni, M., Kupgan, G., Moghadam, F., Tahriri, M., Boughdachi, A., Khoshkenar, P., . . . Ramsey, J. (2017). Development of a DNA-liposome complex for gene delivery applications. *Materials Science and Engineering: C, 75*, 191–197.

Rejeeth, C., & Vivek, R. (2017). Comparison of two silica based nonviral gene therapy vectors for breast carcinoma: Evaluation of the p53 delivery system in Balb/c mice. *Artificial Cells, Nanomedicine, and Biotechnology, 45*(3), 489–494.

Riva, L., & Petrini, C. (2019). A few ethical issues in translational research for gene and cell therapy. *Journal of Translational Medicine, 17*(1), 1–6.

Russell, S., Bennett, J., Wellman, J. A., Chung, D. C., Yu, Z.-F., Tillman, A., . . . McCague, S. (2017). Efficacy and safety of voretigene neparvovec (AAV2-hRPE65v2) in patients with RPE65-mediated inherited retinal dystrophy: A randomised, controlled, open-label, phase 3 trial. *The Lancet, 390*(10097), 849–860.

Sauderson, N. S., Castro, M. G., & Lowenstein, P. R. (2013). Gene therapy: From theoretical potential to clinical implementation. In *Emery and Rimoin's Principles and Practice of Medical Genetics* (pp. 1–32). Elsevier.

Schimmer, J., & Breazzano, S. (2016). Investor outlook: Rising from the ashes; GSK's European approval of strimvelis for ADA-SCID. *Human Gene Therapy Clinical Development, 27*(2), 57–61.

Schuster, S. J., Bishop, M. R., Tam, C. S., Waller, E. K., Borchmann, P., McGuirk, J. P., . . . Westin, J. R. (2019). Tisagenlecleucel in adult relapsed or refractory diffuse large B-cell lymphoma. *New England Journal of Medicine, 380*(1), 45–56.

Sharma, D., Arora, S., Singh, J., & Layek, B. (2021). A review of the tortuous path of nonviral gene delivery and recent progress. *International Journal of Biological Macromolecules.*

Sinclair, A., Islam, S., & Jones, S. (2019). *Gene Therapy: An Overview of Approved and Pipeline Technologies.*

Stirnadel-Farrant, H., Kudari, M., Garman, N., Imrie, J., Chopra, B., Giannelli, S., . . . Aiuti, A. (2018). Gene therapy in rare diseases: The benefits and challenges of developing a patient-centric registry for Strimvelis in ADA-SCID. *Orphanet Journal of Rare Diseases, 13*(1), 1–10.

Suda, H., Murakami, A., Kaga, T., Tomioka, H., & Morishita, R. (2014). Beperminogene perplasmid for the treatment of critical limb ischemia. *Expert Review of Cardiovascular Therapy, 12*(10), 1145–1156.

Sung, Y. K., & Kim, S. (2019). Recent advances in the development of gene delivery systems. *Biomaterials Research, 23*(1), 1–7.

Thrasher, A. J., & Williams, D. A. (2017). Evolving gene therapy in primary immunodeficiency. *Molecular Therapy, 25*(5), 1132–1141.

Wang, D., Tai, P. W., & Gao, G. (2019). Adeno-associated virus vector as a platform for gene therapy delivery. *Nature Reviews Drug Discovery, 18*(5), 358–378.

Xiang, Y., Oo, N. N. L., Lee, J. P., Li, Z., & Loh, X. J. (2017). Recent development of synthetic nonviral systems for sustained gene delivery. *Drug Discovery Today, 22*(9), 1318–1335.

Yazdani, A., Alirezaie, Z., Motamedi, M. J., & Amani, J. (2018). Gene therapy: A new approach in modern medicine. *International Journal of Medical Reviews, 5*(3), 106–117.

Yip, A., & Webster, R. M. (2018). The market for chimeric antigen receptor T cell therapies. *Nature Reviews Drug Discovery, 17*(3), 161–162.

Ylä-Herttuala, S. (2016). ADA-SCID gene therapy endorsed by European medicines agency for marketing authorization. *Molecular Therapy, 24*(6), 1013–1014.

2 Understanding the Technologies Involved in Gene Therapy

Manish P. Patel, Jayvadan K. Patel, Mukesh Patel and Govind Vyas

CONTENTS

2.1 INTRODUCTION

Gene therapy is gaining wide acceptance around the world as personalized medicine. From the unborn child to the patient with a severe pathological condition, gene engineering can be useful. The initial efficacy of gene transfer was observed in bacteria, then in animals and then in humans (Wolff et al. 1994). Gene therapy consists of two major steps: to modify the gene to have the desired character and to transfer the DNA to the targeted organisms. Two methods are used to transfer the DNA to an organism: ex vivo and in vivo, as described in Figure 2.1 (Fraldi et al. 2018; Trainer et al. 1997).

To overcome the effect of the mutated gene or disease-causing gene, there are three prominent methods of gene editing by nucleases: zinc finger nucleases, transcription activator-like effectors nucleases and clustered regularly interspaced short palindromic repeats (Jinek et al. 2012). All three have a general mechanism for cutting and modifying DNA by joining through homologous end joining or nonhomologous end joining (Takata et al. 1998). After gene modification, there is a need to transfer the gene to the targeted cell or tissue, which can be done by two methods:

DOI: 10.1201/9781003186069-2

viral vectors and non-viral vectors. Viral vectors are the viruses that were modified, leaving its pathological condition to causes disease. Non-viral vectors consist of a physical, inorganic and particulate system which transfers the DNA to the cell (Keller et al. 2019).

In this chapter we will review the various vectors used for DNA transfer and gene editing technologies for gene therapy.

2.2 VIRAL VECTORS FOR GENE TRANSFER

Viruses have always had a role in human life in both positive and negative ways, either by causing pandemics or in helping to evade host-defense mechanisms and transfer nucleic acid to desired targeted cells. There have been many detailed studies of the molecular anatomy of viruses. Development and usage of various virus as vectors have taken gene therapy to the next level. High gene loading and easily modifiable properties are the main advantages of virus vectors. There are numerous diseases ranging from metabolic, cardiovascular, muscular and hematologic to infectious diseases in which viral vectors have been used successfully (Lehn et al. 1998).

Numerous viruses can be used as vectors, such as adenoviruses, adeno-associated viruses (AAVs), alphaviruses, flaviviruses, herpes simplex viruses (HSV), measles viruses, rhabdoviruses, retroviruses, lentiviruses, Newcastle disease virus (NDV), poxviruses and picornaviruses (Bouard et al. 2009). Based on the usefulness and various advantages, we have highlighted six main viral vectors: retroviral vectors, adenoviral vectors, HSV vectors, AAV vectors and retroviral vectors.

2.2.1 Retroviral Vectors

Retroviruses have great potential to go inside in healthy cells and replicate. It has two reprints of a single-stranded RNA genome having gag, pol and env as the sequence. When a virus invades the cell, linear double-stranded DNA forms by reverse transcriptase. At the time of mitosis of the attacked cell, viral DNA integrates with its DNA forming a pro-virus. This pro-viral DNA has been studied for use as retroviral vectors for gene transduction. This pro-viral sequence has the capacity to accommodate and carry the desired gene into the targeted cell. These vectors can also enhance gene expression by CMV promoters. There are three major concerns with the usage of retroviral vectors. First, there is need for gene promoters to express their effect, as in many studies it was found that there is high chance of expression failure in vivo. Second, there is less retroviral titer and finally safety concerns, as retroviruses have the potential to cause various cancers and AIDS, which can be life threatening (Kurian et al. 2000).

2.2.2 Adenoviral Vectors

These are widely used for gene transfer, having a proven effect on cancer and cystic fibrosis treatment. It can work on non-dividing cells easily, which leads to gene expression. At 30 to 35 kb in length, they are double-stranded linear DNA viruses.

They are used to remove the E1 gene, which is responsible for causing viral gene expression and replication. Adenoviral vectors work by causing an interaction between the viral fiber protein and cell surface receptor (Graham et al. 1995). The co-receptor further enhances the entry of the vector into the cell. Fiber proteins have a significant role in the interaction of the vector and targeted cell. If we modify the fiber protein, for example, by adding seven lysines to the end of the fiber protein, this allows the bondage of the vector on heparin sulfate moieties. This will enhance the selected and targeted binding, as there are limited moieties to attach to the modified part. This modified virus can bind with higher affinity to cell types that have only low levels of the usual viral receptor protein. Furthermore, we can add specific epitopes or proteins or removal parts for the desired site of action (St George 2003).

2.2.3 Adeno-Associated Virus Vectors

AAVs are tiny, easy to study and non-sovereign. In contrast to the viruses discussed earlier, they are single-stranded DNA (Kotin 1994; Bender et al. 1987). As they cannot work on their own, they need concurrent administration of other viruses in order to carry out replication. The main advantage of the adenovirus is they are not associated in causing any major pathological condition or disease in humans. Their structure has two genes that encode a group of proteins which are responsible for replication and integration. There are 145 nucleotides at the terminal repeat. With the help of virus chromosome number 19 and the rep protein (Kotin et al. 1990), unchanged or unmutated AAVs can cause transduce in DNA into the chromosome of targeted cells without the need of any co-hand. Currently, the growth of AAVs vectors is complicated and hectic because of the need to introduce into the host cell the vector and plasmid encodes such as rep and cap. These encodes are used as helper hands but lack transcription efficiency and so cannot replicate. So, to overcome this problem, an AAV is required with helping codes. The reason for this usage is that they can express in cells which do not undergo mitosis for a required period of time (Flotte et al. 1994). They have less chances of host vector incompatibility, as the structure is simpler than with normal adenovirus vectors.

2.2.4 Herpes Simplex Virus Vector

Most people are familiar with HSV if they have had a cold sore. Out of the many strands, HSV-1 is most researched and used as a vector carrier. It is 152 kb in length and has a coding capacity for 90 proteins for receptor interaction, which is the key to identifying HSV. The foremost characteristic of HSV-1 is its quiescence (Burton et al. 2002). This dormancy character has attracted much research on the virus. It is a virus enveloping icosahedral glycoprotein with receptor binding capacity. Between the capsid core and the viral envelope, there is a tegument, which is responsible for the viral genome. Along with dormancy, it also has a neurotropic effect which can cause a curative effect on neural diseases. In the clinical trial of brain tumors and Parkinson disease, gene therapy with an HSV vector has shown positive effects (Marconi et al. 1996). Currently there are studies of approaches to modify the vectors to increase their efficiency. Pseudo-typing is the first method used for altering a virus by changing the position of the protein in between the strains of gene or between the viral load, It can be an enveloped or non-enveloped vector. The other method is to combine prokaryotic and eukaryotic cells to transfer DNA. One of the efficient methods is to use adaptors that bind with the virus as well as with the target cell. Peptides of avidin and biotin have been used to envelope viruses (Waehler et al. 2007).

2.3 NON-VIRAL VECTORS

Gene delivery systems consists of viral vectors and non-viral vectors. Non-viral vectors are safe, economical, reproducible and have no size limit for DNA transfer through a vector (Gascón et al. 2013). Non-viral vectors in gene delivery systems allow simple and safe administration with low host immunogenicity because of no viral content, although it is to be noted that it is less efficient at implementing and sustaining gene expression of foreign nucleic acids. The non-viral vectors contain naked DNA; they have identical physical and chemical properties as the original gene. It inserts via direct injection either plasmid DNA, naked DNA or by chemical or physical means (Herweijer et al. 2003). In a viral vector, the efficiency of transfecting host cells is relatively high compared to non-viral methods. The drawbacks of viral vectors are immunogenicity and cytotoxicity. The first related fatality of gene therapy in a clinical trial was linked to the inflammatory reaction to the adenovirus viral vector. Insertional mutagenesis is another cause of concern over gene transfer vehicles; for example, abnormal chromosomal integration of viral DNA disrupts the expression of a tumor suppression gene or developed oncogene which leads to malignant transformation of the cells. Because of its reduced pathogenicity, ease of production and low cost, non-viral vectors provide more safety and advantages over viral approaches. The major advantage of non-viral vectors is biosafety. However, the applications of non-viral gene transfer have been ignored in the past because of their poor efficiency in delivery and thus low transient expression of their transgenes.

Due to its diminished immunotoxicity, non-viral vectors have drawn significant attention. From 2004 to 2013 the use of non-viral vectors in clinical trials increased, while that of viral vectors significantly decreased. Developments in efficiency, specificity, gene expression duration and safety profile led to an increased number of non-viral vector products entering into clinical trials. Unfortunately, there are no non-viral vectors currently available which meet the ideal vector properties. This has led research to focus on a suitable efficient vector delivery system (Mandal et al. 2020).

2.3.1 Non-Viral Methods for Transfection

Currently, there are three categories of non-viral systems: inorganic particles, synthetic or natural biodegradable particles and physical methods.

With inorganic particles, different systems for gene delivery are available: calcium phosphate, silica, gold and magnetic. Systems for gene delivery in synthetic or natural biodegradable particles can be categorized into three groups: polymeric-based non-viral vectors: poly(lactic-co-glycolic acid) (PLGA), poly lactic acid (PLA), poly(ethylene imine) (PEI), chitosan, dendrimers, polymethacrylates, cationic lipid-based non-viral vectors: cationic liposomes, cationic emulsions and solid lipid nanoparticles. Peptides also work as non-viral vectors. Examples are poly-L-lysine and peptide-based delivery systems: SAP and protamine. Physical methods are needle injection, ballistic DNA injection, electroporation, sonoporation, photoporation, magnetofection and hydroporation (Gascón et al. 2013).

2.3.1.1 Inorganic Particles

Inorganic nanoparticles are nanostructures that differ in size, shape and porosity and are engineered to evade the reticuloendothelial system or to prevent degradation or denaturation of the molecular payload. Calcium phosphate, silica, gold and several magnetic compounds are the most investigated. Silica-coated nanoparticles are biocompatible structures and have been used for various biological applications, including gene therapy. Mesoporous silica nanoparticles have demonstrated gene transfection efficiency in vitro in glial cells. Magnetic inorganic nanoparticles like Fe_3O_4 and MnO_2 have been used for cancer-targeted delivery of nucleic acids and simultaneous diagnosis via magnetic resonance imaging. Silica nanotubes have been also studied as an efficient gene delivery system and as an imaging agent. Inorganic particles are easy to prepare and surface-functionalized. They express good storage stability and are not subject to microbial attack. To deliver DNA or small interfering RNA (siRNA) in vitro, modified mesoporous silica nanoparticles with poly(ethylene glycol) and methacrylate derivatives are used.

Gold nanoparticles have been studied lately for gene therapy. They can be easily developed, show low toxicity and the surface can be modified using various chemical methods. For example, gold nanorods have been proposed to deliver nucleic acids to tumors. They possess strong absorption bands in the near-infrared (IR) region, and the absorbed light energy is then converted into heat by gold nanorods (the photothermal effect). The near-IR light penetrates deeply into the tissues; hence, the surface of the gold could be modified with double-stranded DNA for a controlled release pattern. After irradiation with near-IR light, single-stranded DNA is released because of thermal denaturation induced by the photothermal effect (Gascón et al. 2013).

2.3.1.2 Physical Methods

- *Needle*: The desired gene is injected into an animal or human. It is helpful to have direct systemic circulation by injecting into the tissue. The only concern is the degradation of the gene in serum (Herweijer et al. 2003).
- *Electroporation*: This is one of the most commonly used methods for increasing passage and permeability of a drug through a transdermal route. An electric field is applied to form a potential difference on the cell structure, causing pore formation by breaking the membrane. Through this pore, a gene can be passed through the skin in the body. This pore will be closed once the potential difference is nullified. Pore formation occurs in 10 nanoseconds. If the pore of the membrane did not close, then it will cause the cell damage, which can be used in cancer treatment. A current of around 700 V/cm is applied in the range of microseconds to milliseconds (Mandal et al. 2020).

- *Photoporation*: Similar to electroporation in its mechanism of action, this involves applying a mono laser pulse to create temporary pores on a cell membrane, which allows transport of the gene into the cell. The controlling parameter for pore formation is the pulse frequency of the laser (Kumar et al. 2021).
- *Gene gun method*: Also termed DNA-coated particle bombardment, this works by using heavy metal particles like tungsten or gold with a diameter of micrometer size. After coating, they are accelerated at high velocity to penetrate the target tissue (Jo et al. 2015).

Another two methods for the transfer of genes is via hydrodynamic pressure and by mechanical massage of the liver, which are hydroporation and mechanical massage, respectively. Generally, hydrodynamic pressure is created by injecting a large amount of DNA, which causes pored in parenchyma cells to form. In the mechanical massage method, there is an increase in the diffusion of hepatic cells enabling the passage of DNA (Herweijer et al. 2007; Su et al. 2012).

2.4 GENE EDITING TECHNIQUES USED IN GENE THERAPY

2.4.1 Zinc Finger Nucleases

Zinc finger nucleases (ZFNs) are custom-designed artificial nucleases that create double-strand breaks at specific sequences, enabling efficient targeted genetic modifications such as corrections, additions, gene knockouts and structural variations. ZFNs were initially developed by Chandrasegaran and colleagues as chimeric restriction enzymes that could induce sequence-specific cleavage at a genomic locus of interest (Jo et al. 2015)

ZFNs are hybrid proteins composed of a non-specific cleavage domain from the type IIS restriction enzyme FokI and a DNA-binding domain made up of Cys2His2 zinc fingers (ZFs) (Carroll et al. 2006). ZFNs are composed of two domains: (i) a DNA-binding domain composed of ZF modules and (ii) the FokI nuclease domain that cleaves the DNA strand (Jo et al. 2015).

The protein modules known as C2H2 ZFs, originally discovered by Klug and coworkers in 1986 (see Ref. 53), are found in the DNA-binding domain of the most abundant family of transcription factors in most eukaryotic genomes. The finger is composed of 30 amino acids folded into a ββα configuration (Porteus et al. 2005). The ZFP region provides a ZFN with the ability to bind a discrete base sequence. This region contains a tandem array of Cys2-His2 fingers, each recognizing approximately 3 bp of DNA (Urnov et al. 2010). The DNA-binding domains of ZFNs consists of three to six individual ZF, repeats enabling 9 to 18 bp DNA sequences to be identified. Thus, ZF domains can be engineered to target specific sequences up to 18 bp. This is generally accepted to be sufficient to target a single locus in a mammalian genome (Akçay et al. 2014).

The FokI domain has been crucial to the success of ZFNs, as it possesses several characteristics that support the goal of targeted cleavage within complex genomes (Urnov et al. 2010). Although it was not recognized initially, the FokI cleavage domain must dimerize to cut DNA. The dimer interface is weak, and the best way to achieve cleavage is to construct two sets of fingers directed to neighboring sequences and join each to a monomeric cleavage domain. When both sets of fingers bind to their recognition sequences, high local concentration facilitates dimerization and cleavage (Carroll 2011).

With the help of ZFNs, the gene of interest can either be knocked in or knocked out. Regardless of the goal, two things are required: the cell line of interest where gene editing is to be performed and a plasmid that contains a nuclease sequence. Once the cell line and integration-defective lentiviral vectors or plasmid encoded with a sequence of nuclease proteins are obtained, the cell needs to be transfected with the plasmid or integration-defective lentiviral vector. This sequence transcribes to form messenger RNA (mRNA) and will be translated then to produce ZFN proteins in the cell. This protein enters the nuclease and binds with the specific target sequence with the help of the DNA binding domain part of the nuclease. After that, it cleaves the specific gene of interest in DNA with the help of the FokI catalytic domain. FokI are only active in a dimerized conformation. Thus, to achieve functionality, two identical domains need to dimerize around one target DNA (Akçay et al. 2014). This cleavage produces a double-strand break (DSB) in DNA. This DSB repair occurs by two pathways in eukaryotic cells: homologous recombination (HR) and non-homologous end joining (NHEJ). During NHEJ repair, the two broken ends of DNA are rapidly and efficiently ligated together, frequently with the introduction of small insertions or deletions at the region, which can lead to gene disruption (Jo et al. 2015).

Targeted gene correction or gene insertion can be achieved by providing homologous donor DNA in combination with the ZFNs. ZFN-based genome editing has been successful in various systems, including *Caenorhabditis elegans, Drosophila melanogaster*, zebrafish, *Xenopus*, rats, mice, plants and human cells (including primary somatic cells, embryonic stem cells and induced pluripotent stem cells) (Jo et al. 2015). It has also proven to be more efficient and precise in creating transgenic animals as human disease models. ZFNs were also used for the generation of genetic disease models also known as "isogeneic human disease models" (Akçay et al. 2014).

The HIV virus requires the expression of co-receptors C-C chemokine receptor type 5 (CCR5) for adhesion onto T cells. Thus, CCR5 is a promising target for the control of HIV entry into the host cell. Humans who are homozygous for a particular variation in the CCR5 gene are naturally resistant to HIV infection by blocking entry of the virus. Additionally, in clinical use the transplantation of ex vivo expanded CCR5 (-/-) primary human CD4+ T cells to HIV patients was found to be beneficial. In light of this evidence, ZFNs were also tested as a potential option for the treatment of HIV infection. The primary aim of this was to disrupt CCR5 in both primary CD4+ human T cells and human hematopoietic stem cells. Reconstitution of the patients' immune systems using stem cells with an engineered "CCR5-negative genome" may render their T cells immune to HIV infection (Akçay et al. 2014).

2.4.2 Transcription Activator–Like Effectors Nucleases

In comparison with the ZF protein and mega-nucleases approach, ZFN technique is a more useful and handier. Its individual parts can be combined to make a protein sequence, which finds unique sites for action in whole compound genomes. It is noted that binding of individual ZFs to DNA can be anticipated, but the binding of a complex combination of ZFs with DNA requires thorough study and a controlled process (Boch et al. 2010). Because of this tedious work requirement and few limitations of ZFNs, there was a need to find a new technique which can be used more easily. Almost 20 years ago, study was initiated on bacterial plant pathogens to investigate the efficiency of genome editing.

Research was carried out on bacterial plant pathogen Xanthomonads which causes diseases on many plants a by Hrp-type III secretion (T3S) system. This secretion system is key in the translocation of effector proteins inside plant cells. It was also noted that the effector has a wide role in supporting bacterial virulence, multiplication and distribution. AvrBs3 or transcription activator-like (TAL) localized on pXV11 group (h2) genes were found in a significant amount in *Xanthomonas* spp. As the name suggests, TAL activates transcription in the cell nucleus. The binding specificity is determined by a modular DNA-binding domain (Boch et al. 2010).

TAL works as a nuclease, an enzyme with cleaving efficiency. Further study was carried out on it its binding efficacy. Transcription activator–like effector nucleases (TALENs) are restriction enzymes that bind to DNA based on its specificity and can be tailored to cut sequences of DNA. They are made by combining TAL binding domains, which allows entry into a cell, and a DNA cleavage domain, which is helpful in gene editing. These can be tailored to bind to any targeted area in the genome to cut any desired specific location (Cermak et al. 2011). In initial studies of transcription activator-like effectors (TALEs) from the pathogenic bacterium *Xanthomonas*, it was found that they can be readily modified to bind virtually any DNA sequence (Boch et al. 2009; Christian et al. 2010).

TALE proteins consist of a central domain which has a key role in DNA binding, a nuclear localization signal and in targeting gene transcription (Schornack et al. 2006) The DNA-binding domain was made up of monomers. Each monomer binds with one nucleotide in the targeted sequence. There are 34 amino acids—monomers at position 12 and 13 are responsible for the recognition of a specific nucleotide due to this high variability (Lamb et al. 2013).

TALENs can be used to modify the gene by undergoing DSBs. After breaking, cells may undergo homologous or non-homologous end joining to repair the break. The steps of genome editing through TALENs is to select the target gene, form the needed TALEN sequence and enter the target cell using the plasmid. Formation of functional nucleases occurs, which enter the nucleus of the cell, initiating the binding and cleavage of the targeted DNA sequence. TALENs can be used to modify the gene or to replace the gene based on the requirement (Miller et al. 2011).

2.4.3 CRISPR-Cas9

Clustered regularly interspaced short palindromic repeats (CRISPR) and accompanying Cas proteins help in the formation of an adaptive CRISPR–Cas defense mechanism in bacteria and singled-cell archaea. This type of defense mechanism, which is DNA-encoded and RNA-mediated, provides for targeting of exogenous nucleic acids, destruction of exogenous nucleic acids and sequence-specific recognition (Barrangou 2015). CRISPR-Cas9 found its beginning in the prokaryote's adaptive immune mechanism which identifies the invading genetic material. After recognizing the invading genetic material, it causes the genetic material to be cleaved into small fragments, which are then integrated into its own DNA. After that, if a subsequent infection by the same material or agent occurs, the following steps will take place to protect the organism: transcription of CRISPR locus is the first process in the mechanism, followed by mRNA processing and the production of small fragment RNA (crRNAs), which aids in the formation of complexes in Cas proteins, and these will protect the organism by identifying foreign nucleic acids and destroying them (Gonçalves et al. 2017).

A useful antiviral defense mechanism has been provided to the host organism due to the interference of CRISPR. CRISPR gives an organism an adaptive defense mechanism, which can reprogram to reject the foreign invasion of DNA molecules that were not exposed to the system beforehand (Marraffini et al. 2010). Editing of DNA sequences of genomes by CRIPSR techniques only requires three important molecules: nuclease (Cas-9), which causes the cleavage of double-stranded DNA; an RNA guide, which helps by guiding the complex to its specific target; and the target DNA (Gonçalves et al. 2017).

At the molecular level, the CRISPR-Cas9 defense system mechanism and function are divided into three stages or steps: DNA-encoded, RNA-mediated and sequence-specific targeting of exogenous nucleic acids. In the first step of the process, which can be called adaptation, fragments of DNA are incorporated from the invading genetic element as additional spacers into CRISPR loci and are programmed to act against the attacking phages and plasmids, which in turn builds up the immune system memory and immunity. This step will allow the organism cell to quickly adapt to the foreign invasion. During the second step, expression, small interfering CRISPR RNAs (crRNAs) are formed by a repeat spacer array when they are transcribed and processed. The third and last step is interference, in which destruction of nucleic acids by sequence-specific targeting and cleavage occurs when guide RNAs direct Cas endonucleases to attack nucleic acids. During the last stage of CRISPR interference, information that has been stored in spacers will be used to repel the invaders (Barrangou 2015; Marraffini et al. 2010).

This technique is precise and simple when compared to other techniques such as TALENs, gene targeting and many more. It provides a versatile tool that advances the editing of the genetic materials by inactivation, exogenous sequence integration and allele substitution. The target DNA is hybridized by the help of guide RNA. The complex is immediately identified by Cas-9, which should mediate the cleavage of DNA and repair in presence of donor DNA. Due to this phase, allele substitution occurs, which is the process of integration of an exogenous sequence into the genome (Gonçalves et al. 2017).

CRISPR Cas-9 technology has changed the field of gene function study and is likely to provide an entire range of new class of therapeutics for many disorders and diseases. Optimization of delivery to a specific target for each disease is required, along with characterization of techniques for specificity and efficacy. Many novel therapeutics can be created for so many diseases that are currently untreatable using the CRISPR-Cas9 system's genome editing technology. For this technology, optimization of delivery and specificity are important for safe and precise clinical translation of this technology (Gori et al. 2015).

Mutation of the hemoglobin gene, which has been known to cause sickle cell anemia, was successful corrected by scientists from the University of Utah and the University of California. Patients who were suffering from sickle cell anemia helped in isolating CD34+ cells, which were then edited by CRISPR-Cas9, and after 16 weeks, it was found that a reduction in the expression levels of the mutated gene was seen and a high level of gene expression of the wild type (DeWitt et al. 2016).

CRISPR-Cas9 technology and techniques can also be employed on plants and animals. It can be used to make plants more resistant to climate change, grow in harsh weather and soil types and to help in increasing the nutritional value of the plant. In animals, the CRISPR-Cas-9 techniques may be employed to make them disease resistant by fixing certain gene mutations. Due to CRISPR-Cas9 technology and techniques, we may witness a large progress in the health of humans in the future. But as every coin has two sides, this technology's threats cannot be ignored. Complete control over the next generation is not possible after genetic code manipulation—only forecasting can be done by scientists and researchers of what is going to happen. A major challenge to the scientist is making sure it is cost-effective for the majority of people, and it may not respond to non-genetic disorders. CRISPR-Cas9 technology and techniques cannot be used and employed daily, so planning and prioritization are vital (Wang et al. 2016).

Table 2.1 describes various clinical trials using the previously mentioned gene editing techniques (Tamura et al. 2020) [45].

TABLE 2.1
List of Clinical Trials Using Gene Editing Techniques (Tamura et al. 2020)

Sr. No.	Clinical Trial No.	Technologies Used	Sponsor
1.	NCT04244656 (I)	CRISPR/Cas9	CRISPR Therapeutics AG
2.	NCT04037566 (I)	CRISPR/Cas9	Xi'An Yufan Biotechnology Co, Ltd.
3.	NCT04035434 (I/II)	CRISPR/Cas9	CRISPR Therapeutics AG
4.	NCT03728322 (I)	CRISPR/Cas9	Allife Medical Science and Technology Co., Ltd.
5.	NCT03745287 (I/II)	CRISPR/Cas9	Vertex Pharmaceuticals Incorporated
6.	NCT03747965 (I)	CRISPR/Cas9	Chinese PLA General Hospital
7.	NCT03655678 (I/II)	CRISPR/Cas9	Vertex Pharmaceuticals, Inc.
8.	NCT03399448 (I)	CRISPR/Cas9	University of Pennsylvania
9.	NCT03538613 (I/II)	CRISPR/Cas9	Intima Bioscience, Inc.
10.	NCT03398967 (I/II)	CRISPR/Cas9	Chinese PLA General Hospital
11.	NCT03545815 (I)	CRISPR/Cas9	Chinese PLA General Hospital
12.	NCT03057912 (I)	CRISPR/Cas9, TALEN	First Affiliated Hospital, Sun Yat-Sen University
13.	NCT03166878 (I/II)	CRISPR/Cas9	Chinese PLA General Hospital
14.	NCT03164135 (N/A)	CRISPR/Cas9	Affiliated Hospital to Academy of Military Medical Sciences

Sr. No.	Clinical Trial No.	Technologies Used	Sponsor
15.	NCT03081715 (N/A)	CRISPR/Cas9	Hangzhou Cancer Hospital
16.	NCT03044743 (I/II)	CRISPR/Cas9	Yang Yang
17.	NCT02867345 (I)	CRISPR/Cas9	Peking University
18.	NCT02867332 (I)	CRISPR/Cas9	Peking University
19.	NCT02793856 (I)	CRISPR/Cas9	Sichuan University
20.	NCT04150497 (I)	TALEN	Cellectis S.A.
21.	NCT03226470 (I)	TALEN	Huazhong University of Science and Technology
22.	NCT03190278 (I)	TALEN	Cellectis S.A.
23.	NCT03653247 (I/II)	ZFN	Bioverativ, a Sanofi company
24.	NCT00842634 (I)	ZFN	University of Pennsylvania
25.	NCT03432364 (I/II)	ZFN	Sangamo Therapeutics
26.	NCT03041324 (I/II)	ZFN	Sangamo Therapeutics
27.	NCT02702115 (I/II)	ZFN	Sangamo Therapeutics
28.	NCT02800369 (I)	ZFN	Huazhong University of Science and Technology
29.	NCT02695160 (I)	ZFN	Sangamo Therapeutics
30.	NCT02500849 (I)	ZFN	City of Hope Medical Center
31.	NCT01252641 (I/II)	ZFN	Sangamo Therapeutics

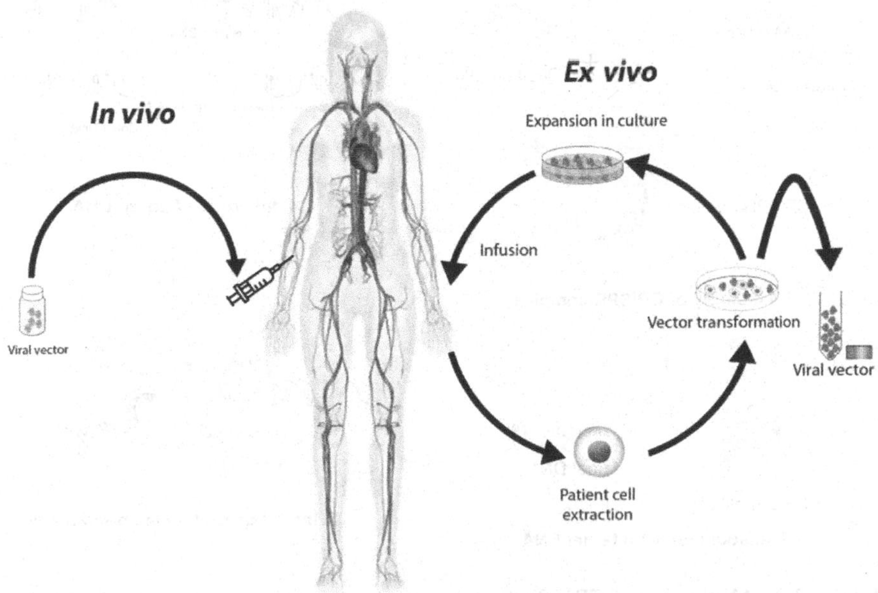

FIGURE 2.1 In vivo and ex vivo vector insertion (Fraldi et al. 2018; Trainer et al. 1997).

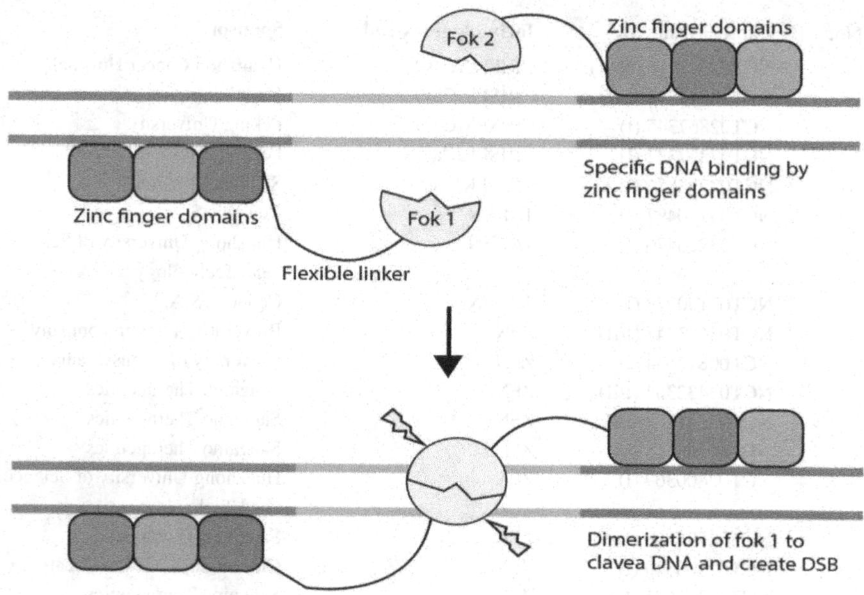

FIGURE 2.2 Working pattern of zinc finger nuclease (Carroll 2011).

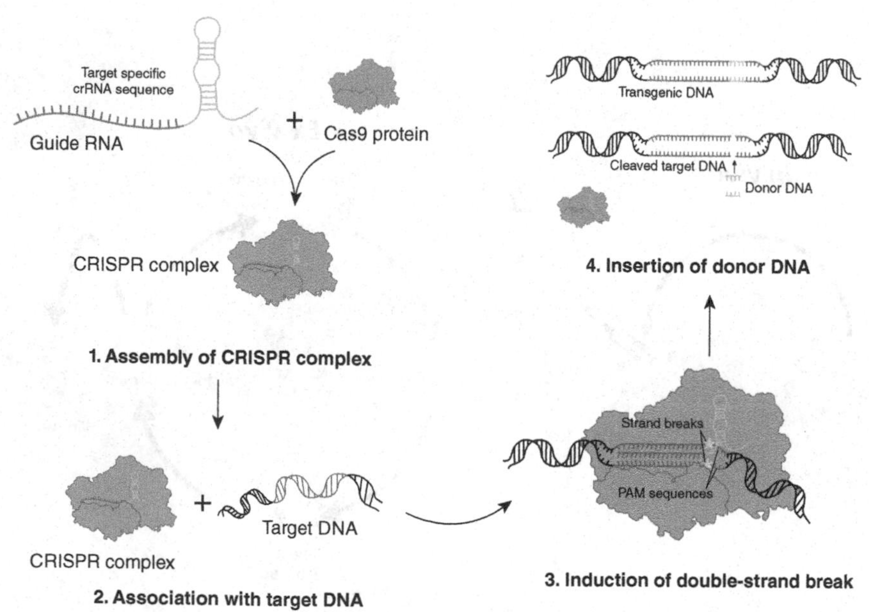

FIGURE 2.3 Mechanism of CRISPR/CAS9 (Costa et al. 2017).

REFERENCES

Akçay, Duygu, and Çetin Kocaefe. "The past, present and future of gene correction therapy." *Acta Medica* 45, no. 1 (2014): 51–54.

Barrangou, Rodolphe. "The roles of CRISPR—Cas systems in adaptive immunity and beyond." *Current opinion in Iimmunology* 32 (2015): 36–41.

Bender, Michael A., Theo D. Palmer, Richard E. Gelinas, and A. Dusty Miller. "Evidence that the packaging signal of Moloney murine leukemia virus extends into the gag region." *Journal of Virology* 61, no. 5 (1987): 1639–1646.

Boch, Jens, and Ulla Bonas. "Xanthomonas AvrBs3 family-type III effectors: Discovery and function." *Annual Review of Phytopathology* 48 (2010): 419–436.

Boch, Jens, Heidi Scholze, Sebastian Schornack, Angelika Landgraf, Simone Hahn, Sabine Kay, Thomas Lahaye, Anja Nickstadt, and Ulla Bonas. "Breaking the code of DNA binding specificity of TAL-type III effectors." *Science* 326, no. 5959 (2009): 1509–1512.

Bouard, D., N. Alazard-Dany, and F-L. Cosset. "Viral vectors: From virology to transgene expression." *British Journal of Pharmacology* 157, no. 2 (2009): 153–165.

Burton, Edward A., David J. Fink, and Joseph C. Glorioso. "Gene delivery using herpes simplex virus vectors." *DNA and Cell Biology* 21, no. 12 (2002): 915–936.

Carroll, Dana. "Genome engineering with zinc-finger nucleases." *Genetics* 188, no. 4 (2011): 773–782.

Carroll, Dana, J. Jason Morton, Kelly J. Beumer, and David J. Segal. "Design, construction and in vitro testing of zinc finger nucleases." *Nature Protocols* 1, no. 3 (2006): 1329–1341.

Cermak, Tomas, Erin L. Doyle, Michelle Christian, Li Wang, Yong Zhang, Clarice Schmidt, Joshua A. Baller, Nikunj V. Somia, Adam J. Bogdanove, and Daniel F. Voytas. "Efficient design and assembly of custom TALEN and other TAL effector-based constructs for DNA targeting." *Nucleic Acids Research* 39, no. 12 (2011): e82–e82.

Christian, Michelle, Tomas Cermak, Erin L. Doyle, Clarice Schmidt, Feng Zhang, Aaron Hummel, Adam J. Bogdanove, and Daniel F. Voytas. "Targeting DNA double-strand breaks with TAL effector nucleases." *Genetics* 186, no. 2 (2010): 757–761.

ClinicalTrials.gov (website: https://www.clinicaltrials.gov/ct2/show/NCT04037566) (accessed on 21st July 2021).

Costa, Joana R., Bruce E. Bejcek, James E. McGee, Adam I. Fogel, Kyle R. Brimacombe, and Robin Ketteler. "Genome editing using engineered nucleases and their use in genomic screening." *Assay Guidance Manual [Internet]* (2017).

DeWitt, Mark A., Wendy Magis, Nicolas L. Bray, Tianjiao Wang, Jennifer R. Berman, Fabrizia Urbinati, Seok-Jin Heo et al. "Selection-free genome editing of the sickle mutation in human adult hematopoietic stem/progenitor cells." *Science Translational Medicine* 8, no. 360 (2016): 360ra134–360ra134.

Flotte, Terence R., Sandra A. Afione, and Pamela L. Zeitlin. "Adeno-associated virus vector gene expression occurs in nondividing cells in the absence of vector DNA integration." *American Journal of Respiratory Cell and Molecular Biology* 11, no. 5 (1994): 517–521.

Fraldi, Alessandro, Marta Serafini, Nicolina Cristina Sorrentino, Bernhard Gentner, Alessandro Aiuti, and Maria Ester Bernardo. "Gene therapy for mucopolysaccharidoses: In vivo and ex vivo approaches." *Italian Journal of Pediatrics* 44, no. 2 (2018): 145–154

Gascón, Alicia Rodríguez, Ana del Pozo-Rodríguez, and María Ángeles Solinís. "Non-viral delivery systems in gene therapy." In *Gene therapy-tools and potential applications*. InTechOpen, 2013.

Gonçalves, Giulliana Augusta Rangel, and Raquel de Melo Alves Paiva. "Gene therapy: Advances, challenges and perspectives." *Einstein (Sao Paulo)* 15 (2017): 369–375.

Gori, Jennifer L., Patrick D. Hsu, Morgan L. Maeder, Shen Shen, G. Grant Welstead, and David Bumcrot. "Delivery and specificity of CRISPR/Cas9 genome editing technologies for human gene therapy." *Human Gene Therapy* 26, no. 7 (2015): 443–451.

Graham, Frank L., and Ludvik Prevec. "Methods for construction of adenovirus vectors." *Molecular Biotechnology* 3, no. 3 (1995): 207–220.

Herweijer, H., and J. A. Wolff. "Progress and prospects: Naked DNA gene transfer and therapy." *Gene Therapy* 10, no. 6 (2003): 453–458.

Herweijer, H., and J. A. Wolff. "Gene therapy progress and prospects: Hydrodynamic gene delivery." *Gene Therapy* 14, no. 2 (2007): 99–107.

Jinek, Martin, Krzysztof Chylinski, Ines Fonfara, Michael Hauer, Jennifer A. Doudna, and Emmanuelle Charpentier. "A programmable dual-RNA—guided DNA endonuclease in adaptive bacterial immunity." *Science* 337, no. 6096 (2012): 816–821.

Jo, Young-Il, Hyongbum Kim, and Suresh Ramakrishna. "Recent developments and clinical studies utilizing engineered zinc finger nuclease technology." *Cellular and Molecular Life Sciences* 72, no. 20 (2015): 3819–3830.

Keller, Andrea-Anneliese, Berith Scheiding, Reinhard Breitling, Andreas Licht, Peter Hemmerich, Stefan Lorkowski, and Siegmund Reissmann. "Transduction and transfection of difficult-to-transfect cells: Systematic attempts for the transfection of protozoa Leishmania." *Journal of Cellular Biochemistry* 120, no. 1 (2019): 14–27.

Kotin, Robert M. "Prospects for the use of adeno-associated virus as a vector for human gene therapy." *Human Gene Therapy* 5, no. 7 (1994): 793–801.

Kotin, Robert M., Marcello Siniscalco, R. Jude Samulski, X. D. Zhu, Lynne Hunter, Catherine A. Laughlin, Susan McLaughlin, Nicholas Muzyczka, Marino Rocchi, and Kenneth I. Berns. "Site-specific integration by adeno-associated virus." *Proceedings of the National Academy of Sciences* 87, no. 6 (1990): 2211–2215.

Kumar, Simple, Andrew Li, Naresh N. Thadhani, and Mark R. Prausnitz. "Optimization of intracellular macromolecule delivery by nanoparticle-mediated Photoporation." *Nanomedicine: Nanotechnology, Biology and Medicine* (2021): 102431.

Kurian, K. M., C. J. Watson, and A. H. Wyllie. "Retroviral vectors." *Molecular Pathology* 53, no. 4 (2000): 173.

Lamb, Brian M., Andrew C. Mercer, and Carlos F. Barbas III. "Directed evolution of the TALE N-terminal domain for recognition of all 5′ bases." *Nucleic Acids Research* 41, no. 21 (2013): 9779–9785.

Lehn, Pierre, Sylvie Fabrega, Noufissa Oudrhiri, and Jean Navarro. "Gene delivery systems: Bridging the gap between recombinant viruses and artificial vectors." *Advanced Drug Delivery Reviews* 30, no. 1–3 (1998): 5–11.

Mandal, Shubhjeet, Piyush Kumar Tiwari, Anees Mohd, and Anchal Deshwal. "Cancer gene therapy and its techniques in cancer biology." *International Journal of Cell Biology and Cellular Processes* 6, no. 1 (2020): 38–54.

Marconi, Peggy, David Krisky, Thomas Oligino, Pietro L. Poliani, Ramesh Ramakrishnan, William F. Goins, David J. Fink, and Joseph C. Glorioso. "Replication-defective herpes simplex virus vectors for gene transfer in vivo." *Proceedings of the National Academy of Sciences of the United States of America* 93, no. 21 (1996): 11319.

Marraffini, Luciano A., and Erik J. Sontheimer. "CRISPR interference: RNA-directed adaptive immunity in bacteria and archaea." *Nature Reviews Genetics* 11, no. 3 (2010): 181–190.

Miller, Jeffrey C., Siyuan Tan, Guijuan Qiao, Kyle A. Barlow, Jianbin Wang, Danny F. Xia, Xiangdong Meng et al. "A TALE nuclease architecture for efficient genome editing." *Nature Biotechnology* 29, no. 2 (2011): 143–148.

Porteus, Matthew H., and Dana Carroll. "Gene targeting using zinc finger nucleases." *Nature Biotechnology* 23, no. 8 (2005): 967–973.

Schornack, Sebastian, Annett Meyer, Patrick Römer, Tina Jordan, and Thomas Lahaye. "Gene-for-gene-mediated recognition of nuclear-targeted AvrBs3-like bacterial effector proteins." *Journal of Plant Physiology* 163, no. 3 (2006): 256–272.

St George, J. A. "Gene therapy progress and prospects: Adenoviral vectors." *Gene Therapy* 10, no. 14 (2003): 1135–1141.

Su, Cheng-Huang, Yih-Jer Wu, Hsueh-Hsiao Wang, and Hung-I. Yeh. "Nonviral gene therapy targeting cardiovascular system." *American Journal of Physiology-Heart and Circulatory Physiology* 303, no. 6 (2012): H629-H638.

Takata, Minoru, Masao S. Sasaki, Eiichiro Sonoda, Ciaran Morrison, Mitsumasa Hashimoto, Hiroshi Utsumi, Yuko Yamaguchi-Iwai, Akira Shinohara, and Shunichi Takeda. "Homologous recombination and non-homologous end-joining pathways of DNA double-strand break repair have overlapping roles in the maintenance of chromosomal integrity in vertebrate cells." *The EMBO Journal* 17, no. 18 (1998): 5497–5508.

Tamura, Ryota, and Masahiro Toda. "Historic overview of genetic engineering technologies for human gene therapy." *Neurologia medico-chirurgica* (2020): ra-2020.

Trainer, Alison H., and M. Yvonne Alexander. "Gene delivery to the epidermis." *Human Molecular Genetics* 6, no. 10 (1997): 1761–1767.

Urnov, Fyodor D., Edward J. Rebar, Michael C. Holmes, H. Steve Zhang, and Philip D. Gregory. "Genome editing with engineered zinc finger nucleases." *Nature Reviews Genetics* 11, no. 9 (2010): 636–646.

Waehler, Reinhard, Stephen J. Russell, and David T. Curiel. "Engineering targeted viral vectors for gene therapy." *Nature Reviews Genetics* 8, no. 8 (2007): 573–587.

Wang, Haifeng, Marie La Russa, and Lei S. Qi. "CRISPR/Cas9 in genome editing and beyond." *Annual Review of Biochemistry* 85 (2016): 227–264.

Wolff, Jon A., and Joshua Lederberg. "An early history of gene transfer and therapy." *Human Gene Therapy* 5, no. 4 (1994): 469–480.

3 Gene Therapy and Gene Correction

Target, Progress and Challenges to Treat Human Diseases

Manish P. Patel, Sagar A. Popat and Jayvadan K. Patel

CONTENTS

DOI: 10.1201/9781003186069-3

3.1 INTRODUCTION

Life starts with the cell because it is the central need of all the basic requirements of the body (Hartwell et al. 1999). Cells contains a double-layer discrete structure called the nucleus, which has rigidly coiled structure called chromosomes. Chromosomes have a slight X-shaped structure and are made up of DNA. The chromosome also known as the carrier of all genes. Genes are the hereditary structures which are found in all the living things on earth starting, from dinosaurs to ants to humans (Venter et al. 2001).

Genes containing DNA are responsible for passing information to the next generation. They are also responsible for protein formation, which are the building blocks of the body. Proteins are made by two processes: conversion of DNA to RNA by transcription and conversion of messenger RNA (mRNA) and transfer RNA (tRNA) to a peptide chain (protein) by translation (Brady 2018).

If there is any fault in a gene, it will directly affect protein production and lead to disfunction of numerous organs and systems of the body (Drummond et al. 2009). Gene mutation is common due to changing environmental factors, changing lifestyles and also sometimes the mating of two minor antimorphic mutating persons, which causes a child with dominant negative mutations to be born, which may lead to many immunogenetic diseases (Sharma et al. 2015).

Numerous diseases are caused by changes in genes (Jackson et al. 2018). Some of the most common are the following:

- Cystic fibrosis (CF) (Riordan et al. 1989)
- Down syndrome (Patterson 2009)
- Sickle cell anemia (Green et al. 1993)
- Huntington disease (Walker 2007)
- Thalassemia (Galanello et al. 2011)
- Muscular dystrophy (Emery et al. 2015)

Much research has been conducted to overcome the problems that arise due to faulty genes, including gene therapy and gene editing. Using these two techniques, functions that are negatively affected by faulty genes can be improved by adding the perfect gene from outside of the body (Cotrim et al. 2008). Gene therapy and correction can be used in almost all diseases and pathological conditions because of recent advancements, but some questions still have yet to be answered in this field of advancement (Cring et al. 2020).

3.2 GENE THERAPY

From embryo formation to death, all life has a designated sequence. Any minor changes in any step may lead to problems. It was clinically observed that 6% of newborns were characterized with congenital heart disease, which mainly occurs due to a genetic abnormality (Movafagh et al. 2008). The abnormalities in a genome that can be identified by a change in the DNA sequence of a gene is called a mutation. This results in the development of a faulty protein, which causes genetic problems by changing normal function (Griffiths et al. 1999).

An abnormal genome is the root cause of genetic diseases and can be caused by only a single gene or multiple genes. If the normally functioning gene is inserted in an abnormal genome, it will replace the faulty gene and potentially cure a disease. This insertion of the healthy gene in place of the malfunctioning gene to obtain normal pathological and physiological function and to ameliorate disease symptoms is called gene therapy (Gonçalves et al. 2017).

Gene therapy not only stabilizes the abnormal function of a gene but also enhances cellular function by modifying the genome, which leads to hybrid functionality by forming immunity, resistance to infection and more (Dickler et al. 1994).

3.3 STRATEGIES FOR TARGETING GENE THERAPY AND GENE CORRECTION

Various methods need to be screened for the gene therapy to obtain an optimized result. Strategies like mode of insertion, vectors used for gene transport and techniques for gene silencing will be discussed in this section.

3.3.1 Mode of Gene Insertion

There are two main strategies to perform gene therapy based on the mode of gene transfer (Fraldi et al. 2018; Trainer et al. 1997):

1. Ex vivo strategy
2. In vivo strategy

In the ex vivo strategy, tissue is removed from the body followed by making a culture of cells in proper aseptic conditions and adding the desired healthy gene to it by transfection and then inserting the tissue in the body at the desired place

With in vivo, the recombinant vector is made by adding the required gene, and it is delivered to the subject at the required place. Delivery of the vector can be done by any suitable method by keeping target of getting less unwanted reaction.

3.3.2 Vectors Used for Delivering Genes

The main challenge in gene therapy is transferring genes to human cells. Advancements in gene therapy research have led to the development of vehicles to achieve this (Bulcha et al. 2021). There are currently two main methods to transfer genes: transduction and transfection. Use of viral vectors in the transfer of genes is called transduction, and the use of vectors other than viruses is called transfection. From a safety point of view, transfection is more reliable, but in terms of efficacy, transduction is one step ahead (Keller et al. 2019).

TABLE 3.1
Viral Vectors for Gene Transfer (Ura et al. 2014; Lundstrom et al. 2018; Hanna et al. 2017)

Sr. No.	Viral Vector	Transduction Capacity	Advantages	Disadvantages
1.	Retroviruses	<6 kb	Long-term expression, can be used with any dividing mammalian cells	Main use in only ex vivo, as does not have good transduction capacity in non-dividing cells
2.	Lentivirus	8–10 kb	Can be used in proliferative and non-proliferative cells	Uncontrolled integration in host cells and insertional mutagenesis
3.	Adenovirus	35 kb	No direct insertion into genome, least serious side effect profile	Highly antigenic, transient expression
4.	Adeno-associated virus	<4 kb	Used as helper virus with herpes virus, no cytotoxic T-cell response	Antibody production/immune response, smallest cargo size, works for only specific genes
5.	Vaccinia virus	25 kb	Broad host range and highest cargo capacity	Very short-term expression

3.3.3 Based on the Type of Cell

Transferring DNA to the human body is an involved process. Based on the requirements and compatibility, gene therapy is divided into two parts: somatic gene therapy and germline gene therapy.

The transfer of well-developed functioning DNA to reproductive cells is called germline gene therapy. The cells that form or participate in the development of sperms or eggs are called reproductive cells. The modifications which are carried out by transferring genes by germline therapy can be advantageous and also observed in the next generation (Tachibana et al. 2013).

If the transfer of DNA segments is done to cells that will not affect the next generation, this is called somatic gene therapy. The changes can be observed clinically in the subject, but the transfer of the changes to the subject's offspring's is null. Somatic gene therapy is currently more efficient in research due to its less ethical issue and less complexity (Gottschalk et al. 1998).

3.3.4 Strategies for Gene Silencing

Genetic disorders can be categorized when there is prominent expression of dominant negative mutating genes and/or abnormal expression of a single gene. There are four techniques to terminate the over-expressive gene, and all four can be summarize as gene silencing. There are four major strategies for gene silencing: antisense oligodeoxynucleotides (ODNs), catalytically active RNA ribozymes, double-stranded small interfering RNAs (siRNA) that induce RNA degradation through RNA interference (RNAi) and transcriptional decoys.

1. **Antisense ODNs:** ODNs are most commonly used for inhibiting protein formation, which leads to decreased expression of the mutated or unwanted harmful gene. They have a shorter structure of 15 to 20 nucleotides and target mRNA by forming a DNA-RNA duplex, which leads to a retardation effect on ribosomes working in translation by interfering with the splicing of pre-mRNA or by recruiting RNase H to cleave the target mRNA (Chen et al. 2005).
2. **Catalytically active RNA ribozymes:** Some ribosomes work as a stimulant to cleave the RNA which is interfering in normal protein formation. The hammerhead hairpin is an example that targets RNA by the base-pairing method. After the cutting of a substrate, they release that sliced part which catalyzes further the RNA strand (Akashi et al. 2005).
3. **Degradation through RNAi:** This is a conserved gene regulatory mechanism in which siRNA duplexes are formed by cleavage of long double-stranded RNA (dsRNA) or short hairpin RNA (shRNA) by the dsRNA-specific RNase III enzyme, dicer. The guide strand of the siRNA duplex is assimilated into a nuclease complex which is known as the RNA-induced silencing complex (RISC). The siRNA guides the complex to the complementary target sites within mRNA, which is halved by the RISC component, forming Argonaute2. Argonaute2 is the main component responsible for degradation (Akashi et al. 2005; Rad et al. 2015).
4. **Decoy:** As name suggests, decoys are used to mislead protein formation. Decoys mimic the various protein transcription path, which leads to stopping the formation of the designated protein. By binding to transcription factors, it prevents the binding of transcription factor complexes to target genes and inhibits transcription (Rad et al. 2015).

3.4 GENE THERAPY TARGETS AND APPROACHES

Gene therapy has great functional affinity and an improvisation strategy for almost every part and system of the human body. Some of the prominent gene therapies are as follows:

1. Childhood blindness and retinal problems
2. Cardiovascular diseases: dyslipidemia, heart failure and hypertension
3. Neurological disorders: Parkinson disease, epilepsy and motor neuron diseases
4. Diabetes type 1 and type 2
5. Metabolic disorders: Lesch Nyhan syndrome and Crigler-Najjar syndrome
6. Cancer.

3.4.1 Childhood Blindness and Retinal Problems

Sight is the most prominent of the senses. Certain gene mutations can lead to a degenerative effect on the human retina (Singh et al. 2018). Leber congenital amaurosis

(LCA) is a disease that is usually verified in newborns and toddlers. With this disease, patients have severely impaired vision and abnormal ocular movements (nystagmus). Dozens of mutated genes cause LCA, but six main ones induce LCA in more than 50% of the population. They are embryonic development (CRX), photoreceptor cell structure (CRB1), phototransduction (GUCY2D), protein trafficking (AIPL1, RPGRIP1) and vitamin A metabolism (RPE65) (Morimura et al. 1998). Out of all these, the RPE65 gene is the main target for gene therapy. RPE65 is a gene that has a prominent function in the development of a protein that is essential for the formation of images in the brain. Mutations in RPE65 can lead to retinitis pigmentosa (RP) and cone-rod dystrophy, which leads to blindness (Morimura et al. 1998).

The RPE65 gene is responsible for the production of 11-cis retinal, which is essential for the production of rhodopsin. The main function of rhodopsin is to initiate electrophysiological events, which lead to vision (Kiser et al. 2014). When the RPE65 gene is mutated, there is faulty production of the RPE65 protein, which hinders the production of 11-cis retinal, delaying visual function and leading to blindness (Astuti et al. 2016).

An RPE65 mutant in a dog was found described by Narfstrom and colleagues (Narfströmet et al. 1989). There was a development of the canine model for treatment research on the RPE 65 mutated gene. In this model, the wild RPE65 gene was inserted in the RPE65 mutated gene in dogs.

Delivery was achieved through subretinal injection of a recombinant adeno-associated virus carrying the RPE65 gene. After insertion, there was enhanced production of subretinal space, retinal pigment epithelium (RPE) cells, photoreceptors, and Muller cells leading to an increase in eyesight (Bennett et al. 2000). Restoration of vision in RPE65 mutant dogs was first reported in 2001 (Acland et al. 2001).

3.4.2 Familial Hypercholesterolemia

If untreated, familial hypercholesterolemia can decrease a person's life span by three decades. The main cause of this heterozygous disease is mutations of the gene responsible for working with low-density lipoprotein (Durrington 2003). The main work of the low-density lipoprotein receptor (LDLR) is to take it in the liver and remove cholesterol from the bile which leads to a normal cholesterol range. To counter these diseases two approaches were developed in gene therapy: ex vivo and in vivo.

- An ex vivo LDLR replacement gene therapy model was developed and used for a non-clinical approach to familial hypercholesterolemia. In this method, Watanabe heritable hyperlipidemic (WHHL) rabbits were used as the subject. Hepatic cells were taken out with the help of hepatectomy and transduced in culture with normal LDLRs. The modified hepatic cells were then transplanted via the portal vein into the liver of the same animal. The result shows that there was a significant decrease in the cholesterol level in the treated subject compared to the untreated one. This therapy has led to testing the same procedure on human subjects (Grossman et al. 1995; Grossman et al. 1994).
- An in vivo approach was also developed for hyperlipidemia treatment. In this approach a vector with a normal working gene was transferred to the

liver of the subject through intravenous injection (Ishibashi et al. 1993; Kozarsky et al. 1994). HDAd-mediated LDLR gene transfer was carried out in subjects with a smaller amount of mutated LDLRs. It shows very encouraging results, having a positive impact on long-term phenotypic correction and also gave assurance of not advancing diet-induced atherosclerosis to subjects (Nomura et al. 2004). The main disadvantage of this therapy is the production of antibodies of LDL receptors.

In the second study, intraportal vein injection was given to subjects (mice). That injection contained AAV2, AAV7, and AAV8 carrying the human LDLR gene separately. It was noted that AAV7 and AAV8 treatment was more useful in normalizing serum lipid for almost seven months. This gene therapy also showed significant protection of LDLR-deficient mice against atherosclerosis.

These approaches were used to decrease the concentration of bad lipids. Moving one step ahead to increase the amount of good lipids can counter the effect of harmful lipids (Lebherz et al. 2004). Apolipoprotein A-I (apoAI) was found to be a major building block of high-density lipoproteins (HDLs). Good cholesterol is helpful in controlling congestive heart diseases and heart blocks. Increasing the HDL cholesterol level by increasing the amount of apoAI has been focused on by researchers for the prevention of atherosclerosis. Long-term hepatic expression of apoAI leads to inhibition of the progression of atherosclerosis and also remodels unstable plaques to a greatly stable phenotype in LDLR-mutated mice (Belalcazar et al. 2003).

3.4.3 Heart Failure

There are many reasons for heart failure. The main cause is insufficient calcium voltage in the heart, and the sarcoplasmic reticulum (SR) has a main role in maintaining the calcium voltage. To avoid heart failure, we need to have a sufficient amount of calcium and appropriate working of the SR (Gwathmey et al. 1990). Various genes have been identified and tested for the proper working of the SR. To evaluate the effect of gene therapy on heart attack, various trials have been conducted.

- The first model was a rat model. The main target of this model was the left ventricle. Three genes were identified for this activity: SERCA 1, SERCA 2 and SERCA 3. Based on the experiment, it was noted that SERCA2a is useful in the heart L voltage calcium channel. The catheter-based injection was chosen, and adenovirus vector was used that expresses SR Ca2+-ATPase. The results show positive improvement in ventricular function in a rat (Miyamoto et al. 2000).
- Other genes tested to sequester calcium include parvalbumin. The main action of parvalbumin is relaxation of the heartbeat. Parvalbumin may offer the unique potential to correct defective relaxation in energetically compromised failing hearts because the relaxation-enhancement effect of parvalbumin arises from an adenosine triphosphate (ATP)–independent mechanism (Szatkowski et al. 2001).

- Another gene tested was phospholamban. Its primary function is to maintain contractility of heart by regulating the SR Ca2+ level in a dephosphorylated state (Hoshijima et al. 2002).

3.4.4 Hypertension

High blood pressure leads to many diseases of various organs. In the central nervous system, it causes stroke; in the kidney, it causes end-stage renal diseases; in the cardiovascular system, it causes congestive heart failure and myocardial infarction (Peck et al. 2013). Many research studies have been carried out which state that the problem of high blood pressure can be due to lifestyle as well as genetics (Patel et al. 2017). Different gene therapies have been tried to cure high blood pressure problems.

- RNA interference, which is also termed post-transcriptional gene silencing (PTGS), works by inhibiting gene expression and is used in gene therapy for hypertension. The renin-angiotensin system is the most useful target for lowering blood pressure is most useful as most marketed hypertension work on RAAS system (Phillips et al. 2005). Antisense ODN was given in a single intracardiac dose with a retrovirus containing an angiotensin II receptor antisense gene. The conclusion was positive, stating that it prolongs blood pressure lowering and also gives protection against cardiac hypertrophy. This gene therapy doesn't increase the amount of nitric oxide, which hints that there is no improvement in endothelial dysfunction (Pachori et al. 2002; Reaves et al. 2003).
- Atrial natriuretic peptide (ANP) is a peptide that is released when there is a condition of wear and tear in the heart and during a heart attack. It also has a potent vasodilatory effect and increases sodium output by the kidney when needed [D'Souza et al. 2004].
- Injection of naked ANP plasmid into SHR- or Ad-expressing ANP into Dahl salt-sensitive rats (Lin et al. 1998) interestingly showed reduced stroke-induced mortality, signifying that important cardiovascular outcomes could be affected (Lin et al. 1999). To achieve long-term ANP expression, Schillinger and colleagues used HDAd-mediated mifepristone-inducible ANP gene transfer with a BHP/2 mouse model and demonstrated decreased blood pressure (BP), increased urinary cGMP output, and decreases in heart weight, which causes a reduction in BP and enhanced natriuresis (Schillinger et al. 2005).

3.4.5 Parkinson Disease

The PARK 8 gene, which is also called leucine-rich repeat kinase 2 (LRRK2h), has a significant role in the development of Parkinson disease. There is a multifunctional protein termed G2019S, which when mutated, leads to deregulation of its catalytic activity, which causes gene malfunction, which can also be transferred to the next generation (Nichols et al. 2005; Paisan-Ruiz et al. 2006).

Another potential and susceptible gene was studied under the PARK1 locus which is located on the lengthy arm of chromosome 4q21-q23. When the study took place to verify the position of the mutated gene, it was concluded that there was a major mutation at position 53 (A53T) in the SNCA gene. The main work of A53T is to form codes for α-synuclein protein synthesis (Polymeropoulos et al. 1997). In another study it was observed that there is a mutation in α-synuclein at A30P (Krüger et al. 1998).

Mutations at A53T and A30P cause increases in the rate of improper α-synuclein protein formation. This leads to the speedy development of Parkinson disease by changing binding efficiency with phospholipids (Choi et al. 2004).

Proteasome is an important enzyme that controls cell cycle progression and apoptosis by degrading unwanted proteins. Mutations in proteasome may lead to changes in normal function of cells causing diseases. The gene carboxy-terminal-hydrolase-L1 (UCH-L1) situated in the PARK5 locus and PARK 2 (parkin) gene has been identified having a connection with the proteasome ubiquitin. The mutation in this gene causes dysregulation of protein formation, leading to increased changes of parkinsonism (Zhang et al. 2000; Leroy et al. 1998; Tanaka et al. 2001).

Treatment trials: Adenosine vectors have been used in large rodent species for treatment studies of Parkinson disease. They have been used to encode the tyrosine hydroxylase (TH) gene. The TH gene helps to increase dopamine levels in the brain by various processes. The vector gene was put into the motor and reward system in the brains of rats with 6-OHDA. 6-OHDA is neurotoxic compound that destroys neurons and their pathways. The results show that there was a reduction in the rate of disease spread (Horellou et al. 1994; Seki et al. 2002). An adenosine vector with the TH gene shows positive expression for 15 days. After insertion, it also shows some serious side effects such as intensive inflammation, damage to glial cells and central nervous system (CNS) tissue damage. After inserting adenosine vectors with TGFβ and glial cell line–derived neurotrophic factor (GDNF) in rats with 6-OHDA, it was observed that there is less chemical-induced damage (Choi-Lundberg et al. 1997).

3.4.6 Epilepsy

N-acetyl-l-aspartate (NAA), if found in abundant amounts in neurons, marks neuronal injury or death in several neurodegenerative diseases. The aspartoacylase (ASPA) gene encodes the enzymes responsible for metabolizing NAA into aspartate and acetate in glial cells. When this metabolizing gene was mutated or deleted, it was observed that there was a tremor in rats, and this conclusion led to the development of a petit mal epilepsy model (Kitada et al. 2000).

To test the efficacy of the ASPA gene, it was injected with the help of a vector into the brain of a 56-day-old rat having tremors. Expressing the gene in rats showed a reduction in the appearance of absence-like seizures (Seki et al. 2002).

A PIMT-based gene model was developed which gave ideas about gene-based therapy for epilepsy in a protein-l-isoaspartyl methyltransferase (PIMT)–deficient mouse (Yamamoto et al. 1998; Kim et al. 1997). The main function of the PIMT enzyme is to repair proteins that have undergone isomerization or deamidation of asparagine residues. If this enzyme is mutated and fails to carry out the normal process, it leads to reduced protein function (Ota et al. 1989).

3.4.7 Motor Neuron Diseases

Diseases where excessive degeneration of motor neurons occurs are called motor neuron diseases. The most common reason for this sort of disease is genetic problems like missense mutation, gene slicing and gene deletion. Examples of motor neuron diseases are familial spastic paraplegia, spinal muscular atrophy, and Kennedy disease (Fischbeck 1997).

Many transgenic mouse models have been created by genetic engineering which express the same activity as humans with a neuron disorder. One model was developed with mice overexpressing mutant superoxide dismutase [Cu-Zn] SOD1. The main function of SOD1 is to destroy free radicals in the body—its mutation has been shown to cause Lou Gehrig's disease, which weakens the muscles and causes physical deformation (Rosen et al. 1993; Wong et al. 1998; Morrison et al. 1998). Inserting parvalbumin in the brain of mutant SOD1 transgenic mice resulted in the delayed onset of motor neuron damage (Beers et al. 2001).

3.4.8 Type 1 Diabetes

Diabetes mellitus, or type 1 diabetes, is a pathological condition that occurs due to a lack of insulin or a resistance to insulin. Due to these two biochemical processes, there is an increase in blood glucose levels, which is termed hyperglycemia. The effect of hyperglycemia on other organs and systems is pathologically dangerous. It can lead to end-stage microvascular and macrovascular damage. Due to this vascular damage, there is organ failure. The main complications are neuropathy, nephropathy, retinopathy and mortality (Sowers et al. 1995; Vinik et al. 2003).

Type 1 diabetes occurs when 70% to 90% of insulin-producing beta cells are damaged or destroyed. Glutamic acid decarboxylase (GAD65) and tyrosine phosphate molecules act as biomarkers for insulin insufficiency. The presence of the anti-GAD65 antibody suggests that a person will need insulin (Notkins et al. 2001).

There have been several experiments with in vivo models in an attempt to cure diabetes. The main work to stop or overcome diabetes complications is to correct the secretion of insulin by regulating beta cells. The approaches for regulations are the delivery of genes to express (1) glucose-regulatable insulin, (2) proteins that stop extra glucose formation and increase glucose uptake and (3) to develop synthesis factors that accelerate the production of normal beta cells (Butler et al. 2007).

The toughest task for curing diabetes with gene therapy is to have glucose responsiveness to insulin transgene expression. That gene will mimic normal beta cells. The strategy is to encode a single-chain insulin gene (Hui et al. 2002).

- Different glucose-responsive promoters have been used that promote the work and efficiency of glucose responsive gene examples, such as promoters from phosphoenolpyruvate carboxykinase (PEPCK) gene elements from the pyruvate kinase gene or glucose-6-phosphatase. These simulate insulin protein production as well as its secretion, giving relief from diabetes (Lu et al. 1998; Thule et al. 2000).

- Other than insulin, many other strategies have also been studied. The glucokinase (Gck) gene has been tested as an antidiabetic gene mainly in rodents. The main function of GCK is to decrease synthesis of glucose in the liver, thereby decreasing hyperglycemic situations (Morral et al. 2003). Many instances have been seen where a higher dose of this gene leads to dyslipidemia and liver dysfunction.
- A mutant form of fructose-2,6-bisphosphatase has been used to activate phosphofructokinase-1 and to simultaneously inhibit fructose1,6-bisphosphatase. The expression of fructose-2,6-bisphosphatase increases Gck levels, increases glucose breakdown and inhibits glucose production in the liver (Wu et al. 2002).
- The Pdx1 gene, which is also called insulin promoter factor 1, is a master developmental factor that promotes the development of pancreas and beta cells. Under-expression or mutation of the Pdx1 gene hinders beta cell production, leading to insufficient amounts of insulin. To verify its accountability in diabetes, it was tested as a gene therapy. When the Pdx1 gene is inserted transgenically in albumin-producing cells in the liver, it was found that there were unwanted side effects like hyperbilirubinemia and severe hepatic dysmorphogenesis (Miyatsuka et al. 2003).
- To overcome side effects of the Pdx1 gene, various endocrine lineage factors have been tried. Factors such as Ngn3, Neurod1 and MafA have been tested singly, in combination and along with Pdx-1. A hybrid adeno-associated virus (AAV) vector has been used to deliver all factors in the liver. It was observed that this gene has enough capacity to lower the glucose level (Song et al. 2007).

3.4.9 Type 2 Diabetes

Type 2 diabetes has a more complicated gene therapy then type 1, as with type 2 diabetes, insulin resistance and beta cell failure occur simultaneously (Wajchenberg et al. 2007).

Hyperglycemia occurs due to the inadequate insulin levels because of peripheral insulin resistance. Type 2 diabetes is a result of lifestyle more than genetic factors (Ozanne et al. 2007). Perhaps the most crucial of these factors is obesity. It was noted that as obesity increases, there is an increase in resistance to insulin, which leads to diabetes mellitus. So studies were carried out to decrease obesity by gene therapy to decrease type 2 diabetes prevalence (Shulman et al. 2000).

The linearity between obesity and diabetes is made due to adipose tissue. Obesity occurs due to excess adipose tissue gathering. Because of that, there is an abnormal increase in circulating free fatty acids. These fatty acids are responsible for inducing insulin resistance by increasing their concentration in metabolic tissues and the liver, which leads to impaired insulin signaling (Kahn et al. 2006; Qatanani et al. 2007).

Adipose tissue works as an endocrine organ by secreting adipokines (such as adiponectin, leptin and resistin), as well as cytokines (such as TNFα and IL-6), both of which have a negative effect on insulin (Qatanani et al. 2007; Kershaw et al. 2004).

3.4.10 Targets for Obesity

- *Peripheral adipose tissue excision*: Kolonin and colleagues have discovered a novel amino acid chain moiety that targets adipose blood vessels specifically via "zip codes" on the blood vessel arrangement. By linking the fat homing peptide with an apoptotic signal called KLAKLAK, adipose tissue can be destroyed. Peptide treatment in obese diabetic mice resulted in a sustained decrease in fatty tissue content, decreased lipid accumulation in muscle and liver and increased energy uptake which leads to more energy use and decreasing adipose tissue (Kolonin et al. 2004).
- *Hunger regulations*: Neuropeptide (NPY), agouti-related peptide (AgRP) and GABA are three neurotransmitters that works in the hypothalamus to stimulate appetite (orexigenic). By decreasing this neurotransmitter, we can suppress hunger, which leads to less food intake and causes less chance of deposition of adipose tissue in large amounts. Leptin is a hormone which keeps a check on hunger. It is secreted from adipose tissue, which inhibits the secretion of neuropeptide Y and also causes activation of pro-opiomelanocortin (POMC) neurons (Kalra et al. 2005; Boghossian et al. 2005). POMC is part of the melanocortin system and produces α-MSH, which has a very important role in appetite suppression.
- *Hepatic gene therapy*: By inhibiting the expression of enzymes required for hepatic gluconeogenesis, we can decrease hepatic glucose production and its output. Phosphoenolpyruvate carboxykinase (PEPCK) is an important enzyme that is used in the metabolic pathway of gluconeogenesis. By decreasing its expression, we can control its rate-limiting step in glucose production. We can use RNAi to degrade messages for protein synthesis or we can repress its translation (Kim et al. 2007).

A specific RNAi is extracted and tested for its activity. When efficacy is confirmed, it is inserted using plasmid-based or viral vector approaches. Gomez-Valades and colleagues used a fluid dynamic mechanism to inject a plasmid for expression of shRNA. shRNA decreases hepatic PEPCK expression and activity. Further results concluded that it decreases glucose production, leading to normalize glucose tolerance in a diabetic subject (Gómez-Valadés et al. 2006).

3.4.11 Inborn Errors of Metabolism

- *Lesch-Nyhan syndrome*: Hypoxanthine-guanine phosphoribosyltransferase (HPRT) is an enzyme that is controlled by the HPRT1 gene. It is useful for recycling the nucleotide, especially purines. Purines are essential for the development of cell growth and other functions. Due to a mutation in the HPRT 1 gene on the X chromosome, HPRT enzyme function decreases, which leads to increases in the amount of uric acid (Torres et al. 2007). The rise in uric acid can be seen in all fluids of the human body as well as in various tissues and joints. There are significant changes in CNS functions, including neuronal damage, mental retardation and self-mutilation. It was found that there was no neurological damage until excessive amphetamine administration and/or when there is prolonged inhibition of adenine phosphoribosyl transferase (APRT) (Kamatani 1996).

Normally the drugs available as antigout drugs can be used to treat high uric acid, but the CNS defects are not cured by this drug, so gene therapy has been considered for this genetically acquired syndrome. The first gene therapy studies were carried out using a retrovirus as a vector. A corrected and normal working HPRT gene was injected in the basal ganglia of an animal by intracerebrally transplanting fibroblasts (Gage et al. 1987). The chronic level of disease can be understood by the amount of enzymatic activity of the HPRT gene in salvaging purines.

- *Crigler-Najjar syndrome*: This is a genetic disorder affecting the breakdown of bilirubin. Due to excessive amounts of bilirubin, neonatal jaundice occurs. There is a high level of unconjugated bilirubin in the brain, which leads to brain damage in infants. This disease is caused by a mutation or deficiency in the UDP glucuronosyltransferase 1 family, specifically the polypeptide A1 (UGT1A) gene that encodes UDP-glucuronosyltransferase 1 (UGT) enzymes (Jansen 1999). These enzymes are important for the metabolism and excretion of bilirubin. Deficiency of these enzymes causes higher amounts of bilirubin, which as mentioned, causes jaundice. By using various vectors like an adenoviral vector, AAV vector, lentiviral and naked plasmid DNA approaches, a corrected gene is inserted in the mutated liver, and results show that it corrects the excessive amount of bilirubin which is present in the rat model for Crigler-Najjar syndrome (Jia et al. 2005; Seppen et al. 2006; Van Der Wegen et al. 2006).

3.5 APPROVED GENE THERAPY PRODUCTS

TABLE 3.2
FDA and EMA Approved Gene Therapies (Crin et al. 2020)

Sr. No.	Gene Therapy	Vector Used	Cost (approval year)
1	Glybera	Adeno-Associated Virus	$1 million (2012)
2	IMLYGIC	Herpes Simplex Virus	$65,000 (2015)
3	Luxturna	Adeno-Associated Virus	$850,000 (2017)
4	ZOLGENSMA	Adeno-Associated Virus	$2.1 million (2019)

3.6 GENE CORRECTION

It is common to identify the function of a non-working gene, normal gene or mutating gene and replace or edit the required gene with a new modified gene through a vector or modified nucleus to obtain a novel form of functioning or to enhance the functionality of that gene.

The technology that gives us the tools for repairing or mutating DNA for the purpose of discovering gene functions or to engineer new genetic variants is called gene correction (Storici et al. 2014). There are thousands of genes in our body, each with a different function. Thus, it is very important to understand the role of particular genes in our body.

The working of a gene can be understood by two methods: over-expression and loss of function. In the former approach, we have to insert the gene in excess amounts in the target cell and observe the response by the body. Over-expression can be achieved by transferring the gene with the help of a vector (Prelich et al. 2012). In the latter approach, the gene partially or fully loses its ability to do its desired work. By analyzing the changes in the body or any changes in the working efficiency of any part, we can find out the role of the gene (Capecchi 2005).

Both these techniques give us an idea of the phenotypic changes occurring due to genotype modification. In over-expression and in loss of function, gene correction is a major tool. Gene correction and genome editing are synonyms for each other. Specifically, genome editing is engineering of genes in which precise genome modifications are brought about using artificially engineered nucleases in transgenic animals or in a desired living being (Porteus et al. 2016). Engineered nucleases are used to introduce DNA insertions, deletions or replacements at sequence-specific sites.

To gain sequence specificity in the nuclease action, proteins that are site-specific in binding are used, which can cleave off the desired site. These proteins are developed by the following methods: (1) zinc-finger nucleases (ZFNs), (2) transcription activator–like effector (TALE) and (3) clustered regulatory interspaced short palindromic repeats (CRISPR/Cas) (Gaj et al. 2013).

3.6.1 Zinc-Finger Nucleases

ZFNs are already being approved for clinical trial testing (Muenzer et al. 2019). Initially ZFNs were developed based on the ability of zinc-finger transcription factors to recognize a DNA sequence. Zinc-finger proteins have a sequence for DNA-binding activity, which are specific for each gene (Bibikova et al. 2001). The first study was carried out to produce a chimeric protein by hybridizing the zinc-finger domain with a nuclease. It produced a sequence-specific double-strand break (Rouet et al. 1994).

After this study was carried out, it was concluded that ZFNs can be used for both the DNA binding domain and DNA cleavage domain. It was observed that the cleavage domain was not target specific. So, by using ZFNs in the binding domain, we can direct the cleavage domain to the desired locus. The ZFN binding domain can be characterized by the Cys2His2 motif. This motif is most abundant in eukaryotic transcription factors and can be found in each unit of the binding domain. The single

DNA binding domain of ZNF contains three to six zinc finger structures. Each zinc finger structure can connect with three base pairs of DNA. So, we can target an 18–base pair structure with a single ZNF binding domain. Synthesis of ZFN nuclease is carried out by the type IIS restriction endonuclease Fok 1. Fok 1 contains DNA binding at the N-terminal and DNA cleavage at the C-terminal. As discussed earlier, DNA cleavage is not site specific. To direct it to a specific locus, the N terminal is used. Thus, there is a need to dimerize ZFN domains, as type 2 endonuclease is only active in the dimerized form. Binding of two dimerize domains around a single DNA is essential to achieve functionality (Bibikova et al. 2001).

ZFNs have targeted many plants, animals, flies, fish and various mammalian cell lines for genome engineering. ZFNs also have the useful advantage of generation of mutation as same as organism, which can be used as model for further study. ZFNs were also evaluated as a possible cure for HIV infection. C chemokine receptor 5 (CCR5) is a promising target for the control of HIV entry, as HIV requires expression of a co-receptor of CCR5 for adhesion to T cells (Maier et al. 2013). ZNFs were tested in an attempt to disrupt CCR5 in CD4+ human T cells and human hematopoietic stem cells. A phase 1 clinical trial in humans was concluded evaluating the ZNF approach for HIV treatment (Holt et al. 2010; Perez et al. 2008).

Currently two more notable phase 1 clinical trials are going on. The main concept of the trials is to isolate T cells from patients, followed by treating the cells with ZFNs to block CCR5 receptor expression. By blocking its expression, there will be no adhesion, which will provide protection against HIV infection. Then after treatment, T cells are injected back into the patients (Cai et al. 2014).

The binding domain of ZFNs will bind with DNA by the help of alpha helix insertion into the major groove of the helix of DNA, and each finger primarily binds to a triplet within the DNA substrate. Injecting mRNA that can encode ZFNs in fertilized zebrafish eggs has made it possible to get mutated fish through non-homologous end-joining recombination mechanisms (Gaj et al. 2013).

The notable effect of ZFNs was the reduction of the number of off-target cleavage sites and ability to incorporate more amount mRNA without increased toxicity. It was observed that ZFNs can carry out mutations by just injecting the sample in a micro amount. Based on such developments, we can say that ZFN-mediated transgenesis mutation is on the verge of becoming a highly attractive alternative to many cell and nuclear transfer technologies.

3.6.2 Clustered Regulatory Interspaced Short Palindromic Repeats

In the early 1980s a highly complex structure with a variable sequence entangled with a continuous sequence were identified in the genome of *Escherichia coli* (Ishino et al. 2018). Initially there was no clue about the working and function of this complex structure. Later it was noted that the sequences other than the repeated ones were of extra-chromosomal origin. It was acting as an immune memory against phages and plasmids. This gave rise to the concept of clustered regularly interspaced short palindromic repeats (CRISPR) with associated proteins (Cas). CRISPR has become a vital tool for genome editing (Deltcheva et al. 2011).

When any virus or antibody enters the body, CRISPR will cleave the invading genetic materials into small fragments. After fragmentation, with the help of virus-encoded integrase, the viral DNA will be inserted in the host genome. When the same infectious organism attacks again, the sequential cycle starts by transcription of the CRISPR locus followed by mRNA processing, which leads to small fragmentation of CRISPR RNAs (crRNAs). This fragmentated crRNAs will form a complex with Cas proteins, and this complex will anchor to identify alien nucleic acids and destroy them to stop the infection from spreading again (Wiedenheft et al. 2011).

CRISPR-associated protein 9, also called Cas9, is an enzyme that is responsible for the modification of DNA. Based on its site recognition function, it can carry out single-strand nicking or double-strand breaking (Jinek et al. 2012). The Cas9 endonuclease has a prominent role in the cleavage of DNA. Cong and colleagues demonstrated that CRISPR Cas9 can be used as am engineering tool to create double-stranded DNA break. The Cas9 endonuclease also can be used to create a double-stranded break on a targeted site, which can lead to chromosomal changes (Isaac et al. 2016).

After the double-stranded break occurs, it is repaired by either non-homologous end joining (NHEJ) or homology-directed repair (HDR) based on the potency of the DNA (Ran F et al. 2013). Both techniques enhance understanding of disease by helping in the identification of causative genes. It can also be used as direct therapeutic option by silencing genes to dominant gain-of-function mutations or to correct disease-causing mutations. The process of creating and repairing double-stranded breaks in DNA by NHEJ can be utilized to stop and break the transcription of alleles that cause mutations or any dominant negative effect.

Another study was carried out that is based on CRISPR-mediated NHEJ. It was tested on mice expressing human mutant myocilin on their anterior angle. CRISPR was used to knock down its transcription, which resulted in decreased intraocular pressure, giving protection from glaucomatous changes (Jain A et al. 2017). There have been many investigations of CRISPR on various diseases like tumor cells (Jackow J et al. 2019), on inherited retinopathies (Burnight E et al. 2017), on autoimmune disease with the help of DNA methyltransferases such as DNMT3A (Vojta A et al. 2016) and many more.

3.6.3 Transcription Activator-Like Effectors

Transcription activator–like effectors (TALEs) are a group of DNA binding proteins. They were discovered from the plant pathogen of *Xanthomonas* bacteria (Boch et al. 2010). Each TALE contains 33 to 35 amino acids, which are major building blocks. Amino acid at the twelfth and thirteenth residue are most valuable for DNA binding specificity, and they are called repeat-variable di-residues (RVDs) (Cermak et al. 2011).

The cracking of the code of this repeat residue lead to the generation of engineered TALE proteins. This protein targets a desired sequence in the host genome and provides specificity to the Fok1 restriction enzyme to create a double-stranded break at the target site (Li et al. 2011). When a pair of TALENs binds to their desired specific sites with the required orientation and spacing, nuclease domains will create a dimerized form. After this, TALENs will intervene and the sequence is cleaved. TALENs have the disadvantage of an uneven rate of modification and a low detection range (Akçay et al. 2014).

3.7 CHALLENGES

The manufacturing of viral vectors used in gene therapy needs to comply with the cGMP as per section 501(a)(2)(B) of the Federal Food, Drug, and Cosmetic Act (FD&C Act) and as in 21 CFR parts 210 and 211. Large investments are needed to establish a GMP manufacturing operation site which fully complies with norms (Van der Loo et al. 2016).

3.7.1 Based on Safety of Therapy

Viral vectors are most prominent in gene therapy. Its expression sequence can be engineered with different elements to enhance target specificity and increase transgenic expression (Marshall 2001; Schepelmann et al. 2006), and different options are available for viral vectors. But beside these advantages, there are some drawbacks. The insertion of viral vectors can cause an immunogenic reaction, for example, the adenovirus vector and herpes viral vector (Ginn et al. 2018). Some viral vectors have a very high potential for oncogenesis (Fears et al. 2018).

Gene therapy using viral vectors remains risky and is still under scrutiny to ensure safety and efficacy during clinical trials. Less information is available about the risk assessment and safety protocol of gene therapy to institutional biosafety committees (IBCs) and health care providers (Ghosh et al. 2020).

A few experiments also show that sometimes vectors are not able to achieve efficient gene transfer into dormancy cells, like human CD34+ cells that reside in the Go phase of the cell cycle. This is major problem in some important diseases of the blood. Some of the major drawbacks affecting gene therapy negatively in sickle cell diseases and thalassemia includes (1) insufficient transduction efficiency to targeted cells, (2) non-linear expression of the transgene, (3) expression at the deviated site raising safety issues and 4) lack of long-term expression of the transgene (Papanikolaou et al. 2010).

In the treatment of type I and type III glycogen storage diseases (GSDs), there were some limitations of AAV-mediated gene transfer like immune response, reduced persistence of vector genomes in diseases underlying liver degeneration, and genotoxicity of host genomes, and there is a significant need for high vector doses to target non-permissive tissue. Hepatocyte degeneration is also reported in GSD1 and GSD2 gene treatment (Jauze et al. 2019). It was observed that ubiquitously expressed promoters like CAG and CMV cause toxicity in the retina after subretinal injection (Xiong et al. 2019).

There were already safety issues with off-target cutting by genome editing, and there have been recent concerns regarding the immunogenicity of the Cas9 protein. One study investigating nonalcoholic steatohepatitis on Pten using the SpCas9 method resulted in the induction of humoral immunity (Wang et al. 2015).

Treatment of Wiskott-Aldrich syndrome using a γ-retrovirus expressing WASP resulted in leukemia in seven out of nine patients who underwent this therapy (Cring et al. 2020). The development of leukemia was also noted after retroviral treatment in small children during treatment of X-linked immunodeficiency using SCID-X1 (Hacein-Bey-Abina S et al. 2003).

There have been reports of many complexities of host–vector interactions in gene therapy, and species-specific differences have also been observed. This leads to indecisive results in preclinical trials and clinical trials alike. Toxicities like severe hepatotoxicity, a decrease in platelet count, renal disease, development of anemia and the development of hemolytic uremic syndrome have been observed in some of the subjects in gene therapy trials for Duchenne muscular dystrophy (Wilson et al. 2020).

Sometimes an immune reaction is also the result of an engineered transgene rather than the capsid itself. Using a recombinant AAV vector (rAAV2) to deliver β-galactosidase intramuscularly to wild-type canines has shown activation of humoral immunity. When the same study was carried out through an empty vector, there was no immune response (Yuasa et al. 2007).

3.7.2 Ethical Issues

As we have seen, there are two types of gene therapy based on cells (i.e. somatic and germline). In germline therapy, changes in reproductive cells are transferred to the next generation. There are many concerns about these genetic changes. Is it helpful to society, or it will be used as tool of show off? The main concern is about the changes we are doing to things that occur naturally. There are also advantages of germline therapy in treating or in controlling major diseases that can be spread to the next generation, like baldness, heart disease, and many more by pre-genetic modification (Rabino 2003).

There is continuous observation by bioethics committees when any new technique is developed and applied for approval in gene therapy or gene correction. The role of the committees is to assess the risk and negative impact of these techniques on human subjects and also the need to verify and rectify ethical issues, if any, and approve a technique without hurting any sentiment (Gonçalves et al. 2017).

Ethics committees have different mindsets throughout the world. Starting in China and Japan followed by the United Kingdom, these nations have approved clinical research on human embryo editing techniques, but on the other hand America has yet to approve changes to egg cells through gene editing techniques (Callaway 2016).

In 2015, putting all ethical question aside, a few Chinese researchers modified the egg cells of a human being with the help of the CRISPR-Cas9 method to see its effect on curing HIV. The result was promising in terms of treatment, but it was also concluded that there is a need for pre-clinical testing in this area before experimenting on human subjects (Tebas et al. 2014).

3.7.3 Financial Challenges

The very first challenge encountered in treating genetically heterogeneous diseases is identifying the specific genes responsible for the underlying disease. With advancement and hard work, a great deal of progress has been made to allow for cheaper and more approachable methods to identify particular disease-causing mutations. The high-throughput sequencing method has reduced the cost of whole-genome and exome sequencing to $1,000 (Reuter et al. 2015). After target gene identification, there are many process that a gene undergoes before reaching the patient. Starting with gene modification, identifying the perfect vector for pre-clinical trials, clinical trials, various data and many more. The cost and difficulty level of testing gene therapy is as high as with a new drug molecule. The cost of clinical trials and other regulatory required data findings to bring a new drug to market ranges between $161 million and $2 billion (Sertkaya et al. 2014).

The high cost of gene therapy development directly affects its marketing cost. Due to very high price, it is not affordable for every patient, and even if obtained, there is a high burden of health insurance repayment. Neparvovec-rzyl, which is a Food and Drug Administration (FDA)–approved gene therapy for RPE65 used in retinal dystrophy, cost $850,000 in 2017. So, the issue of high cost is definitely a concern (Darrow et al. 2019).

Another FDA-approved gene therapy, eteplirsen, which is used in Duchenne muscular dystrophy, costs around $300,000 per patient per year. Due to a very minor increase in dystrophin levels, a few insurance companies will not cover the cost of this medicine, so patients need to pay for this on their own (Aartsma-Rus et al. 2017).

This, gene therapy and gene correction techniques have efficacy and safety challenges, ethical issues and economical challenges.

REFERENCES

Aartsma-Rus, Annemieke, and Arthur M. Krieg. "FDA approves eteplirsen for Duchenne muscular dystrophy: The next chapter in the eteplirsen saga." *Nucleic Acid Therapeutics* 27, no. 1 (2017): 1–3.

Acland, Gregory M., Gustavo D. Aguirre, Jharna Ray, Qi Zhang, Tomas S. Aleman, Artur V. Cideciyan, Susan E. Pearce-Kelling et al. "Gene therapy restores vision in a canine model of childhood blindness." *Nature Genetics* 28, no. 1 (2001): 92–95.

Akashi, Hideo, Sahohime Matsumoto, and Kazunari Taira. "Gene discovery by ribozyme and siRNA libraries." *Nature Reviews Molecular Cell Biology* 6, no. 5 (2005): 413–422

Akçay, Duygu, and Çetin Kocaefe. "The past, present and future of gene correction therapy." *Acta Medica* 45, no. 1 (2014): 51–54.

Astuti, Galuh D. N., Mette Bertelsen, Markus N. Preising, Muhammad Ajmal, Birgit Lorenz, Sultana M. H. Faradz, Raheel Qamar, Rob W. J. Collin, Thomas Rosenberg, and Frans P. M. Cremers. "Comprehensive genotyping reveals RPE65 as the most frequently mutated gene in Leber congenital amaurosis in Denmark." *European Journal of Human Genetics* 24, no. 7 (2016): 1071–1079

Beers, David R., Bao-Kuang Ho, Laszlo Siklós, Maria E. Alexianu, Dennis R. Mosier, A. Habib Mohamed, Yasushi Otsuka et al. "Parvalbumin overexpression alters immune-mediated increases in intracellular calcium, and delays disease onset in a transgenic model of familial amyotrophic lateral sclerosis." *Journal of Neurochemistry* 79, no. 3 (2001): 499–509.

Belalcazar, L. Maria, Aksam Merched, Boyd Carr, Kazuhiro Oka, Kuang-Hua Chen, Lucio Pastore, Arthur Beaudet, and Lawrence Chan. "Long-term stable expression of human apolipoprotein AI mediated by helper-dependent adenovirus gene transfer inhibits atherosclerosis progression and remodels atherosclerotic plaques in a mouse model of familial hypercholesterolemia." *Circulation* 107, no. 21 (2003): 2726–2732.

Bennett, Jean, Vibha Anand, Gregory M. Acland, and Albert M. Maguire. "[50] Cross-species comparison of in vivo reporter gene expression after recombinant adeno-associated virus-mediated retinal transduction." *Methods in Enzymology* 316 (2000): 777–789.

Bibikova, Marina, Dana Carroll, David J. Segal, Jonathan K. Trautman, Jeff Smith, Yang-Gyun Kim, and Srinivasan Chandrasegaran. "Stimulation of homologous recombination through targeted cleavage by chimeric nucleases." *Molecular and Cellular Biology* 21, no. 1 (2001): 289–297.

Boch, Jens, and Ulla Bonas. "Xanthomonas AvrBs3 family-type III effectors: Discovery and function." *Annual Review of Phytopathology* 48 (2010): 419–436.

Boghossian, Stéphane, Anne Lecklin, Rita Torto, Pushpa S. Kalra, and Satya P. Kalra. "Suppression of fat deposition for the life time with gene therapy." *Peptides* 26, no. 8 (2005): 1512–1519.

Brady, Timothy P. "Genes and protein synthesis—updating our understanding." *The American Biology Teacher* 80, no. 9 (2018): 642–648.

Bulcha, Jote T., Yi Wang, Hong Ma, Phillip W. L. Tai, and Guangping Gao. "Viral vector platforms within the gene therapy landscape." *Signal Transduction and Targeted Therapy* 6, no. 1 (2021): 1–24.

Burnight, E., M. Gupta, L. Wiley, K. Anfinson, A. Tran, R. Triboulet, et al. "Using CRISPR-Cas9 to generate gene-corrected autologous iPSCs for the treatment of inherited retinal degeneration." *Molecular Therapy* 25, (2017): 1999–2013.

Butler, A. E., R. Galasso, J. J. Meier, R. Basu, R. A. Rizza, and P. C. Butler. "Modestly increased beta cell apoptosis but no increased beta cell replication in recent-onset type 1 diabetic patients who died of diabetic ketoacidosis." *Diabetologia* 50, no. 11 (2007): 2323–2331.

Cai, Mi, and Yi Yang. "Targeted genome editing tools for disease modeling and gene therapy." *Current Gene Therapy* 14, no. 1 (2014): 2–9.

Callaway, Ewen. "Second Chinese team reports gene editing in human embryos." *Nature News* (2016).

Capecchi, Mario R. "Gene targeting in mice: Functional analysis of the mammalian genome for the twenty-first century." *Nature Reviews Genetics* 6, no. 6 (2005): 507–512.

Cermak, Tomas, Erin L. Doyle, Michelle Christian, Li Wang, Yong Zhang, Clarice Schmidt, Joshua A. Baller, Nikunj V. Somia, Adam J. Bogdanove, and Daniel F. Voytas. "Efficient design and assembly of custom TALEN and other TAL effector-based constructs for DNA targeting." *Nucleic Acids Research* 39, no. 12 (2011): e82–e82.

Chen, Xiaolan, Nancy Dudgeon, Long Shen, and Jui H. Wang. "Chemical modification of gene silencing oligonucleotides for drug discovery and development." *Drug Discovery Today* 10, no. 8 (2005): 587–593.

Choi, Woong, Shahin Zibaee, Ross Jakes, Louise C. Serpell, Bazbek Davletov, R. Anthony Crowther, and Michel Goedert. "Mutation E46K increases phospholipid binding and assembly into filaments of human α-synuclein." *FEBS Letters* 576, no. 3 (2004): 363–368.

Choi-Lundberg, Derek L., Qing Lin, Yung-Nien Chang, Yawen L. Chiang, Carl M. Hay, Hasan Mohajeri, Beverly L. Davidson, and Martha C. Bohn. "Dopaminergic neurons protected from degeneration by GDNF gene therapy." *Science* 275, no. 5301 (1997): 838–841.

Cotrim, Ana P., and Bruce J. Baum. "Gene therapy: Some history, applications, problems, and prospects." *Toxicologic Pathology* 36, no. 1 (2008): 97–103.

Cring, Matthew R., and Val C. Sheffield. "Gene therapy and gene correction: Targets, progress, and challenges for treating human diseases." *Gene Therapy* (2020): 1–10.

Darrow, Jonathan J. "Luxturna: FDA documents reveal the value of a costly gene therapy." *Drug Discovery Today* 24, no. 4 (2019): 949–954.

Deltcheva, Elitza, Krzysztof Chylinski, Cynthia M. Sharma, Karine Gonzales, Yanjie Chao, Zaid A. Pirzada, Maria R. Eckert, Jörg Vogel, and Emmanuelle Charpentier. "CRISPR RNA maturation by trans-encoded small RNA and host factor RNase III." *Nature* 471, no. 7340 (2011): 602–607.

Dickler, Howard B., and Elaine Collier. "Gene therapy in the treatment of disease." *Journal of Allergy and Clinical Immunology* 94, no. 6 (1994): 942–951.

Drummond, D. Allan, and Claus O. Wilke. "The evolutionary consequences of erroneous protein synthesis." *Nature Reviews Genetics* 10, no. 10 (2009): 715–724

D'Souza, Savio P., Martin Davis, and Gary F. Baxter. "Autocrine and paracrine actions of natriuretic peptides in the heart." *Pharmacology & Therapeutics* 101, no. 2 (2004): 113–129.

Durrington, Paul. "Dyslipidaemia." *The Lancet* 362, no. 9385 (2003): 717–731.

Emery, Alan E. H., Francesco Muntoni, and Rosaline C. M. Quinlivan. *Duchenne Muscular Dystrophy*. Oxford: Oxford University Press, 2015.

Fears, Robin, and Volker Ter Meulen. "Assessing security implications of genome editing: Emerging points from an international workshop." *Frontiers in Bioengineering and Biotechnology* 6 (2018): 34.

Fischbeck, K. H. "Kennedy disease." *Journal of Inherited Metabolic Disease* 20, no. 2 (1997): 152–158.

Fraldi, Alessandro, Marta Serafini, Nicolina Cristina Sorrentino, Bernhard Gentner, Alessandro Aiuti, and Maria Ester Bernardo. "Gene therapy for mucopolysaccharidoses: In vivo and ex vivo approaches." *Italian Journal of Pediatrics* 44, no. 2 (2018): 145–154.

Gage, F. H., J. A. Wolff, M. B. Rosenberg, L. Xu, J-K. Yee, C. Shults, and T. Friedmann. "Grafting genetically modified cells to the brain: Possibilities for the future." *Neuroscience* 23, no. 3 (1987): 795–807.

Gaj, Thomas, Charles A. Gersbach, and Carlos F. Barbas III. "ZFN, TALEN, and CRISPR/Cas-based methods for genome engineering." *Trends in Biotechnology* 31, no. 7 (2013): 397–405.

Galanello, Renzo, and Antonio Cao. "Alpha-thalassemia." *Genetics in Medicine* 13, no. 2 (2011): 83–88.

Ghosh, Sumit, Alex M. Brown, Chris Jenkins, and Katie Campbell. "Viral vector systems for gene therapy: A comprehensive literature review of progress and biosafety challenges." *Applied Biosafety* 25, no. 1 (2020): 7–18.

Ginn, Samantha L., Anais K. Amaya, Ian E. Alexander, Michael Edelstein, and Mohammad R. Abedi. "Gene therapy clinical trials worldwide to 2017: An update." *The Journal of Gene Medicine* 20, no. 5 (2018): e3015.

Gómez-Valadés, Alicia G., Anna Vidal-Alabró, Maria Molas, Jordi Boada, Jordi Bermúdez, Ramon Bartrons, and José C. Perales. "Overcoming diabetes-induced hyperglycemia through inhibition of hepatic phosphoenolpyruvate carboxykinase (GTP) with RNAi." *Molecular Therapy* 13, no. 2 (2006): 401–410.

Gonçalves, Giulliana Augusta Rangel, and Raquel de Melo Alves Paiva. "Gene therapy: Advances, challenges and perspectives." *Einstein (Sao Paulo)* 15, no. 3 (2017): 369–375

Gottschalk, U., and S. Chan. "Somatic gene therapy. Present situation and future perspective." *Arzneimittel-forschung* 48, no. 11 (1998): 1111–1120.

Green, Nancy S., Mary E. Fabry, Lazar Kaptue-Noche, and Ronald L. Nagel. "Senegal haplotype is associated with higher HbF than Benin and Cameroon haplotypes in African children with sickle cell anemia." *American Journal of Hematology* 44, no. 2 (1993): 145–146.

Griffiths, A. J. F., Gelbart, W. M., Miller, J. H., et al. *Modern Genetic Analysis*. New York: W. H. Freeman, 1999. Protein Function and Malfunction in Cells.

Grossman, Mariann, Daniel J. Rader, David W. M. Muller, Daniel M. Kolansky, Karen Kozarsky, Bernard J. Clark, Evan A. Stein et al. "A pilot study of ex vivo gene therapy for homozygous familial hypercholesterolaemia." *Nature Medicine* 1, no. 11 (1995): 1148–1154.

Grossman, Mariann, Steven E. Raper, Karen Kozarsky, Evan A. Stein, John F. Engelhardt, David Muller, Paul J. Lupien, and James M. Wilson. "Successful ex vivo gene therapy directed to liver in a patient with familial hypercholesterolaemia." *Nature Genetics* 6, no. 4 (1994): 335–341.

Gwathmey, J. K., M. T. Slawsky, R. J. Hajjar, G. M. Briggs, and J. P. Morgan. "Role of intracellular calcium handling in force-interval relationships of human ventricular myocardium." *The Journal of Clinical Investigation* 85, no. 5 (1990): 1599–1613.

Hacein-Bey-Abina S, Von Kalle C, Schmidt M, McCormack M, Wulffraat N, Leboulch P, et al. LMO2-associated clonal T cell proliferation in two patients after gene therapy for SCID-X1. *Science* 302 (2003): 415–419.

Hanna, Eve, Cécile Rémuzat, Pascal Auquier, and Mondher Toumi. "Gene therapies development: Slow progress and promising prospect." *Journal of Market Access & Health Policy* 5, no. 1 (2017): 1265293.

Hartwell, Leland H., John J. Hopfield, Stanislas Leibler, and Andrew W. Murray. "From molecular to modular cell biology." *Nature* 402, no. 6761 (1999): C47-C52.

Holt, Nathalia, Jianbin Wang, Kenneth Kim, Geoffrey Friedman, Xingchao Wang, Vanessa Taupin, Gay M. Crooks et al. "Human hematopoietic stem/progenitor cells modified by zinc-finger nucleases targeted to CCR5 control HIV-1 in vivo." *Nature Biotechnology* 28, no. 8 (2010): 839–847.

Horellou, Philippe, Emmanuelle Vigne, Marie-Noëlle Castel, Pascal Barnéoud, Philippe Colin, Michel Perricaudet, Pia Delaère, and Jacques Mallet. "Direct intracerebral gene transfer of an adenoviral vector expressing tyrosine hydroxylase in a rat model of Parkinson's disease." *Neuroreport* 6, no. 1 (1994): 49–53.

Hoshijima, Masahiko, Yasuhiro Ikeda, Yoshitaka Iwanaga, Susumu Minamisawa, Moto-O. Date, Yusu Gu, Mitsuo Iwatate et al. "Chronic suppression of heart-failure progression by a pseudophosphorylated mutant of phospholamban via in vivo cardiac rAAV gene delivery." *Nature Medicine* 8, no. 8 (2002): 864–871.

Hui, Hongxiang, and Riccardo Perfetti. "Pancreas duodenum homeobox-1 regulates pancreas development during embryogenesis and islet cell function in adulthood." *European Journal of Endocrinology* 146, no. 2 (2002): 129–141.

Isaac, R. Stefan, Fuguo Jiang, Jennifer A. Doudna, Wendell A. Lim, Geeta J. Narlikar, and Ricardo Almeida. "Nucleosome breathing and remodeling constrain CRISPR-Cas9 function." *Elife* 5 (2016): e13450.

Ishibashi, Shun, Michael S. Brown, Joseph L. Goldstein, Robert D. Gerard, Robert E. Hammer, and Joachim Herz. "Hypercholesterolemia in low density lipoprotein receptor knockout mice and its reversal by adenovirus-mediated gene delivery." *The Journal of Clinical Investigation* 92, no. 2 (1993): 883–893.

Ishino, Yoshizumi, Mart Krupovic, and Patrick Forterre. "History of CRISPR-Cas from encounter with a mysterious repeated sequence to genome editing technology." *Journal of Bacteriology* 200, no. 7 (2018).

Jackow, J., Z. Guo, C. Hansen, H. Abaci, Y. Doucet, J. Shin, et al. "CRISPR/Cas9-based targeted genome editing for correction of recessive dystrophic epidermolysis bullosa using iPS cells." *PNAS* 116 (2019): 26846–26852.

Jackson, Maria, Leah Marks, Gerhard HW May, and Joanna B. Wilson. "The genetic basis of disease." *Essays in Biochemistry* 62, no. 5 (2018): 643–723.

Jain, A., G. Zode, R. Kasetti, F. Ran, W. Yan, T. Sharma, et al. "CRISPR-Cas9—based treatment of myocilin-associated glaucoma." *PNAS* 114 (2017): 11199–204.

Jansen, P. L. M. "Diagnosis and management of Crigler-Najjar syndrome." *European Journal of Pediatrics* 158, no. 2 (1999): S089–S094.

Jauze, Louisa, Laure Monteillet, Gilles Mithieux, Fabienne Rajas, and Giuseppe Ronzitti. "Challenges of gene therapy for the treatment of glycogen storage diseases type I and type III." *Human Gene Therapy* 30, no. 10 (2019): 1263–1273.

Jia, Zhen, and István Dankó. "Single hepatic venous injection of liver-specific naked plasmid vector expressing human UGT1A1 leads to long-term correction of hyperbilirubinemia and prevention of chronic bilirubin toxicity in Gunn rats." *Human Gene Therapy* 16, no. 8 (2005): 985–995.

Jinek, M., K. Chylinski, I. Fonfara, M. Hauer, J. A. Doudna, and E. Charpentier. "A programmable dual-RNA-guided DNA endonuclease in adaptive bacterial immunity." *Science* 2012; 337: 816–821.

Kahn, Steven E., Rebecca L. Hull, and Kristina M. Utzschneider. "Mechanisms linking obesity to insulin resistance and type 2 diabetes." *Nature* 444, no. 7121 (2006): 840–846.

Kalra, Satya P., and Pushpa S. Kalra. "Gene-transfer technology: A preventive neurotherapy to curb obesity, ameliorate metabolic syndrome and extend life expectancy." *Trends in Pharmacological Sciences* 26, no. 10 (2005): 488–495.

Kamatani, N. "Adenine phosphoribosyltransferase (APRT) deficiency." *Nihon rinsho. Japanese Journal of Clinical Medicine* 54, no. 12 (1996): 3321–3327.

Keller, Andrea-Anneliese, Berith Scheiding, Reinhard Breitling, Andreas Licht, Peter Hemmerich, Stefan Lorkowski, and Siegmund Reissmann. "Transduction and transfection of difficult-to-transfect cells: Systematic attempts for the transfection of protozoa Leishmania." *Journal of Cellular Biochemistry* 120, no. 1 (2019): 14–27.

Kershaw, Erin E., and Jeffrey S. Flier. "Adipose tissue as an endocrine organ." *The Journal of Clinical Endocrinology & Metabolism* 89, no. 6 (2004): 2548–2556.

Kim, Daniel H., and John J. Rossi. "Strategies for silencing human disease using RNA interference." *Nature Reviews Genetics* 8, no. 3 (2007): 173–184.

Kim, Edward, Jonathan D. Lowenson, Duncan C. MacLaren, Steven Clarke, and Stephen G. Young. "Deficiency of a protein-repair enzyme results in the accumulation of altered proteins, retardation of growth, and fatal seizures in mice." *Proceedings of the National Academy of Sciences* 94, no. 12 (1997): 6132–6137.

Kiser, Philip D., Marcin Golczak, and Krzysztof Palczewski. "Chemistry of the retinoid (visual) cycle." *Chemical Reviews* 114, no. 1 (2014): 194–232.

Kitada, Kazuhiro, Tomohide Akimitsu, Yosuke Shigematsu, Akira Kondo, Toshiro Maihara, Norihide Yokoi, Takashi Kuramoto, Masashi Sasa, and Tadao Serikawa. "Accumulation of N-acetyl-L-aspartate in the brain of the tremor rat, a mutant exhibiting absence-like seizure and spongiform degeneration in the central nervous system." *Journal of Neurochemistry* 74, no. 6 (2000): 2512–2519.

Kolonin, Mikhail G., Pradip K. Saha, Lawrence Chan, Renata Pasqualini, and Wadih Arap. "Reversal of obesity by targeted ablation of adipose tissue." *Nature Medicine* 10, no. 6 (2004): 625–632.

Kozarsky, Karen F., Dawn R. McKinley, Linda L. Austin, Steven E. Raper, Leslie D. Stratford-Perricaudet, and James M. Wilson. "In vivo correction of low density lipoprotein receptor deficiency in the Watanabe heritable hyperlipidemic rabbit with recombinant adenoviruses." *Journal of Biological Chemistry* 269, no. 18 (1994): 13695–13702.

Krüger, Rejko, Wilfried Kuhn, Thomas Müller, Dirk Woitalla, Manuel Graeber, Sigfried Kösel, Horst Przuntek, Jörg T. Epplen, Ludger Schols, and Olaf Riess. "AlaSOPro mutation in the gene encoding α-synuclein in Parkinson's disease." *Nature Genetics* 18, no. 2 (1998): 106–108.

Lebherz, Corinna, Guangping Gao, Jean-Pierre Louboutin, John Millar, Daniel Rader, and James M. Wilson. "Gene therapy with novel adeno-associated virus vectors substantially diminishes atherosclerosis in a murine model of familial hypercholesterolemia." *The Journal of Gene Medicine: A Cross-disciplinary Journal for research on the Science of Gene Transfer and its Clinical Applications* 6, no. 6 (2004): 663–672.

Leroy, Elisabeth, Dimitri Anastasopoulos, Spiridon Konitsiotis, Christian Lavedan, and Mihael H. Polymeropoulos. "Deletions in the Parkin gene and genetic heterogeneity in a Greek family with early onset Parkinson's disease." *Human Genetics* 103, no. 4 (1998): 424–427.

Li, Ting, Sheng Huang, Xuefeng Zhao, David A. Wright, Susan Carpenter, Martin H. Spalding, Donald P. Weeks, and Bing Yang. "Modularly assembled designer TAL effector nucleases for targeted gene knockout and gene replacement in eukaryotes." *Nucleic Acids Research* 39, no. 14 (2011): 6315–6325.

Lin, Kuei-Fu, Julie Chao, and Lee Chao. "Atrial natriuretic peptide gene delivery attenuates hypertension, cardiac hypertrophy, and renal injury in salt-sensitive rats." *Human Gene Therapy* 9, no. 10 (1998): 1429–1438.

Lin, Kuei-Fu, Julie Chao, and Lee Chao. "Atrial natriuretic peptide gene delivery reduces stroke-induced mortality rate in Dahl salt-sensitive rats." *Hypertension* 33, no. 1 (1999): 219–224.

Lu, D., H. Tamemoto, H. Shibata, I. Saito, and T. Takeuchi. "Regulatable production of insulin from primary-cultured hepatocytes: Insulin production is up-regulated by glucagon and cAMP and down-regulated by insulin." *Gene Therapy* 5, no. 7 (1998): 888–895.

Lundstrom, Kenneth. "Viral vectors in gene therapy." *Diseases* 6, no. 2 (2018): 42.

Maier, Dawn A., Andrea L. Brennan, Shuguang Jiang, Gwendolyn K. Binder-Scholl, Gary Lee, Gabriela Plesa, Zhaohui Zheng et al. "Efficient clinical scale gene modification via zinc finger nuclease—targeted disruption of the HIV co-receptor CCR5." *Human Gene Therapy* 24, no. 3 (2013): 245–258.

Marshall, Eliot. "Viral vectors still pack surprises." (2001): 1640–1640.

Miyamoto, Michael I., Federica Del Monte, Ulrich Schmidt, Thomas S. DiSalvo, Zhao Bin Kang, Takashi Matsui, J. Luis Guerrero, Judith K. Gwathmey, Anthony Rosenzweig, and Roger J. Hajjar. "Adenoviral gene transfer of SERCA2a improves left-ventricular function in aortic-banded rats in transition to heart failure." *Proceedings of the National Academy of Sciences* 97, no. 2 (2000): 793–798.

Miyatsuka, T., H. Kaneto, Y. Kajimoto, S. Hirota, Y. Arakawa, Y. Fujitani, Y. Umayahara et al. "Ectopically expressed PDX-1 in liver initiates endocrine and exocrine pancreas differentiation but causes dysmorphogenesis." *Biochemical and Biophysical Research Communications* 310, no. 3 (2003): 1017–1025.

Morimura, Hiroyuki, Gerald A. Fishman, Sandeep A. Grover, Anne B. Fulton, Eliot L. Berson, and Thaddeus P. Dryja. "Mutations in the RPE65 gene in patients with autosomal recessive retinitis pigmentosa or leber congenital amaurosis." *Proceedings of the National Academy of Sciences* 95, no. 6 (1998): 3088–3093.

Morral, Núria. "Novel targets and therapeutic strategies for type 2 diabetes." *Trends in Endocrinology & Metabolism* 14, no. 4 (2003): 169–175.

Morrison, Brett M., John H. Morrison, and Jon W. Gordon. "Superoxide dismutase and neurofilament transgenic models of amyotrophic lateral sclerosis." *Journal of Experimental Zoology* 282, no. 1-2 (1998): 32–47.

Movafagh, A., Z. Pear Zadeh, M. HajiseyedJavadi, F. M. Mohammed, S. M. H. Ghaderian, M. H. Heidari, and R. Ghasemi Barghi. "Occurrence of congenital anomalies and genetic diseases in a population of Ghazvin Province, Iran: A study of 33380 cases." *Pakistan Journal of Medical Sciences* 24, no. 1 (2008): 80.

Muenzer, Joseph, Carlos E. Prada, Barbara Burton, Heather A. Lau, Can Ficicioglu, Cheryl Wong Po Foo, Sagar A. Vaidya, Chester B. Whitley, and Paul Harmatz. "CHAMPIONS: A phase 1/2 clinical trial with dose escalation of SB-913 ZFN-mediated in vivo human genome editing for treatment of MPS II (Hunter syndrome)." *Molecular Genetics and Metabolism* 126 (2019): S104.

Narfström, K., A. N. D. E. R. S. Wrigstad, and S. E. Nilsson. "The Briard dog: A new animal model of congenital stationary night blindness." *British Journal of Ophthalmology* 73, no. 9 (1989): 750–756.

Nichols, William C., Nathan Pankratz, Dena Hernandez, Coro Paisán-Ruíz, Shushant Jain, Cheryl A. Halter, Veronika E. Michaels et al. "Genetic screening for a single common LRRK2 mutation in familial Parkinson's disease." *The Lancet* 365, no. 9457 (2005): 410–412.

Nomura, S., A. Merched, E. Nour, C. Dieker, K. Oka, and L. Chan. "Low-density lipoprotein receptor gene therapy using helper-dependent adenovirus produces long-term protection against atherosclerosis in a mouse model of familial hypercholesterolemia." *Gene Therapy* 11, no. 20 (2004): 1540–1548.

Notkins, Abner Louis, and Åke Lernmark. "Autoimmune type 1 diabetes: Resolved and unresolved issues." *The Journal of Clinical Investigation* 108, no. 9 (2001): 1247–1252.

Ota, Irene M., and Steven Clarke. "Calcium affects the spontaneous degradation of aspartyl/asparaginyl residues in calmodulin." *Biochemistry* 28, no. 9 (1989): 4020–4027.

Ozanne, Susan E., and Miguel Constância. "Mechanisms of disease: The developmental origins of disease and the role of the epigenotype." *Nature Clinical Practice Endocrinology & Metabolism* 3, no. 7 (2007): 539–546.

Pachori, Alok S., Mohammed T. Numan, Carlos M. Ferrario, Debra M. Diz, Mohan K. Raizada, and Michael J. Katovich. "Blood pressure—independent attenuation of cardiac hypertrophy by AT1R-AS gene therapy." *Hypertension* 39, no. 5 (2002): 969–975.

Paisan-Ruiz, C., E. W. Evans, S. Jain, G. Xiromerisiou, J. R. Gibbs, J. Eerola, V. Gourbali et al. "Testing association between LRRK2 and Parkinson's disease and investigating linkage disequilibrium." *Journal of Medical Genetics* 43, no. 2 (2006): e09–e09.

Papanikolaou, Eleni, and Nicholas P Anagnou. "Major challenges for gene therapy of thalassemia and sickle cell disease." *Current Gene Therapy* 10, no. 5 (2010): 404–412.

Patel, Riyaz S., Stefano Masi, and Stefano Taddei. "Understanding the role of genetics in hypertension." *European Heart Journal* 38, no. 29 (2017): 2309–2312.

Patterson, David. "Molecular genetic analysis of Down syndrome." *Human Genetics* 126, no. 1 (2009): 195–214.

Peck, Robert N., Ethan Green, Jacob Mtabaji, Charles Majinge, Luke R. Smart, Jennifer A. Downs, and Daniel W. Fitzgerald. "Hypertension-related diseases as a common cause of hospital mortality in Tanzania: A 3-year prospective study." *Journal of Hypertension* 31, no. 9 (2013): 1806.

Perez, Elena E., Jianbin Wang, Jeffrey C. Miller, Yann Jouvenot, Kenneth A. Kim, Olga Liu, Nathaniel Wang et al. "Establishment of HIV-1 resistance in CD4+ T cells by genome editing using zinc-finger nucleases." *Nature Biotechnology* 26, no. 7 (2008): 808–816.

Phillips, M. Ian, and Birgitta Kimura. "Gene therapy for hypertension: Antisense inhibition of the renin-angiotensin system." *Methods in Molecular Medicine* 108 (2005): 363–379.

Polymeropoulos, Mihael H., Christian Lavedan, Elisabeth Leroy, Susan E. Ide, Anindya Dehejia, Amalia Dutra, Brian Pike et al. "Mutation in the α-synuclein gene identified in families with Parkinson's disease." *Science* 276, no. 5321 (1997): 2045–2047.

Porteus, Matthew. "Genome editing: A new approach to human therapeutics." *Annual Review of Pharmacology and Toxicology* 56 (2016): 163–190.

Prelich, Gregory. "Gene overexpression: Uses, mechanisms, and interpretation." *Genetics* 190, no. 3 (2012): 841–854.

Qatanani, Mohammed, and Mitchell A. Lazar. "Mechanisms of obesity-associated insulin resistance: Many choices on the menu." *Genes & Development* 21, no. 12 (2007): 1443–1455.

Rabino, Isaac. "Gene therapy: Ethical issues." *Theoretical Medicine and Bioethics* 24, no. 1 (2003): 31–58.

Rad, Seyed Mohammad Ali Hosseini, Lida Langroudi, Fatemeh Kouhkan, Laleh Yazdani, Alireza Nouri Koupaee, Sara Asgharpour, Zahra Shojaei, Taravat Bamdad, and Ehsan Arefian. "Transcription factor decoy: A pre-transcriptional approach for gene downregulation purpose in cancer." *Tumor Biology* 36, no. 7 (2015): 4871–4881.

Ran, F., P. Hsu, J. Wright, V. Agarwala, D. Scott, and F. Zhang. "Genome engineering using the CRISPR-Cas9 system." *Nature Protocols* 8 (2013): 2281–2308.

Reaves, Phyllis Y., Caren R. Beck, Hong-Wei Wang, Mohan K. Raizada, and Michael J. Katovich. "Endothelial-independent prevention of high blood pressure in L-name-treated rats by angiotensin II type I receptor antisense gene therapy." *Experimental Physiology* 88, no. 4 (2003): 467–473.

Reuter, Jason A., Damek V. Spacek, and Michael P. Snyder. "High-throughput sequencing technologies." *Molecular Cell* 58, no. 4 (2015): 586–597.

Riordan, John R., Johanna M. Rommens, Bat-sheva Kerem, Noa Alon, Richard Rozmahel, Zbyszko Grzelczak, Julian Zielenski, Si Lok, Natasa Plavsic, and Jia-Ling Chou. "Identification of the cystic fibrosis gene: Cloning and characterization of complementary DNA." *Science* 245, no. 4922 (1989): 1066–1073.

Rosen, Daniel R., Teepu Siddique, David Patterson, Denise A. Figlewicz, Peter Sapp, Afif Hentati, Deirdre Donaldson et al. "Mutations in Cu/Zn superoxide dismutase gene are associated with familial amyotrophic lateral sclerosis." *Nature* 362, no. 6415 (1993): 59–62.

Rouet, Philippe, Fatima Smih, and Maria Jasin. "Introduction of double-strand breaks into the genome of mouse cells by expression of a rare-cutting endonuclease." *Molecular and Cellular Biology* 14, no. 12 (1994): 8096–8106.

Schepelmann, Silke, and Caroline J. Springer. "Viral vectors for gene-directed enzyme prodrug therapy." *Current Gene Therapy* 6, no. 6 (2006): 647–670.

Schillinger, K. J., S. Y. Tsai, G. E. Taffet, A. K. Reddy, A. J. Marian, M. L. Entman, K. Oka, L. Chan, and B. W. O'Malley. "Regulatable atrial natriuretic peptide gene therapy for hypertension." *Proceedings of the National Academy of Sciences of the United States of America* 102 (2005): 13789–13794.

Seki, Takahiro, Hiroaki Matsubayashi, Taku Amano, Kazuhiro Kitada, Tadao Serikawa, Norio Sakai, and Masashi Sasa. "Adenoviral gene transfer of aspartoacylase into the tremor rat, a genetic model of epilepsy, as a trial of gene therapy for inherited epileptic disorder." *Neuroscience Letters* 328, no. 3 (2002): 249–252.

Seppen, Jurgen, Conny Bakker, Berry De Jong, Cindy Kunne, Karin Van Den Oever, Kristin Vandenberghe, Rudi De Waart, Jaap Twisk, and Piter Bosma. "Adeno-associated virus vector serotypes mediate sustained correction of bilirubin UDP glucuronosyltransferase deficiency in rats." *Molecular Therapy* 13, no. 6 (2006): 1085–1092.

Sertkaya, Aylin, Anna Birkenbach, Ayesha Berlind, and John Eyraud. "Examination of clinical trial costs and barriers for drug development." *Report, US Department of Health and Human Services, Office of the Assistant Secretary for Planning and Evaluation, Washington, DC* 7 (2014).

Sharma, S., S. M. Javadekar, M. Pandey, M. Srivastava, R. Kumari, and S. C. Raghavan. "Homology and enzymatic requirements of microhomology-dependent alternative end joining." *Cell Death & Disease* 6, no. 3 (2015): e1697–e1697.

Shulman, Gerald I. "Cellular mechanisms of insulin resistance." *The Journal of Clinical Investigation* 106, no. 2 (2000): 171–176.

Singh, Mahavir, and Suresh C. Tyagi. "Genes and genetics in eye diseases: A genomic medicine approach for investigating hereditary and inflammatory ocular disorders." *International Journal of Ophthalmology* 11, no. 1 (2018): 117.

Song, Young-Duk, Eun-Jig Lee, Parham Yashar, Liza E. Pfaff, So-Youn Kim, and J. Larry Jameson. "Islet cell differentiation in liver by combinatorial expression of transcription factors neurogenin-3, BETA2, and RIPE3b1." *Biochemical and Biophysical Research Communications* 354, no. 2 (2007): 334–339.

Sowers, James R., and Murray Epstein. "Diabetes mellitus and associated hypertension, vascular disease, and nephropathy: An update." *Hypertension* 26, no. 6 (1995): 869–879.

Storici, Francesca, ed. *Gene Correction: Methods and Protocols*. Humana Press, 2014.

Szatkowski, Michael L., Margaret V. Westfall, Carlen A. Gomez, Philip A. Wahr, Daniel E. Michele, Christiana DelloRusso, Immanuel I. Turner, Katie E. Hong, Faris P. Albayya, and Joseph M. Metzger. "In vivo acceleration of heart relaxation performance by parvalbumin gene delivery." *The Journal of Clinical Investigation* 107, no. 2 (2001): 191–198.

Tachibana, Masahito, Paula Amato, Michelle Sparman, Joy Woodward, Dario Melguizo Sanchis, Hong Ma, Nuria Marti Gutierrez et al. "Towards germline gene therapy of inherited mitochondrial diseases." *Nature* 493, no. 7434 (2013): 627–631.

Tanaka, Yuji, Simone Engelender, Shuichi Igarashi, Raghuram K. Rao, Tracy Wanner, Rudolph E. Tanzi, Akira Sawa, Valina L. Dawson, Ted M. Dawson, and Christopher A. Ross. "Inducible expression of mutant α-synuclein decreases proteasome activity and increases sensitivity to mitochondria-dependent apoptosis." *Human Molecular Genetics* 10, no. 9 (2001): 919–926.

Tebas, Pablo, David Stein, Winson W. Tang, Ian Frank, Shelley Q. Wang, Gary Lee, S. Kaye Spratt et al. "Gene editing of CCR5 in autologous CD4 T cells of persons infected with HIV." *New England Journal of Medicine* 370, no. 10 (2014): 901–910.

Thule, P. M., J. Liu, and L. S. Phillips. "Glucose regulated production of human insulin in rat hepatocytes." *Gene Therapy* 7, no. 3 (2000): 205–214.

Torres, Rosa J., and Juan G. Puig. "Hypoxanthine-guanine phosophoribosyltransferase (HPRT) deficiency: Lesch-Nyhan syndrome." *Orphanet Journal of Rare Diseases* 2, no. 1 (2007): 1–10.

Trainer, Alison H., and M. Yvonne Alexander. "Gene delivery to the epidermis." *Human Molecular Genetics* 6, no. 10 (1997): 1761–1767.

Ura, Takehiro, Kenji Okuda, and Masaru Shimada. "Developments in viral vector-based vaccines." *Vaccines* 2, no. 3 (2014): 624–641.

van der Loo, Johannes CM, and J. Fraser Wright. "Progress and challenges in viral vector manufacturing." *Human Molecular Genetics* 25, no. R1 (2016): R42–R52.

Van Der Wegen, Pascal, Rogier Louwen, Ali M. Imam, Ruvalic M. Buijs-Offerman, Maarten Sinaasappel, Frank Grosveld, and Bob J. Scholte. "Successful treatment of UGT1A1 deficiency in a rat model of Crigler—Najjar disease by intravenous administration of a liver-specific lentiviral vector." *Molecular Therapy* 13, no. 2 (2006): 374–381.

Venter, J. C., M. D. Adams, E. W. Myers, P. W. Li, R. J. Mural, G. G. Sutton, H. O. Smith, M. Yandell, C. A. Evans, R. A. Holt, J. D. Gocayne, P. Amanatides, R. M. Ballew, D. H. Huson, J. R. Wortman, Q. Zhang, C. D. Kodira, X. H. Zheng, L. Chen, M. Skupski, G. Subramanian, P. D. Thomas, J. Zhang, G. L. Gabor Miklos, C. Nelson, S. Broder, A. G. Clark, J. Nadeau, V. A. McKusick, N. Zinder, A. J. Levine, R. J. Roberts, M. Simon, C. Slayman, M. Hunkapiller, R. Bolanos, A. Delcher, I. Dew, D. Fasulo, M. Flanigan, L. Florea, A. Halpern, S. Hannenhalli, S. Kravitz, S. Levy, C. Mobarry, K. Reinert, K. Remington. . . . . "The sequence of the human genome." *Science* 291 (2001): 1304–1351.

Vinik, Aaron I., Raelene E. Maser, Braxton D. Mitchell, and Roy Freeman. "Diabetic autonomic neuropathy." *Diabetes Care* 26, no. 5 (2003): 1553–1579.

Vojta, A., P. Dobrinic, V. Tadic, L. Bockor, P. Korac, B. Julg, et al. "Repurposing the CRISPR-Cas9 system for targeted DNA methylation." *Nucleic Acid Research* 44 (2016): 5615–5628.

Wajchenberg, Bernardo L. "β-cell failure in diabetes and preservation by clinical treatment." *Endocrine Reviews* 28, no. 2 (2007): 187–218.

Walker, Francis O. "Huntington's disease." *The Lancet* 369, no. 9557 (2007): 218–228.

Wang, Dan, Haiwei Mou, Shaoyong Li, Yingxiang Li, Soren Hough, Karen Tran, Jia Li et al. "Adenovirus-mediated somatic genome editing of Pten by CRISPR/Cas9 in mouse liver in spite of Cas9-specific immune responses." *Human Gene Therapy* 26, no. 7 (2015): 432–442.

Wiedenheft, Blake, Gabriel C. Lander, Kaihong Zhou, Matthijs M. Jore, Stan JJ Brouns, John van der Oost, Jennifer A. Doudna, and Eva Nogales. "Structures of the RNA-guided surveillance complex from a bacterial immune system." *Nature* 477, no. 7365 (2011): 486–489.

Wilson, James M., and Terence R. Flotte. "Moving forward after two deaths in a gene therapy trial of myotubular myopathy: To learn from these tragedies, the scientific community must commit to full transparency and cooperation." *Genetic Engineering & Biotechnology News* 40, no. 8 (2020): 14–16.

Wong, Philip C., David R. Borchelt, Michael K. Lee, Carlos A. Pardo, Gopal Thinakaran, Lee J. Martin, Sangram S. Sisodia, and Donald L. Price. "Familial amyotrophic lateral sclerosis and Alzheimer's disease." *Molecular and Cellular Mechanisms of Neuronal Plasticity* (1998): 145–159.

Wu, Chaodong, David A. Okar, Christopher B. Newgard, and Alex J. Lange. "Increasing fructose 2, 6-bisphosphate overcomes hepatic insulin resistance of type 2 diabetes." *American Journal of Physiology-Endocrinology and Metabolism* 282, no. 1 (2002): E38–E45.

Xiong, Wenjun, David M. Wu, Yunlu Xue, Sean K. Wang, Michelle J. Chung, Xuke Ji, Parimal Rana, Sophia R. Zhao, Shuyi Mai, and Constance L. Cepko. "AAV cis-regulatory sequences are correlated with ocular toxicity." *Proceedings of the National Academy of Sciences* 116, no. 12 (2019): 5785–5794.

Yamamoto, Akihiro, Hideyuki Takagi, Daisuke Kitamura, Hozumi Tatsuoka, Hirotake Nakano, Hitoshi Kawano, Hidehito Kuroyanagi et al. "Deficiency in protein L-isoaspartyl methyltransferase results in a fatal progressive epilepsy." *Journal of Neuroscience* 18, no. 6 (1998): 2063–2074.

Yuasa, K., M. Yoshimura, N. Urasawa, S. Ohshima, J. M. Howell, A. Nakamura, T. Hijikata, Y. Miyagoe-Suzuki, and S. Takeda. "Injection of a recombinant AAV serotype 2 into canine skeletal muscles evokes strong immune responses against transgene products." *Gene Therapy* 14, no. 17 (2007): 1249–1260.

Zhang, Yi, Valina L. Dawson, and Ted M. Dawson. "Oxidative stress and genetics in the pathogenesis of Parkinson's disease." *Neurobiology of Disease* 7, no. 4 (2000): 240–250.

4 Clinical Applications of siRNA

Seth Kwabena Amponsah, Ismaila Adams and Kwasi Agyei Bugyei

CONTENTS

4.1 INTRODUCTION

With technological advancements, there exist novel therapeutic interventions that are used to manage and treat diseases, some of which include gene therapy. The potential for gene therapy is enormous, as it targets disease-causing genes based on their sequence. Gene therapy helps to achieve accurate and customized treatment in a number of life-threatening disorders. Gene expression can be down-regulated, up-regulated or corrected by delivering specific nucleic acids to targeted tissues (1). Small interfering ribonucleic acid (siRNA), microRNA (miRNA), and inhibitory antisense oligonucleotides (ASOs) are examples of molecules used to inhibit genes (2). On the other hand, plasmid deoxyribonucleic acid (pDNA), messenger RNA (mRNA), small activating RNA (saRNA) and splicing-modulatory ASOs can also be used to increase gene expression (2–3).

RNA interference (RNAi) is a phenomenon of sequence-specific gene silencing. RNAi can be used to investigate the physiological and pathophysiological mechanisms of diseases (4–5). Since the discovery of RNAi, significant progress has been made in understanding and exploiting gene-silencing mechanisms, particularly with the use of siRNA. RNAi modalities such as siRNA and miRNA can knock down expression of target genes in a sequence-specific manner (6) and subsequently silence a number of disease-related genes.

RNAi is thought to have promising therapeutic applications, and clinicians are eager to apply this new treatment strategy. There have been a number of studies on RNAi; however, only a few clinical trial reports have been published (7). Nonetheless,

DOI: 10.1201/9781003186069-4

there has been significant clinical advancement with RNAi (8–9). Among the modalities of RNAi, siRNA holds prospects in therapy. However, certain intracellular and extracellular barriers limit its extensive clinical application. Naked and unmodified siRNA possess unsatisfactory stability and poor pharmacokinetic characteristics (9). To maximize efficacy and reduce side effects, scientists have developed different delivery systems for siRNA. Alnylam Pharmaceuticals has received clearance for two siRNA therapies, Onpattro (patisiran) and Givlaari (givosiran), after about two decades of development (9). Indeed, siRNA has reached a watershed moment in the treatment and management of diseases and will continue to do so in the future. In this chapter, we discuss current clinical applications of siRNA.

4.2 BIOCHEMISTRY OF siRNA

siRNAs are short synthetic RNA duplexes that are made up of two 21-mer oligonucleotide strands with 19 nucleotides of complementary bases and a 2-nucleotide overhang at each 3' end (10). There can be cleavage of longer double-stranded RNA (dsRNA) into siRNA (11). The enzyme responsible for this processing is an RNase III–like enzyme known as dicer (12). A nuclease-containing multiprotein complex known as RNA-induced silencing complex (RISC) in the cytoplasm binds to the siRNAs as they are produced. siRNA strands are split inside the RISC (13). The strand with the more stable 5' end is integrated into the active RISC complex. The RISC complex is then guided and aligned on target mRNA by the antisense single-stranded siRNA component. Finally, the mRNA is cleaved by the catalytic RISC protein, a member of the argonaute family (Ago2) (13). This entire mechanism is summarized in Figure 4.1.

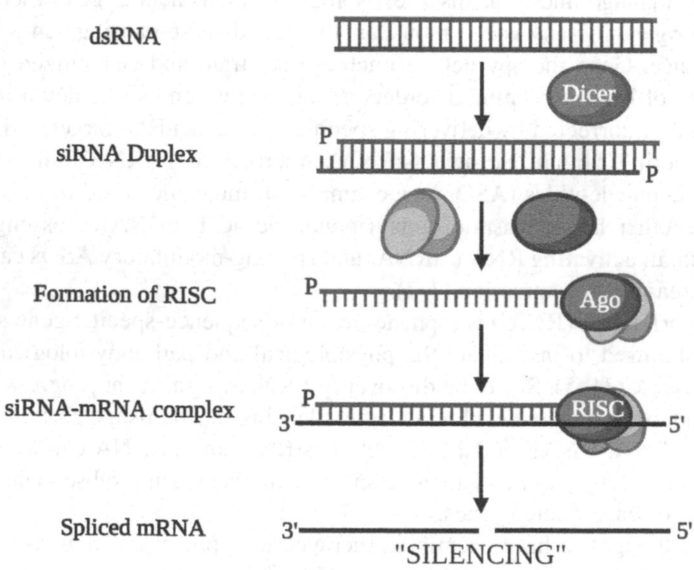

FIGURE 4.1 Biochemistry of siRNA.

4.3 RECENT CLINICAL APPLICATIONS OF siRNA

4.3.1 Cancers

siRNA-based delivery systems hold promise in cancer therapy so far as their safety is guaranteed. These delivery systems can target any cancer-related gene (14). The use of siRNAs in cancer therapy allows precise targeting of cancer-related genes such as epidermal growth factor receptor (EGFR), tumor protein p53 (p53), histone deacetylase (HDAC) or integrin subunit beta 1 (Itgbl). Targeting these genes has the tendency to decrease tumor cell proliferation, metastasis and drug resistance (15–16).

EGFRs are good targets for inhibiting tumor angiogenesis. Some carcinogenic EGFR genes have been coupled with siRNA in lung cancer models, and this has led to significant therapeutic impact (17). Additionally, the use of siRNA to target p53 for the treatment of lung cancers has recently received a lot of attention (18). Lung cancers can be treated with a combination of miR-34a (which restores p53 downstream) and siRNA (19). This combination has the tendency to increase apoptosis in cells and decrease tumor volume (19). HDAC regulates protein expression by interacting with cancer-related genes and preventing tumor development. In an orthotropic xenograft model, HDAC siRNA/lipid nanoparticles were found to be beneficial in decreasing the development of liver tumors (20). Furthermore, Itgbl is important for hepatoma cell proliferation. Experiments have demonstrated that siRNAs targeting Itgbl can slow the progression of hepatocellular carcinoma (21–22). In hepatocellular and breast cancer cells, human telomerase reverse transcriptase (hTERT) is abundantly expressed and active (23). Telomerase activity can be reduced by using hTERT-siRNA that targets bioreducible polyethylenimine (SS-PEI) (24). It is therefore not surprising that about one-third of siRNA-based medicinal interventions target cancers (25).

4.3.1.1 Lung Cancer

RNAi can be delivered to lung cancer cells using nanocarriers (26). For example, chitosan-derived carbon, a highly effective fluorescent nanoparticle coupled to a functionalized siRNA, was found to target tumor cell overexpression in the polo-like kinase 1 (PlK1) gene (27). In vivo and in vitro studies have demonstrated that these nanoparticles efficiently lower Plk1 expression and increase apoptosis (28). Due to selective silencing of oncogenes and multidrug resistance–related genes, nanoparticle-mediated RNAi are now favorable alternatives to traditional chemotherapy (29–30). Research into microRNA in the diagnosis, prognosis and treatment of lung cancer is ongoing. These studies aim at overcoming barriers of nanoparticle-mediated siRNA therapy (31–33).

4.3.1.2 Colorectal Cancer

Colorectal cancer is a common digestive system malignancy (34). Surgery, radiation and chemotherapeutic interventions are unable to increase survival among patients with colorectal cancer beyond five years (35). Given that colonic epithelial cells undergo neoplastic transformation, RNAi has been recommended as a treatment approach. RNAi offers greater efficacy and reduced toxicity. However, due to transfection, limited specificity, low immune response and superfluous gene insertion, only a handful of RNAi-based treatments have undergone clinical trials (28). New molecular targets for RNAi are still being studied (36). Novel intracellular targeting technologies, such as siRNA, and new nano-delivery systems have been reported to have high anticancer potential and few side effects (37). Furthermore, colon cancer causes carcinogenesis via a number of molecular mechanisms, including overexpression of EGFR (38). Dimerized EGFR is known to deliver mitotic signals to tumor cells, causing cell proliferation and resistance to apoptosis. As a result, siRNA knockout of EGFR has been proposed as a plausible treatment option for colon cancer (39).

4.3.1.3 Breast Cancer

Breast cancer is the most prevalent malignancy among women (40). Different genetic alterations can cause varied breast cancer subtypes, case outcome and therapy responsiveness (41). In this context, gene therapy is a possible therapeutic option for breast cancer. Genetic alteration of target cells with RNAi interventions such as siRNAs and miRNAs have been reported as having great potential in breast cancer treatment (28).

RNAi-based therapies for human epidermal growth factor receptor 2+ (HER2+) breast cancers have been investigated. Two clinical trials targeting HER2 have yielded positive results (42). Furthermore, targeted siRNA has been investigated as a possible means to overcome chemoresistance in cancer therapy (43–44).

4.3.1.4 Pancreatic Cancer

Pancreatic cancer is an aggressive malignant tumor that is generally asymptomatic in its early stages. Pancreatic ductal adenocarcinoma is known to account for about 90% of all pancreatic cancer cases (45). Despite availability of therapeutic options for pancreatic ductal adenocarcinoma, the five-year survival rate remains poor (46–47). Data suggest that when radiation and chemotherapy are coupled with RNAi, pancreatic cancer cells become less resistant to these treatments (28).

Kirsten rat sarcoma viral oncogene (KRAS) is a mutant oncogene found in a variety of human malignancies, including pancreatic, colon and lung cancer (48). A number of studies have used siRNA to silence KRAS (49–50). Additionally, there are miRNA-based treatment options for pancreatic cancers (51). Despite the potential for siRNA treatments, there are challenges such as difficulty in crossing biological barriers, limited cell uptake and degradation (52). Nanotechnology may be an option in solving the aforementioned challenges (53).

4.3.2 Eye Diseases

siRNA therapy has proven effective in the treatment of eye diseases. Indeed, the first therapeutic use of RNAi was to treat wet age-related macular degeneration (54). Since then, RNAi-based treatments have been used for diabetic retinopathy, retinitis pigmentosa, corneal neovascularization, fibrotic eye diseases and glaucoma (54–55). The eye is currently considered a good target for RNAi therapy mainly because it is found in a confined compartment. However, delivery strategies that protect siRNAs from degradation would help improve its efficacy (56).

Sylentis Company (Madrid, Spain) has developed an siRNA treatment for glaucoma that targets β_2-adrenoceptors (57). This long-lasting reduction of intraocular pressure by siRNA may be one of the most promising new approaches in glaucoma treatment. siRNAs can penetrate the corneal limbus and reduce intraocular pressure (54). Other targets have also been proposed, although they have not yet been tested in humans. siRNA silencing of Ras homolog family member A (RhoA) in the trabecular meshwork effectively decreased intraocular pressure in a mouse model (58). Cochlin is another potential target for siRNA in glaucoma therapy (59). siRNA-based treatments to prevent apoptosis and provide ocular neuroprotection have also been proposed (54).

The primary cause of age-related macular degeneration and diabetic retinopathy is angiogenesis (60). The ability of siRNAs to target vascular endothelial growth factor (VEGF) and prevent neovascularization has been proven (61). The most frequent approach is to inject naked siRNA into the posterior region of the eye across the corneal scleral barrier (62). This approach delivers medication to the target. siRNAs targeting β_2-adrenergic receptors (SYL040012) were evaluated in animal models (57). Findings revealed that SYL040012 expression was suppressed and aqueous humor production was decreased. In phase II studies in individuals with eye disorders, the effectiveness, safety and tolerability of this siRNA therapy have been positive (63).

4.3.3 Liver Disease

RNAi-mediated gene silencing has been used to treat liver conditions in numerous proof-of-concept studies and clinical trials (64). The very specific down-regulation of gene expression that siRNA has over other antisense-based treatments is key.

At the molecular level, liver diseases are caused by either gain of function of specific genes (such as the addition of foreign genes) or loss of function of any of the many genes involved in normal liver metabolism (65). When gain of function is the primary cause of disease, RNAi applications are straightforward. However, when loss of function is the primary cause, altering homeostatic balance of cellular pathways may be the option (66). Both methods have been studied with equal effectiveness in a range of liver disorders, and a large number of current clinical trials have also been conducted (67). Lipid nanoparticle formulations have been developed as agents for delivering siRNAs to hepatocytes, resulting in a stable and long-lasting decrease in genetic expression (68).

The promise of RNAi as a therapeutic intervention for hereditary diseases caused by gain-of-function mutations in the liver has recently been shown (69). For instance, preclinical and clinical research have been conducted into conformational disorders such as amyloidosis and some forms of alpha-1 antitrypsin deficiency (70). PiZ (p.E342K), a frequent pathogenic allele, can cause protein misfolding and aggregation inside the hepatocyte, resulting in liver damage (71). Heterozygous individuals carrying a single copy of the PiZ allele show no apparent liver disease. RNAi technologies can interfere with the expression of the gene p.E342K, which causes protein misfolding and liver damage (72).

Dynamic PolyConjugate (Arrowhead Pharmaceuticals), which targets the endosomal pathway, is able to lower circulating alpha-1 antitrypsin levels by almost 80% (73). Alnylam Pharmaceuticals has also tried siRNA that is directly coupled to *N*-acetylgalactosamine (GalNAc). The company also has developed transthyretin siRNA to treat amyloidosis (73).

Liver porphyrias are good examples of hereditary liver diseases. Specific enzymes have been successfully targeted by siRNA to reduce the production of toxic porphyrins (74). The heme-producing enzyme delta-aminolevulinate synthase (ALAS) is the first and rate-limiting enzyme of heme synthesis. ALAS1 has been proposed as a good target for RNAi therapeutics in acute hepatic porphyria (74).

Hepatitis B and C are viral infections that, if left untreated, can lead to cirrhosis and cancer of the liver (75). The complexity of the life cycle of hepatitis B virus (HBV), its integration into the host genome and its effect on the host immune system all contribute to challenges in appropriate treatment. The use of an RNAi-based technology has multiple potential benefits and may be able to harness natural mechanisms in the treatment of chronic hepatitis B (76). The molecular biology of HBV means that it is amenable to RNAi (77).

RNAi could be used to develop new therapies for chronic hepatitis B, but there are several important aspects to consider. There are concerns about immunogenicity and the possibility of mutations when utilizing viral vectors (78). RNAi can also accumulate in non-target tissue after systemic treatment, causing toxicity in healthy tissues (79).

ARC-520 (produced by Arrowhead Pharmaceuticals) is a polymer-based technology that facilitates endosomal escape and cytoplasmic distribution of RNAi (9). Arrowhead Pharmaceuticals was the first to publish results of RNAi as a possible candidate in the treatment of chronic hepatitis B (73). The liver is also one of the main locations for Ebola virus replication, and siRNAs may be beneficial in the treatment of Ebola virus disease (80).

4.3.4 Respiratory Diseases

Several studies have shown the use of siRNA in the treatment of respiratory diseases (26, 81–83). Some of these diseases include influenza, cystic fibrosis and asthma. Influenza infection can be treated by using siRNA against conserved sections of the influenza virus gene or nucleocapsid gene (84). Infections with parainfluenza virus were also shown to be successfully treated with siRNA (85).

Cystic fibrosis, a hereditary disease that impairs lung function, has been found to be managed adequately using siRNA therapeutic agents (86). The epithelial sodium channel (EnaC) is thought to be a promising target for RNAi treatment in cystic fibrosis (87). In allergic-impaired mice, siRNAs were found to decrease airway resistance (88). Cationic polymers like polyethyleneimines are frequently employed to deliver siRNA to the lungs. When siRNA targeting the influenza virus gene was combined with polyethyleneimine, viral titers in the lungs of mice infected with influenza were dramatically reduced (89). Polyethyleneimine employed as an siRNA vector reduced the development of cancer in a lung metastasis model (89).

4.4 CONCLUSION

Researchers and pharmaceutical companies are exploring the use of siRNA in the treatment of diseases, as summarized in Table 4.1. SiRNA-based therapy has its innate advantages, some of which include providing treatment options for several

TABLE 4.1
Clinical Applications of siRNA

Disease	siRNA target(s)	References
Colorectal cancer	Epidermal growth factor receptor, Ras	(17, 49)
Lung cancer	p53	(19)
Breast cancer	Human epidermal growth factor receptor 2+	(42)
Glaucoma	Ras, cochlin, β_2-adrenergic receptors	(54–55)
Amyloidosis	Transthyretin	(7, 68)
Hepatitis B	Hepatitis B viral proteins	(78)
Cystic fibrosis	Epithelial sodium channel (EnaC)	(87)

cancer types. Despite successes with siRNA, there are challenges in some aspects of its delivery systems. If these delivery systems are optimized, siRNA-based therapy has the potential to revolutionize disease treatment.

REFERENCES

1. Goswami R, Subramanian G, Silayeva L, Newkirk I, Doctor D, Chawla K, et al. Gene therapy leaves a vicious cycle. *Front Oncol* [Internet]. 2019 Apr 24 [cited 2021 Jul 24];9(Apr):297. Available from: www.frontiersin.org
2. Chery J. RNA therapeutics: RNAi and antisense mechanisms and clinical applications. *Postdoc J* [Internet]. 2016 Jul 20 [cited 2021 Jul 24];4(7):35. Available from: /pmc/articles/PMC4995773/
3. Bennett CF, Swayze EE. RNA targeting therapeutics: Molecular mechanisms of antisense oligonucleotides as a therapeutic platform. *Annu Rev Pharmacol Toxicol.* 2010 Feb 10;50:259–293.
4. Fuchs U, Damm-Welk C, Borkhardt A. Silencing of disease-related genes by small interfering RNAs. *Curr Mol Med.* 2005 Mar 18;4(5):507–517.
5. Cheng JC, Moore TB, Sakamoto KM. RNA interference and human disease. *Mol Genet Metab* [Internet]. 2003 [cited 2021 Jul 24];80(1–2):121–128. Available from: https://pubmed.ncbi.nlm.nih.gov/14567961/
6. Leung RKM, Whittaker PA. RNA interference: From gene silencing to gene-specific therapeutics. *Pharmacol Ther* [Internet]. 2005 Aug [cited 2021 Jul 24];107(2):222–239. Available from: /pmc/articles/PMC7112686/
7. Kubowicz P, Zelaszczyk D, Pekala E. RNAi in Clinical Studies. *Curr Med Chem.* 2013 Apr 8;20(14):1801–1816.
8. Chernikov IV., Vlassov VV., Chernolovskaya EL. Current development of siRNA bioconjugates: From research to the clinic. *Front Pharmacol.* 2019;10(Apr):444.
9. Hu B, Zhong L, Weng Y, Peng L, Huang Y, Zhao Y, et al. Therapeutic siRNA: State of the art. *Signal Transduct Target Ther* [Internet]. 2020 Jun 19 [cited 2021 Jul 24];5(1):1–25. Available from: https://www.nature.com/articles/s41392-020-0207-x
10. Elbashir SM, Lendeckel W, Tuschl T. RNA interference is mediated by 21- and 22-nucleotide RNAs. *Genes Dev* [Internet]. 2001 Jan 15 [cited 2021 Jul 24];15(2):188–200. Available from: /pmc/articles/PMC312613/
11. Agrawal N, Dasaradhi PVN, Mohmmed A, Malhotra P, Bhatnagar RK, Mukherjee SK. RNA Interference: Biology, mechanism, and applications. *Microbiol Mol Biol Rev* [Internet]. 2003 Dec [cited 2021 Jul 24];67(4):657–685. Available from: /pmc/articles/PMC309050/

12. Ji X. The mechanism of RNase III action: How Dicer dices. *Curr Top Microbiol Immunol* [Internet]. 2008 [cited 2021 Jul 24];320:99–116. Available from: https://pubmed.ncbi.nlm.nih.gov/18268841/
13. Leuschner PJF, Ameres SL, Kueng S, Martinez J. Cleavage of the siRNA passenger strand during RISC assembly in human cells. *EMBO Rep* [Internet]. 2006 Mar [cited 2021 Jul 24];7(3):314–320. Available from: /pmc/articles/PMC1456892/
14. Xu C fei, Wang J. Delivery systems for siRNA drug development in cancer therapy. *Asian J Pharm Sci.* 2015 Feb 1;10(1):1–12.
15. Mahmoodi Chalbatani G, Dana H, Gharagouzloo E, Grijalvo S, Eritja R, Logsdon CD, et al. Small interfering RNAs (siRNAs) in cancer therapy: A nano-based approach. *Int J Nanomedicine* [Internet]. 2019 [cited 2021 Jul 24];14:3111–128. Available from: /pmc/articles/PMC6504672/
16. Mansoori B, Shotorbani SS, Baradaran B. RNA interference and its role in cancer therapy. Adv Pharm Bull [Internet]. 2014 [cited 2021 Jul 24];4(4):313–321. Available from: /pmc/articles/PMC4137419/
17. Yamanaka S, Gu Z, Sato M, Fujisaki R, Inomata K, Sakurada A, et al. siRNA targeting against EGFR, a promising candidate for a novel therapeutic application to lung adenocarcinoma. *Pathobiology* [Internet]. 2008 Mar [cited 2021 Jul 24];75(1):2–8. Available from: https://pubmed.ncbi.nlm.nih.gov/18334834/
18. Ubby I, Krueger C, Rosato R, Qian W, Chang J, Sabapathy K. Cancer therapeutic targeting using mutant—p53-specific siRNAs. *Oncogene* [Internet]. 2019 Jan 14 [cited 2021 Jul 24];38(18):3415–3427. Available from: https://www.nature.com/articles/s41388-018-0652-y
19. Xue W, Dahlman JE, Tammela T, Khan OF, Sood S, Dave A, et al. Small RNA combination therapy for lung cancer. *Proc Natl Acad Sci U S A* [Internet]. 2014 Aug 26 [cited 2021 Jul 24];111(34):E3553. Available from: /pmc/articles/PMC4151750/
20. Lee YH, Seo D, Choi KJ, Andersen JB, Won MA, Kitade M, et al. Antitumor effects in hepatocarcinoma of isoform-selective inhibition of HDAC2. *Cancer Res* [Internet]. 2014 Sep 1 [cited 2021 Jul 24];74(17):4752–4761. Available from: /pmc/articles/PMC4155016/
21. Hajiasgharzadeh K, Somi MH, Shanehbandi D, Mokhtarzadeh A, Baradaran B. Small interfering RNA—mediated gene suppression as a therapeutic intervention in hepatocellular carcinoma. *J Cell Physiol* [Internet]. 2019 Apr 1 [cited 2021 Jul 24];234(4):3263–3276. Available from: https://onlinelibrary.wiley.com/doi/full/10.1002/jcp.27015
22. Bogorad RL, Yin H, Zeigerer A, Nonaka H, Ruda VM, Zerial M, et al. Nanoparticle-formulated siRNA targeting integrins inhibits hepatocellular carcinoma progression in mice. *Nat Commun* [Internet]. 2014 May 21 [cited 2021 Jul 24];5:3869. Available from: /pmc/articles/PMC4107318/
23. Leão R, Apolónio JD, Lee D, Figueiredo A, Tabori U, Castelo-Branco P. Mechanisms of human telomerase reverse transcriptase (hTERT) regulation: Clinical impacts in cancer. *J Biomed Sci* [Internet]. 2018 Mar 12 [cited 2021 Jul 24];25(1):1–12. Available from: https://jbiomedsci.biomedcentral.com/articles/10.1186/s12929-018-0422-8
24. Xia W, Wang P, Lin C, Li Z, Gao X, Wang G, et al. Bioreducible polyethylenimine-delivered siRNA targeting human telomerase reverse transcriptase inhibits HepG2 cell growth in vitro and in vivo. *J Control Release.* 2012 Feb 10;157(3):427–436.
25. Guo W, Chen W, Yu W, Huang W, Deng W. Small interfering RNA-based molecular therapy of cancers. *Chin J Cancer* [Internet]. 2013 [cited 2021 Jul 24];32(9):488–493. Available from: /pmc/articles/PMC3845562/
26. Fujita Y, Kuwano K, Ochiya T. Development of small RNA delivery systems for lung cancer therapy. *Int J Mol Sci* [Internet]. 2015 Mar 6 [cited 2021 Jul 24];16(3):5254–5270. Available from: /pmc/articles/PMC4394474/

27. Zhang L, Zheng W, Tang R, Wang N, Zhang W, Jiang X. Gene regulation with carbon-based siRNA conjugates for cancer therapy. *Biomaterials*. 2016 Oct 1;104:269–278.
28. Tian Z, Liang G, Cui K, Liang Y, Wang Q, Lv S, et al. Insight into the prospects for RNAi therapy of cancer. *Front Pharmacol*. 2021 Mar 16;12:308.
29. Kim YD, Park TE, Singh B, Maharjan S, Choi YJ, Choung PH, et al. Nanoparticle-mediated delivery of siRNA for effective lung cancer therapy. *Nanomedicine* [Internet]. 2015 Apr 1 [cited 2021 Jul 24];10(7):1165–1188. Available from: https://pubmed.ncbi.nlm.nih.gov/25929572/
30. Babu A, Munshi A, Ramesh R. Combinatorial therapeutic approaches with RNAi and anticancer drugs using nanodrug delivery systems. *Drug Dev Ind Pharm*. 2017 Sep 2;43(9):1391–401.
31. Iqbal MA, Arora S, Prakasam G, Calin GA, Syed MA. MicroRNA in lung cancer: Role, mechanisms, pathways and therapeutic relevance. *Mol Aspects Med*. 2019 Dec 1;70:3–20.
32. Zhu X, Kudo M, Huang X, Sui H, Tian H, Croce CM, et al. Frontiers of MicroRNA signature in non-small cell lung cancer. *Front Cell Dev Biol*. 2021 Apr 7;9:771.
33. Wu KL, Tsai YM, Lien CT, Kuo PL, Hung JY. The roles of microRNA in lung cancer. *Int J Mol Sci* [Internet]. 2019 Apr 1 [cited 2021 Jul 24];20(7). Available from: /pmc/articles/PMC6480472/
34. Katona BW, Lynch JP. Mechanisms of gastrointestinal malignancies. *Physiol Gastrointest Tract Sixth Ed*. 2018 Jan 1;2–2:1615–1642.
35. Miller KD, Nogueira L, Mariotto AB, Rowland JH, Yabroff KR, Alfano CM, et al. Cancer treatment and survivorship statistics, 2019. *CA Cancer J Clin* [Internet]. 2019 Sep 1 [cited 2021 Jul 24];69(5):363–385. Available from: https://acsjournals.onlinelibrary.wiley.com/doi/full/10.3322/caac.21565
36. Swaminathan G, Shigna A, Kumar A, Byroju VV, Durgempudi VR, Dinesh Kumar L. RNA interference and nanotechnology: A promising alliance for next generation cancer therapeutics. *Front Nanotechnol*. 2021 Jun 9;0:42.
37. Sezgin-Bayindir Z, Losada-Barreiro S, Bravo-Díaz C, Sova M, Kristl J, Saso L. Nanotechnology-based drug delivery to improve the therapeutic benefits of NRF2 modulators in cancer therapy. *Antioxidants* [Internet]. 2021 Apr 27;10(5):685. Available from: https://www.mdpi.com/2076-3921/10/5/685
38. Pabla B, Bissonnette M, Konda VJ. Colon cancer and the epidermal growth factor receptor: Current treatment paradigms, the importance of diet, and the role of chemoprevention. http://www.wjgnet.com/ [Internet]. 2015 Oct 10 [cited 2021 Jul 27];6(5):133–141. Available from: https://www.wjgnet.com/2218-4333/full/v6/i5/133.htm
39. Kim JS, Kim MW, Kang SJ, Jeong HY, Park S Il, Lee YK, et al. Tumor-specific delivery of therapeutic siRNAs by anti-EGFR immunonanoparticles. *Int J Nanomedicine* [Internet]. 2018 [cited 2021 Jul 27];13:4817. Available from: /pmc/articles/PMC6118344/
40. Momenimovahed Z, Salehiniya H. Epidemiological characteristics of and risk factors for breast cancer in the world. *Breast Cancer Targets Ther* [Internet]. 2019 [cited 2021 Jul 24];11:151–164. Available from: /pmc/articles/PMC6462164/
41. Testa U, Castelli G, Pelosi E. Breast cancer: A molecularly heterogenous disease needing subtype-specific treatments. *Med Sci* [Internet]. 2020 Mar 23 [cited 2021 Jul 24];8(1):18. Available from: /pmc/articles/PMC7151639/
42. Ngamcherdtrakul W, Castro DJ, Gu S, Morry J, Reda M, Gray JW, et al. Current development of targeted oligonucleotide-based cancer therapies: Perspective on HER2-positive breast cancer treatment. *Cancer Treat Rev* [Internet]. 2016 Apr 1 [cited 2021 Jul 24];45:19–29. Available from: http://www.cancertreatmentreviews.com/article/S0305737216000207/fulltext
43. Subhan MA, Attia SA, Torchilin VP. Advances in siRNA delivery strategies for the treatment of MDR cancer. *Life Sci* [Internet]. 2021 Jun 1 [cited 2021 Jul 24];274. Available from: https://pubmed.ncbi.nlm.nih.gov/33713664/

44. Lee SJ, Kim MJ, Kwon IC, Roberts TM. Delivery strategies and potential targets for siRNA in major cancer types. *Adv Drug Deliv Rev* [Internet]. 2016 [cited 2021 Jul 24];104:2–15. Available from: /pmc/articles/PMC4958528/
45. Kleeff J, Korc M, Apte M, La Vecchia C, Johnson CD, Biankin AV, et al. Pancreatic cancer. *Nat Rev Dis Prim* [Internet]. 2016 Apr 21 [cited 2021 Jul 24];2. Available from: https://pubmed.ncbi.nlm.nih.gov/27158978/
46. Adamska A, Domenichini A, Falasca M. Pancreatic ductal adenocarcinoma: Current and evolving therapies. *Int J Mol Sci* [Internet]. 2017 Jul 1 [cited 2021 Jul 24];18(7). Available from: /pmc/articles/PMC5535831/
47. Lambert A, Schwarz L, Borbath I, Henry A, Van Laethem JL, Malka D, et al. An update on treatment options for pancreatic adenocarcinoma. *Ther Adv Med Oncol* [Internet]. 2019 [cited 2021 Jul 24];11. Available from: /pmc/articles/PMC6763942/
48. Liu P, Wang Y, Li X. Targeting the untargetable KRAS in cancer therapy. *Acta Pharm Sin B*. 2019 Sep 1;9(5):871–9.
49. Strand MS, Krasnick BA, Pan H, Zhang X, Bi Y, Brooks C, et al. Precision delivery of RAS-inhibiting siRNA to KRAS driven cancer via peptide-based nanoparticles. *Oncotarget* [Internet]. 2019 [cited 2021 Jul 24];10(46):4761–4775. Available from: /pmc/articles/PMC6677667/
50. Papke B, Azam SH, Feng AY, Gutierrez-Ford C, Huggins H, Pallan PS, et al. Silencing of oncogenic KRAS by mutant-selective small interfering RNA. *ACS Pharmacol Transl Sci* [Internet]. 2021 Apr 9 [cited 2021 Jul 24];4(2):703–712. Available from: https://pubs.acs.org/doi/abs/10.1021/acsptsci.0c00165
51. Daoud AZ, Mulholland EJ, Cole G, McCarthy HO. MicroRNAs in pancreatic cancer: Biomarkers, prognostic, and therapeutic modulators. *BMC Cancer* [Internet]. 2019 Nov 21 [cited 2021 Jul 24];19(1):1–13. Available from: https://bmccancer.biomedcentral.com/articles/10.1186/s12885-019-6284-y
52. Sajid MI, Moazzam M, Tiwari RK, Kato S, Cho KY. Overcoming barriers for siRNA therapeutics: From bench to bedside. *Pharmaceuticals* [Internet]. 2020 Oct 1 [cited 2021 Jul 24];13(10):1–25. Available from: /pmc/articles/PMC7600125/
53. Shi J, Kantoff PW, Wooster R, Farokhzad OC. Cancer nanomedicine: Progress, challenges and opportunities. *Nat Rev Cancer* [Internet]. 2017 Jan 1 [cited 2021 Jul 24];17(1):20–37. Available from: /pmc/articles/PMC5575742/
54. Guzman-Aranguez A, Loma P, Pintor J. Small-interfering RNAs (siRNAs) as a promising tool for ocular therapy. *Br J Pharmacol* [Internet]. 2013 Oct [cited 2021 Jul 24];170(4):730–747. Available from: /pmc/articles/PMC3799589/
55. Naik S, Shreya AB, Raychaudhuri R, Pandey A, Lewis SA, Hazarika M, et al. Small interfering RNAs (siRNAs) based gene silencing strategies for the treatment of glaucoma: Recent advancements and future perspectives. *Life Sci*. 2021 Jan 1;264:118712.
56. Lam JKW, Chow MYT, Zhang Y, Leung SWS. siRNA versus miRNA as therapeutics for gene silencing. *Mol Ther—Nucleic Acids*. 2015 Jan 1;4(9):e252.
57. Martínez T, González MV, Roehl I, Wright N, Pañeda C, Jiménez AI. In vitro and in vivo efficacy of SYL040012, a novel siRNA compound for treatment of glaucoma. *Mol Ther* [Internet]. 2014 [cited 2021 Jul 24];22(1):81–91. Available from: /pmc/articles/PMC3978804/
58. Liu Q, Wu K, Qiu X, Yang Y, Lin X, Yu M. siRNA silencing of gene expression in trabecular meshwork: RhoA siRNA reduces IOP in mice. *Curr Mol Med*. 2012;12(8):1015–1027.
59. Goel M, Sienkiewicz AE, Picciani R, Wang J, Lee RK, Bhattacharya SK. Cochlin, intraocular pressure regulation and mechanosensing. *PLoS One* [Internet]. 2012 Apr 4 [cited 2021 Jul 24];7(4):34309. Available from: /pmc/articles/PMC3319572/
60. Penn JS, Madan A, Caldwell RB, Bartoli M, Caldwell RW, Hartnett ME. Vascular endothelial growth factor in eye disease. *Prog Retin Eye Res* [Internet]. 2008 Jul [cited 2021 Jul 24];27(4):331–371. Available from: https://pubmed.ncbi.nlm.nih.gov/18653375/

61. Chang JH, Garg NK, Lunde E, Han KY, Jain S, Azar DT. Corneal neovascularization: An anti-VEGF therapy review. *Surv Ophthalmol* [Internet]. 2012 Sep [cited 2021 Jul 24];57(5):415–429. Available from: /pmc/articles/PMC3709023/
62. Thakur A, Fitzpatrick S, Zaman A, Kugathasan K, Muirhead B, Hortelano G, et al. Strategies for ocular siRNA delivery: Potential and limitations of non-viral nanocarriers. *J Biol Eng* [Internet]. 2012 Jun 11 [cited 2021 Jul 24];6:7. Available from: /pmc/articles/PMC3533807/
63. Benitez-Del-Castillo JM, Moreno-Montañés J, Jiménez-Alfaro I, Muñoz-Negrete FJ, Turman K, Palumaa K, et al. Safety and efficacy clinical trials for SYL1001, a novel short interfering RNA for the treatment of dry eye disease. *Investig Ophthalmol Vis Sci* [Internet]. 2016 Nov 1 [cited 2021 Jul 24];57(14):6447–6454. Available from: www.clinicaltrials.gov
64. Bumcrot D, Manoharan M, Koteliansky V, Sah DWY. RNAi therapeutics: A potential new class of pharmaceutical drugs. *Nat Chem Biol* [Internet]. 2006 [cited 2021 Jul 24];2(12):711–719. Available from: https://www.nature.com/articles/nchembio839
65. Worman HJ. Molecular biology and the diagnosis and treatment of liver diseases. *World J Gastroenterol* [Internet]. 1998 [cited 2021 Jul 24];4(3):185. Available from: /pmc/articles/PMC4723453/
66. Sledz CA, Williams BRG. RNA interference in biology and disease. *Blood* [Internet]. 2005 Aug 1 [cited 2021 Jul 24];106(3):787–794. Available from: /pmc/articles/PMC1895153/
67. Kim KH, Park KK. Small RNA- And DNA-based gene therapy for the treatment of liver cirrhosis, where we are? *World J Gastroenterol* [Internet]. 2014 Oct 28 [cited 2021 Jul 24];20(40):14696–705. Available from: /pmc/articles/PMC4209535/
68. Yonezawa S, Koide H, Asai T. Recent advances in siRNA delivery mediated by lipid-based nanoparticles. *Adv Drug Deliv Rev* [Internet]. 2020 Jan 1 [cited 2021 Jul 24];154–155:64–78. Available from: /pmc/articles/PMC7406478/
69. Ambesajir A, Kaushik A, Kaushik JJ, Petros ST. RNA interference: A futuristic tool and its therapeutic applications. *Saudi J Biol Sci* [Internet]. 2012 Oct [cited 2021 Jul 24];19(4):395–403. Available from: /pmc/articles/PMC3730950/
70. Lomas DA. New therapeutic targets for alpha-1 antitrypsin deficiency. *Chronic Obstr Pulm Dis* [Internet]. 2018 [cited 2021 Jul 24];5(4):233–243. Available from: /pmc/articles/PMC6361470/
71. Mitchell EL, Khan Z. Liver disease in alpha-1 antitrypsin deficiency: Current approaches and future directions. *Curr Pathobiol Rep* [Internet]. 2017 Sep 1 [cited 2021 Jul 24];5(3):243–252. Available from: /pmc/articles/PMC5780543/
72. Gonzalez-Rodriguez A, Valverde A. RNA interference as a therapeutic strategy for the treatment of liver diseases. *Curr Pharm Des* [Internet]. 2015 Oct 15 [cited 2021 Jul 24];21(31):4574–4786. Available from: https://pubmed.ncbi.nlm.nih.gov/26486144/
73. Hu B, Weng Y, Xia XH, Liang X jie, Huang Y. Clinical advances of siRNA therapeutics. *J Gene Med* [Internet]. 2019 Jul 1 [cited 2021 Jul 25];21(7):e3097. Available from: https://onlinelibrary.wiley.com/doi/full/10.1002/jgm.3097
74. Lai C, Martin-Higueras C, Salido E. siRNA therapeutics to treat liver disorders. *Saf Effic Gene-Based Ther Inherit Disord* [Internet]. 2017 May 22 [cited 2021 Jul 25];159–190. Available from: https://link.springer.com/chapter/10.1007/978-3-319-53457-2_8
75. Ringehan M, McKeating JA, Protzer U. Viral hepatitis and liver cancer. *Philos Trans R Soc B Biol Sci* [Internet]. 2017 Oct 19 [cited 2021 Jul 25];372(1732). Available from: /pmc/articles/PMC5597741/
76. van den Berg F, Limani SW, Mnyandu N, Maepa MB, Ely A, Arbuthnot P. Advances with RNAi-based therapy for hepatitis B virus infection. *Viruses* [Internet]. 2020 Aug 1 [cited 2021 Jul 25];12(8). Available from: /pmc/articles/PMC7472220/

77. Nayagam JS, Cargill ZC, Agarwal K. The role of RNA interference in functional cure strategies for chronic hepatitis B. *Curr Hepatol Reports* [Internet]. 2020 Oct 28 [cited 2021 Jul 25];19(4):362–369. Available from: https://link.springer.com/article/10.1007/s11901-020-00548-4
78. Chen Y, Cheng G, Mahato RI. RNAi for treating hepatitis B viral infection. *Pharm Res* [Internet]. 2008 Jan [cited 2021 Jul 25];25(1):72–86. Available from: /pmc/articles/PMC2217617/
79. Wittrup A, Lieberman J. Knocking down disease: A progress report on siRNA therapeutics. *Nat Rev Genet* [Internet]. 2015 Aug 18 [cited 2021 Jul 25];16(9):543–552. Available from: /pmc/articles/PMC4756474/
80. Thi EP, Mire CE, Lee ACH, Geisbert JB, Zhou JZ, Agans KN, et al. Lipid nanoparticle siRNA treatment of Ebola-virus-Makona-infected nonhuman primates. *Nature* [Internet]. 2015 Apr 22 [cited 2021 Jul 24];521(7552):362–365. Available from: https://www.nature.com/articles/nature14442
81. Fujita Y, Takeshita F, Kuwano K, Ochiya T. RNAi therapeutic platforms for lung diseases. *Pharmaceuticals* [Internet]. 2013 Feb 6 [cited 2021 Jul 24];6(2):223–250. Available from: /pmc/articles/PMC3816685/
82. Kandil R, Merkel OM. Pulmonary delivery of siRNA as a novel treatment for lung diseases. *Ther Deliv* [Internet]. 2019 Apr 17 [cited 2021 Jul 24];10(4):203–206. Available from: https://www.future-science.com/doi/abs/10.4155/tde-2019-0009
83. Ding L, Tang S, Wyatt TA, Knoell DL, Oupický D. Pulmonary siRNA delivery for lung disease: Review of recent progress and challenges. *J Control Release*. 2021 Feb 10;330:977–991.
84. Ge Q, Eisen HN, Chen J. Use of siRNAs to prevent and treat influenza virus infection. *Virus Res* [Internet]. 2004 Jun 1 [cited 2021 Jul 24];102(1):37–42. Available from: https://pubmed.ncbi.nlm.nih.gov/15068878/
85. Fulton A, Peters ST, Perkins GA, Jarosinski KW, Damiani A, Brosnahan M, et al. Effective treatment of respiratory alphaherpesvirus infection using RNA interference. *PLoS One* [Internet]. 2009 Jan 5 [cited 2021 Jul 24];4(1):e4118. Available from: https://journals.plos.org/plosone/article?id=10.1371/journal.pone.0004118
86. Da Silva Sanchez A, Paunovska K, Cristian A, Dahlman JE. Treating cystic fibrosis with mRNA and CRISPR. *Hum Gene Ther* [Internet]. 2020 Sep 16 [cited 2021 Jul 24];31(17–18):940–955. Available from: https://www.liebertpub.com/doi/abs/10.1089/hum.2020.137
87. Tagalakis AD, Munye MM, Ivanova R, Chen H, Smith CM, Aldossary AM, et al. Effective silencing of ENaC by siRNA delivered with epithelial-targeted nanocomplexes in human cystic fibrosis cells and in mouse lung. *Thorax* [Internet]. 2018 Sep 1 [cited 2021 Jul 24];73(9):847–856. Available from: https://thorax.bmj.com/content/73/9/847
88. Lively TN, Kossen K, Balhorn A, Koya T, Zinnen S, Takeda K, et al. Effect of chemically modified IL-13 short interfering RNA on development of airway hyperresponsiveness in mice. *J Allergy Clin Immunol* [Internet]. 2008 Jan [cited 2021 Jul 24];121(1):88–94. Available from: /pmc/articles/PMC7112280/
89. Chen Y, Huang L. Tumor-targeted delivery of siRNA by non-viral vector: Safe and effective cancer therapy. *Expert Opin Drug Deliv* [Internet]. 2008 Dec [cited 2021 Jul 24];5(12):1301–1311. Available from: /pmc/articles/PMC5515368/

5 Human Genomics Projects, Gene Therapy and Precision Medicine

Sakshi Thassu and Yashwant V. Pathak

CONTENTS

5.1 INTRODUCTION

After the completion of the Human Genome Project (HGP), lots of expectations arose from the impact it would have on genomics in healthcare. At the time, HGP was a "monumental achievement" (5). We went from seeing the double helix to 3 billion nucleotides in only 50 years (5). With this achievement, precision medicine (PM) was born. PM is

> the tailoring of medical treatment to the individual characteristics of each patient . . . to classify individuals into subpopulation that differ in their susceptibility to a particular disease or their response toa specific treatment. Preventative or therapeutic interventions can then be concentration on those who will benefit, sparing expense and side effects for those who will not (1).

Although the term "precision medicine" is relatively new, the concept has been a part of healthcare for many years (6). An example is a blood transfusion. One person

DOI: 10.1201/9781003186069-5

needs blood, but only a specific type (A, B, AB or O). This person is given blood by a donor that matches the recipient (6).

PM has so much potential; however, every revolutionary idea requires time before it is fully adopted into medicine. To accelerate this, the incorporation of fundamental changes is needed in the infrastructure and mechanisms for data collection, storage and sharing (2). More specifically the

> health information technology community will need to design secure and interoperable genomics-enabled systems for actionable use in both health care and community settings. Policy makers will need to address the return of results, privacy, confidentiality, and education while developing regulations and economic incentives that can align all stakeholders toward the same outcomes (3).

In addition, changes need to be made in policy, government funding and cooperation of patients and other players in the ecosystem.

Finally, if PM is efficacious with its goals, "it is likely, in the future, periodic molecular and digital profiling will shift health care strategies from acute intervention and disease management to a focus on assessing health and proactive management of disease risks and prevention" (3).

5.2 PRECISION MEDICINE

In 2015 President Obama announced a government-funded PM initiative that enrolled over 1 million people in what was called "All of US" (7). This initiative expected participants to share the data generated or captured over more than 10 years from sequencing, electronic medical records, personal reported information and digital health technologies. The data will be the subject of analyses to drive both a completely novel scientific agenda for the understanding of disease biology and pathogenesis and an agenda for data- and precision-driven healthcare for individuals and for populations (3).

5.2.1 What Is Precision Medicine?

The National Research Council (NRC) adopted the definition of PM as the

> tailoring of medical treatment to the individual characteristics of each patient . . . to classify individuals into subpopulation that differ in their susceptibility to a particular disease or their response toa specific treatment. Preventative or therapeutic interventions can then be concentration on those who will benefit, sparing expense and side effects for those who will not (1).

When trying to understand the meaning of PM, many people may get confused by the term "personalized medicine." The latter refers to an approach to patients that considers their genetic makeup but with attention to their preferences, beliefs, attitudes, knowledge and social context, whereas PM describes a model for healthcare delivery that relies heavily on data, analytics and information (3). There can be a lot of overlap with these two terms, and according to the NRC, "personalized medicine" is an older term with a meaning similar to "precision medicine." However, there was concern that the word "personalized" could be misinterpreted to imply that treatments and preventions are being developed uniquely for each individual. The NRC therefore preferred the term "precision medicine" to "personalized medicine." However, some people still use the two terms interchangeably (8).

The rise of PM is due to the following four points (3). The first would be the dramatic decline in cost and increase in throughput of DNA sequencing (9). The human genome consists of the four building blocks, or bases, with the abbreviations of G, A, T and C. This has all of our biological information stored there. In humans, the genome has approximately 3 billion bases compared to the bacteria *Escherichia coli*, with 5 million bases (9). As you can imagine, the human genome would take longer to sequence and the price would be much larger than for bacteria. We now have better methods to sequence, which make it much faster than the early 1990s during the HGP. In 2016 the cost to sequence was below 1000 dollars, while the initial genome in 1999 cost approximately 300 million dollars (9). The decrease in cost and increase in technology have helped sequencing become more widespread and has made it more accessible from years prior.

The second is the near-ubiquitous adoption of electronic medical records (EMRs) across the United States (10). The use of EMRs occurs in most hospitals and at the state level. Basic EMR adoption was above 80% for 35 states in 2015, whereas no states in 2011 had a basic EMR (9). The use of EMRs allows more continuous records of heathcare and a base for data to be stored and an avenue for information to be shared with a patient electronically.

The third is the growth of digital health as a source of continuous and rich personal data (11). According to transparency market research, the global digital heath market will reach 536.6 billion dollars by 2025. Ever since the introduction of information technology into the healthcare industry, there has been a need for the improvement and development of healthcare IT infrastructure and mobile platforms (11). Digital heath is the future of healthcare, and it goes hand in hand with new and upcoming technological advancements.

The fourth is other genome-based technology platforms. For example, assays for RNA, proteins and metabolites are also increasingly being used to classify disease states (as diagnostic tests) and to predict future clinical outcomes (as prognostic tests) (3).

> Together these four developments form the basis of 1) a new molecular taxonomy of disease, 2) provide more precise ways to screen for and to detect disease at its earliest molecular manifestations, often pre-clinically, and 3) allow the selection of certain drugs guided by a patient's underlying genetic makeup (3).

5.2.1.1 What Does Precision Medicine Look Like?

Think of PM like an ecosystem in the wild with multiple connected parts working together (see Figure 5.1). The players involved are patients, providers/clinicians, clinical laboratories and researchers. It also involves EMRs, research and other curated databases.

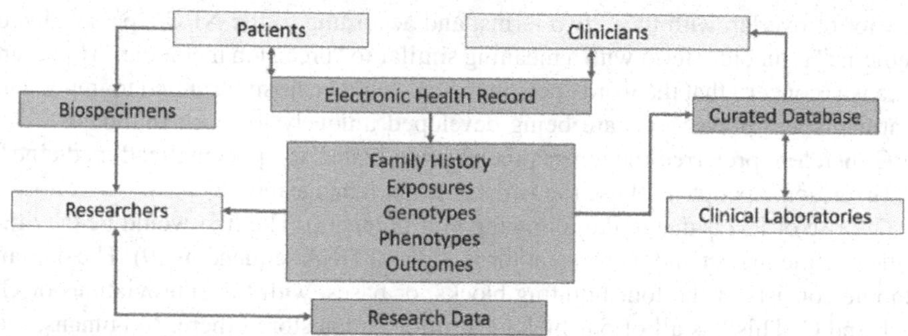

FIGURE 5.1 A diagram of the precision medicine ecosystem (3). (Adapted from reference 10.)

It starts with the patients/research participants who agree to provide biospecimens and share their data (both clinical and research) to the researchers (3). While the researchers take the biospecimens and generate new findings from the data derived from samples linked to digital phenotypes, family history and environmental exposures are captured as part of clinical care (3). While researchers input information into the ecosystem, they can also learn from previously stored data. Clinical laboratories leverage data and inform the clinical community as they assess genomic variation and its impact on human health (12). Clinicians look at the assembly of data from multiple players in the ecosystem and determine its use with both patients and public health (12).

There are several other branches in this ecosystem. One is the government, namely its research and regulation of the healthcare industry regarding development and commercialization (3). Schools and societies, on the other hand, are responsible for training future healthcare professionals, and lastly the payers are responsible for financing and evaluation (3).

Interpretation of the data is key at each level of the ecosystem (2). Information from each of the players can be interpreted based on a specific set of assumptions (2). For example, genetic and clinical data together provide the best patient outcome; however, the quality of patient care is based on the quality of the data (2). When this ecosystem is "optimized, the infrastructure that supports the precision-medicine ecosystem efficiently manages and integrates the flow of material, knowledge and data needed to generate, validate, store, refine and apply clinical interpretations" (2).

5.2.2 Data Science in Precision Medicine

One of the many goals in creating successful PM is the addition of an enormous amount of genomic data into the healthcare infrastructure to provide the best patient care possible. The future of healthcare is a unique intersection of digital heath, data science and PM. Vast amounts of biological, radiological and other bioinformatics datasets are being collected with multidimensional implications both in research and clinical support (3). The immense amount of data that will be collected lend itself to inimitable opportunity to use new techniques such as machine learning, natural language processing and artificial intelligence (3). The advantages are "increasing the efficiency and effectiveness of disease prevention, diagnosis, and treatment through new analytical methods" (3).

Another factor to keep in mind are the multiple players in the ecosystem that are creating, interpreting and deciding how to use the data. For example, healthcare providers need the data when they are trying to determine a particular clinical workflow. On the other hand, patients will need to define preferences about the use and sharing of their genomic data with researchers and others beyond the delivery system in which they receive care (3). These are just two examples of the players in the PM ecosystem.

The outcome of integrating high-quality data into the healthcare system results in the best information for patient care and research. Currently, the government and private sector are working on creating data repositories, but they are not yet available for use (3). A standardized dataset has several uses outside its original purpose. For example, data from the "EMR coupled with gene sequencing information is a powerful tool for identifying genetic variants associated with disease and for understanding individual response to therapeutics" (13). The sharing of data also plays a role. When one heath system shares 100 genomes and patient records with 10 others who also do so (3), that one heath system gains 900 for the cost of 100 (3). There is power in the amount of data available. If it could be summed across a large group of people, a lot of information could be gleaned about population and public health in the area (3).

Both the present and future health systems and infrastructure will need to offer providers tools and systems that help to further the goals of PM and medicine overall (3).

5.2.3 Precision Medicine Policy

The development of a healthcare policy is a difficult dilemma. There are several challenges, such as the evolving nature of healthcare technology. It moves and changes at such a rapid pace, and PM is developing alongside it. For PM to be truly integrated, there must be concrete policy development. The following are five challenges that we currently face (14).

5.2.3.1 Evidence Generation

To provide the best output, we need the best input. This metaphor also applies to data. To get the best patient outcomes, we need high-quality data from genetic testing. The current market is constantly flooded with new technology. There are currently more than 70,000 unique genetic testing products on the market, and an average of 10 new products are added each day (15), specifically, at a compound annual rate of 28% (16).

5.2.3.2 Data Sharing and Infrastructure Needs

As discussed in previous sections, the large amount of data must be shared via enhanced data systems among several players at different points in the PM healthcare ecosystem (14). These data also need the building blocks of infrastructure to support viewing and altering the data along the way.

5.2.3.3 Incorporating Genomic and Other Molecular Data Into Clinical Care and Research

With any innovation, it takes a long time to be adopted, and PM is no different. So many sections of healthcare, technology, government initiatives and policy need to be on the same page for this to become a success (3). This issue also exists in other countries such as France, who committed $700 million to fun sequencing center or China, with $10 billion (15).

5.2.3.4 Diagnostics, Drug Discovery and Economics of PM

Implementation cannot occur if PM does not provide a demonstrated value or if payers and consumers are unwilling to pay for them (3). The logical follow-up is if PM lives up to its costs, should payers be reimbursed for PM testing? In most cases, there is limited or variable coverage of PM testing (17).

From an economic viewpoint, many gaps need to be evaluated in the future, but the current economic evaluations of PM in general are increasing (3). "Studies found that PM interventions are generally similar in cost-effectiveness as other types of health care interventions, with a majority of interventions found to be cost-effective relative to standard practice but only a minority of studies finding PM to be cost-saving" (3).

5.2.3.5 Participant Engagement and Trust

One of the most important players are the patients who use PM, without which it would not be able to reach its potential. The recent lack of trust in healthcare providers and data breaches have many consumers or patients concerned about sharing their genetic information. Concerns about how data are used, stored and secured are all valid and necessary when thinking about adopting PM.

These five challenges make the implementation of PM in the realm of policy difficult. The policy development process requires a concrete system to be in place that supports the changes a policy proposes. Standardization of data and technology are also necessary, as well as evidence and research to back the claims made. "Policy makers will have to address the return of results, privacy, confidentiality, and education while developing regulations and economic incentives that can align all stakeholders toward the same outcomes" (3). PM has several areas of improvement before it can be adopted into both medicine and policy.

5.3 WHAT IS THE CURRENT STATE OF PRECISION MEDICINE?

The integration of PM into heathcare has been stagnant and not on pace with the discoveries of science. According to Health Aff et al., there is a genuine lack of research on the implementation of PM; however, two new initiatives, as well as others, are addressing the need for evidence generation.

5.3.1 Clinical Sequencing Evidence—Generating Research (CSER2)

CSER2 builds upon its predecessor and "will support the development of methods needed to integrate genome sequencing into the practice of medicine, improve the discovery and interpretation of genomic variants and investigate the impact of genome sequencing on healthcare outcomes" (3).

CSER2's goal is to fast-track the use of genomic sequencing in clinical care settings, as well as beyond. This project has three main concerns to investigate:

> 1) define, generate and analyze evidence regarding the clinical utility of genome sequencing; 2) research the critical interactions among patients, family members, health practitioners, and clinical laboratories that influence implementation of clinical genome sequencing; and 3) identify and address real-world barriers to integrating genomic, clinical, and healthcare utilization data within a healthcare system to build a shared evidence base for clinical decision-making (3).

CSER2 grants also focus on recruiting diverse racial and ethnic groups and historically underrepresented groups in genomics research, as well as including payer perspectives (18–19).

5.3.2 Implementing Genomics in Practice (IGNITE)

This grant was established in 2013 with around 30 million dollars in funding (3), "with a goal to support the development, investigation and dissemination of genomic medicine practice models that seamlessly integrate genomic data into the electronic health record and that deploy tools for point of care decision making" (3).

The projects under this grant vary widely, such as "including exploring genetic markers for disease risk prediction and prevention or refining disease diagnosis using sequence-based mutation discovery" (3) They also have projects targeting underserved populations and minorities (20).

The main challenges they will tackle are as follows:

1) Implementation science requires both a transdisciplinary team and an implementation framework. Thus, to enable genomic medicine implementation teams with the right expertise need to be assembled. Implementation frameworks should be established that guide intervention deployment, assessment, and analyses. IGNITE adopted and adapted the consolidated framework for implementation research (21) in creating a network focused on developing lessons for the larger community (3).
2) It is important to optimize the setting and personnel to carry out the implementation research in the clinic. Pre-implementation research is often overlooked as a critical element to ensure that researchers understand and consider the priorities, concerns and educational needs of these key stakeholders before implementation begins (3).
3) Genomic medicine research is information technology (IT) intensive. Broad implementation of genomic medicine requires that IT solutions work with an EMR to either incorporate genomic information into it extract phenotypic

data from it. Thus, IT leadership at the implementing institution needs to prioritize its incorporation (3).

5.4 PRECISION MEDICINE AND THE WORLD

Across the world there are many national initiatives for the implementation of PM, from Japan, and Singapore to Estonia (4 Table 5.2). One example is in Canada, where they have research projects focused on applying genomics to PM (4 Table 5.2). Many of these efforts worldwide are being done without any external collaboration, "risking the duplication of efforts and slowing the pace of discovery and translation" (22). As with the US system, a similar struggle with implementation occurs worldwide.

5.5 CONCLUSION

"In many ways, genomics has served as the foundation for 'precision medicine.' However, precision medicine is much more than genomic medicine. It focuses on individual differences in genes, environment, and lifestyle, allowing the design of targeted disease interventions" (23).

For PM to reach its full potential, it will need a multipronged approach towards its scientific, clinical and policy agenda. How genetic data are shared, stored and secured are essential for PM to move forward. "The precision medicine ecosystem's stakeholders—participants, patients, providers, payers and regulators—each will require evidence of value in terms of quality of life, quality of medical care and efficiency and effectiveness optimized for cost (3)." If PM is successful, medical care will shift to prevention and early detection (3). Patients stand to benefit with optimized health outcomes in such a genomics- and data-enabled learning precision health system (3). "Precision medicine is not uniquely American and requires global leadership and perseverance to see it through to its rightful place in health and society" (3).

5.6 FUTURE OF PRECISION MEDICINE

5.6.1 Genomic Medicine and PM

After the completion of the HGP, science now has a greater understanding of the complexities of the genetic component of disease, "including the roadblocks between association signals and the development of meaningful therapies" (5). For example, we have a more comprehensive catalog of molecular lesions underlying cancer and can use more targeted therapies. We also are making some progress on understanding the genetic mechanisms of almost all Mendelian disorders (5).

So far, this field has made immense strides in the cost of sequencing and genetic testing (5). The HGP promised radical changes with very high expectations regarding PM and genomic medicine. However, those were not met.

New goals and expectations are needed. The future includes advancements in next-generation sequencing and gene editing; however, this is not enough. More breakthroughs are coming, as earlier examples show, but they will come slowly. The HGP is not enough to keep up with the needs of PM and genomic medicine. More investment in science, research and technologies is needed for the success on this long journey (5).

Four challenges that will propel the future of genomic medicine and the development of PM are the following:

> 1. understanding, at least at some basic level, the function of every gene in the human genome; 2. scaling the identification of causal variants, genes and mechanisms for existing GWAS signals from a handful to thousands; 3. a spatially-resolved molecular atlas of all human cell types, from birth to death, e.g. including their chromatin landscape, gene expression and protein expression signatures; 4. developing accurate, quantitative models for predicting the impact of arbitrary sequence variants on gene expression and/or protein function in any one of these cell types (5).

These challenges promote further research, funding and solutions to help increase the adoption of PM.

Another consideration due to the advancing technology is the ever-changing PM tests. There is ambiguity in how the Food and Drug Administration (FDA) regulates PM tests (3). Currently "laboratory-developed tests (LDTs)" do not require FDA approval, but the future is uncertain (24). Another challenge for the FDA will be how they choose to regulate these new tests that use new sequencing technologies (24).

With the advent of at-home sequencings and highly advanced genomic sequencings, a significant population of people will have their genomes sequenced in some way (5). This extends to microorganisms as well. Access to sequencing data of pathogens can illuminate the relationship between infectious diseases and chronic illnesses (23). "Investigations of the human microbiome seem to be promising in assessing the role of infectious diseases in a wide variety of diseases, including obesity and diabetes" (23). The role of the microbiome is a subject of a host of different research studies and is becoming increasingly important in terms of public health (23).

An individual's genetic information lasts throughout their lifetime (5). This implies that advancing technology and understanding of the genome will continue to provide benefits into perpetuity as science learns more. For example, "sequencing in some form is likely to become routine for all cancers, and possibly for prospective parents and the unborn as well. We may even be recurrently sequenced, e.g. routine monitoring of cell-free DNA for cancer or other conditions" (5). "Combined with other advances (e.g. polygenic risk scores, gene therapy, immunotherapy, etc.), our collective genomes will serve as the basis not only for advancing our understanding of disease, but also for the development of new preventative and therapeutic strategies."

As with any technology that discusses the human genome and any changes that PM and advancing genomic therapies may bring about, ethical considerations can be raised. The following are some examples:

1. In the past human genomics has been "overly weighted" towards a set population to that population's sole benefit (5).
2. The popularity of ancestry tests and who has access to the data raise privacy concerns (5).

3. Scientists have made unnecessary genetic modifications in research experiments (5).
4. Non-disease trait selection in embryos (5).

These arc just a fcw of thc concerns with the ever-evolving field of PM and genomic advancements. In light of this, we must be sure to minimize any harm towards our fellow human beings.

5.7 PHARMACOGENOMICS

"Pharamacogenomics is a part of precision medicine. "Pharmacogenomics is the study of how genes affect a person's response to particular drugs. This relatively new field combines pharmacology (the science of drugs) and genomics (the study of genes and their functions) to develop effective, safe medications and doses that are tailored to variations in a person's genes" (8). Pharmacogenomic is still developing, but its applications are far and wide (8).

5.8 PUBLIC HEALTH AND PRECISION MEDICINE

With the advancement of PM, its applications can extend towards populations in what we will call "precision public heath" (25–26). The US Precision Medicine Initiative, launched in 2015, created a national cohort of around 1 million people enrolled in the "All of US" research program "to evaluate genetic and environmental determinants of various diseases" (23). This inherently required a public health perspective "to help ensure generalizability to the population, focus on preventive interventions, and increase the efficiency and precision with which interventions are implemented" (23). For example, the 1 million people enrolled in the initiative could have various diseases processes. "These individuals and their relatives could help evaluate [the] best individual and system-wide implementation strategies to reduce risk" (23).

The main goal of precision public health is to provide the correct heath intervention to the right population at the right time (23).

> Precision public health involves the collection of more accurate population- and individual-level data on genes, exposures, behaviors, and other social/economic health determinants; enhancing public health action for improving health in subpopulations in need of recommended prevention measures; and addressing and reducing health disparities in the population by using more precision data for action. (23)

This can also include the analysis of the biological and environmental determinants of health by tracking heath and disease geographically to measure the social and environmental determinants of heath (23).

Overall, the path toward precision public health is promising. There are several challenges that plague both precision medicine and public health, the biggest one being "how to best use large-scale data, including genomic and environmental information, in order to better understand determinants of population health and target interventions that can improve health outcomes in subpopulations" (23). With public heath there is not one solution for a multidimensional problem—other changes and interventions are needed. However, with precision public health, there is hope with the development of a more tailored approach towards high-risk groups (23).

REFERENCES

1. National Research Council, Committee on A Framework for Developing a New Taxonomy of Disease. *Toward Precision Medicine: Building a Knowledge Network for Biomedical Research and a New Taxonomy of Disease*. Washington, DC: National Academies Press; 2011.
2. *Nature*. 2015 October 15; 526(7573):336–342. https://doi.org/10.1038/nature15816.
3. Ginsburg GS, Phillips KA. Precision medicine: From science to value. *Health Affairs (Project Hope)* 2018; 37(5):694–701. https://doi.org/10.1377/hlthaff.2017.1624
4. Cell. 2019 March 21; 177(1):45–57. https://doi.org/10.1016/j.cell.2019.02.003.
5. Shendure J, et al. Genomic medicine-progress, pitfalls, and promise. *Cell* 2019;177(1): 45–57. https://doi.org/10.1016/j.cell.2019.02.003
6. https://medlineplus.gov/genetics/understanding/precisionmedicine/definition/
7. https://allofus.nih.gov
8. https://medlineplus.gov/genetics/understanding/precisionmedicine/precisionvspersonalized/
9. https://www.genome.gov/about-genomics/fact-sheets/Sequencing-Human-Genome-cost
10. https://dashboard.healthit.gov/evaluations/data-briefs/non-federal-acute-care-hospital-ehr-adoption-2008-2015.php
11. https://www.globenewswire.com/news-release/2017/09/22/1131466/0/en/Digital-Health-Market-will-Reach-USD-536-6-Billion-by-2025-Transparency-Market-Research.html
12. Aronson SJ, Rehm HL. Building the foundation for genomics in precision medicine. *Nature*. 2015 October 15; 526(7573):336–342.
13. Rasmussen-Torvik LJ, Stallings SC, Gordon AS, Almoguera B, Basford MA, Bielinski SJ, et al. Design and anticipated outcomes of the eMERGE-PGx project: A multicenter pilot for preemptive pharmacogenomics in electronic health record systems. *Clin Pharmacol Ther*. 2014 October; 96(4):482–489. [PubMed: 24960519]
14. https://pubmed.ncbi.nlm.nih.gov/29240076/
15. Bergin, J. *DNA Sequencing: Emerging Technologies and Applications*. Wellesley, MA: BCC Research; 2016 May.
16. Phillips KA, Deverka PA, Hooker G, Douglas MP. Genetic test availability, spending, and market trends. Where are we now? Where are we going? *Health Affairs*. 2018 this issue.
17. Phillips KA, Deverka PA, Trosman JR, Douglas MP, Chambers JD, Weldon CB, et al. Payer coverage policies for multigene tests. *Nature Biotechnology*. 2017; 35(7): 614–617.
18. *NIH Accelerates the Use of Genomics in Clinical Care: New Funding Awards Focus on Diverse and Underserved Populations*. 2017.
19. *Clinical Sequencing Evidence-Generating Research (CSER2)*. 2017.
21. http://www.cfirguide.org/
20. https://grants.nih.gov/grants/guide/rfa-files/RFA-HG-17-010.html
22. Manolio TA, Abramowicz M, Al-Mulia F, Anderson W, Balling R, Berger AC, et al. Global implementation of genomic medicine: We are not alone. *Sci Transl Med*. 2015 June 3; 7(290):290ps13.
23. Khoury, Muin J et al. From public health genomics to precision public health: A 20-year journey. *Genetics in Medicine: Official Journal of the American College of Medical Genetics* 2018; 20(6):574–582. https://doi.org/10.1038/gim.2017.211

24. *The Personalized Medicine Report: 2017 Opportunity, Challenges, and the Future: Personalized Medicine Coalition*. 2017.
25. Khoury MJ, Galea S. Will precision medicine improve population health? *JAMA*. 2016; 316(13):1357–1358. [PubMed: 27541310]
26. Khoury MJ, Iademarco MF, Riley WT. Precision public health for the era of precision medicine. *Am J Prev Med*. 2016; 50(3):398–401. [PubMed: 26547538]
27. Dzau VJ, Ginsburg GS. Realizing the full potential of precision medicine in health and health care. *JAMA*. 2016; 316(16):1659–1660. [PubMed: 27669484]

6 The Current State of Non-Viral Vector–Based mRNA Medicine Using Various Nanotechnology Applications

Kshama Patel, Preetam Dasika and Yashwant V. Pathak

CONTENTS

DOI: 10.1201/9781003186069-6

6.1 INTRODUCTION

6.1.1 Messenger Ribonucleic Acid

The study of messenger ribonucleic acid (mRNA) dates as far back as the early 1980s, in the form of a struggling Hungarian biochemist looking to make a revolutionary discovery with her findings.[1] Katalin Kariko saw the potential of mRNA harnessed to fight disease and other innumerable illnesses. Logically, it made sense to her that by being able to override the protein production plants of the body, any number of changes could be induced. One of the first documented cases of successful synthetic mRNA was by researchers at the University of Wisconsin, who managed to re-create protein expression in the skeletal muscle of mice which didn't inherently create a physical change.[2] Instead, the protein generated was a superficial conformation that could be tracked by chemical expression vectors; the particular RNA and DNA vectors used by the researchers contained genes for chloramphenicol acetyltransferase, luciferase, and beta-galactosidase.[2] According to the report, the activity of luciferase was present in the skeletal muscle of the mice for an additional two months at the least.[2] Surprisingly, no carrier or delivery system was used to obtain these results.[2] The reason that delivery systems are often used in the modern application of mRNA is because the human body recognizes synthetic mRNA as foreign. This was reflected in Kariko's work, spanning nearly a decade, where she and immunologist Drew Weissman developed a hybridized version of mRNA that was structured with modified nucleosides in order to circumvent the body's immune response to the synthetic strand.[1] After a series of scientific publications were made in 2005 regarding this discovery, researchers of the technology saw that the foundations were ready to bring mRNA to the forefront of biochemical sciences. No other application was as coveted by then as the vaccine.

The three biggest names today in mRNA technology involving vaccines are Pfizer Incorporated, Moderna Therapeutics, and BioNTech (of which Katalin Kariko is currently the senior vice president). It is nothing short of a race between these companies to produce a working solution to restore the balance of global public health and prove that their solutions, through the usage of mRNA technology, will revolutionize pharmacy, medicine, and biochemistry. However, mRNA would have remained an experimental study without the incorporation of another revered field of technology: nanotechnology.

6.1.2 Nanotechnology

Nanotechnology was first introduced as a concept by Richard Feynman in 1959 and then put into use and defined by a Japanese scientist by the name of Norio Taniguchi in 1974, 15 years later.[3] It was not until 1989 that it became widely popularized for its potential applications after Don Eigler and Erhard Schweizer spelled out the IBM logo by manipulating 35 individual xenon atoms using a scanning tunneling microscope (invented by Gerd Binnig and Heinrich Rohrer in 1982). Through nanotechnology, several nanostructures and nanomaterials were discovered or created and played a pivotal role in particular delivery systems for non-viral mRNA vectorization. Some of these structures are nanotubes, fullerenes, graphene, dendrimers, and liposomes.[3] Since its practical importance was realized, a multitude of different fields have utilized the technology, especially biology. For the purpose of this chapter, the topics will generally trend toward more medicinal, pharmaceutic, and therapeutic areas of study.

In its relation to mRNA, nanotechnology is primarily seen as a method of modifying synthetic strands and a way to develop delivery systems that allow mRNA treatments to be vectorized in a non-viral manner.

6.2 SYNOPSIS

This chapter covers the past and most modern states of mRNA-based medicine to date, as well as the progression of the numerous forms of nanotechnology that have been used or are currently being used to administer this form of medicine. The two are essentially a coalescent field of study and are rarely separable when considering the widespread public distribution of mRNA-based treatments in pharmaceutical, therapeutic, and preventative contexts. However, mRNA and nanotechnology have an outstanding potential to go further beyond that, based on current research. The comprehensive development of both fields of study have come an incredibly long way and are only going to be increasing in the frequency of their innovations and developments. As of now, the utilization of synthetic mRNA has garnered a dedicated following of scientists and professionals who suggest that it could become incredibly prevalent in the future of a variety of healthcare careers, but even currently mRNA has an incredible array of uses.

6.3 ANTIBODIES

Antibodies are proteins that specialize in neutralizing foreign invaders to the body. Antibodies retain a quaternary level of structure at the highest point of conformation in their natured protein state. They are considered a part of humoral immunity, which concerns itself with the macromolecules and proteins found within the fluid outside of cells—generally, body fluids like plasma and the interstitial region of organs.[4] Antibodies function by way of a trigger-based system, the trigger being an antigen that spikes the activity of antibody-generating B-cells.[4] Because of the way this system works, it can be easily exploited for greater effectiveness when coming into contact with a real antigen such as COVID-19.

6.3.1 Antibody Generation

Every viral strain has a composition of a protein capsid and genetic material in the form of RNA or DNA.[4] The identifying structure that the B-cells use to identify a foreign invader in the body are the surface proteins of the invader.[4] The surface proteins are what viral strains use to bind and infuse their genetic material into a host cell, and if the memory B-cells are unfamiliar with the surface proteins of a particular viral strain, the antibody B-cells will take longer to synthesize an antibody and neutralize the invading virus.[4] This is where mRNA has become an incredibly relevant innovation for modern disease control.

6.3.2 Induction by Synthetic mRNA

The nanotechnology involved in delivering the synthetic mRNA strand in this case is a vesicle with a lipid bilayer called a liposome.[4] The synthetic mRNA is contained within the liposome and is transferred by absorption into B-cells. What this synthetic mRNA prompts the B-cell to do is express a "spike protein," which mimics the protein capsule of the virus.[4] This principle is what currently developed mRNA vaccines are using to combat the current COVID-19 pandemic. By triggering the B-cells into synthesizing antibodies, they are taught to recognize features of a specific virus—almost like virally vectorized vaccinations, minus the weakened or dead germ sample.[5]

6.3.3 Active and Passive Immunity

The initial delivery of the synthetic mRNA encoded for the spike protein can be considered a form of passive humoral immunity with respect to an individual's antibody generation.[5] The most appropriate way to consider the effect of mRNA vaccines on antibody generation is initial passive immunization through a non-viral vector. This doesn't mean, however, that active immunization won't take place. The primary delivery of the synthetic strand will generate antibodies that stand ready for an invader, but will eventually subside in their levels in an individual if there is no infection to handle or the individual has recovered from a persisting infection.[5] Depending on the number of lipid bilayers in the liposome used to deliver the synthetic mRNA, the expression of the spike protein can be delayed.[5]

6.4 GENERAL THERAPEUTICS

In addition to being used to target and neutralize a variety of viral infections in terms of mRNA, the synthetic strands of mRNA can be used in treatments that seek to mitigate the symptoms that are present with chronic and genetic illnesses and potentially some autoimmune disorders.[6] Much of the novel treatments that encompass this utilization of mRNA technology are still emerging and undergoing clinical development, but a framework has been established for how such therapeutics can be used and delivered in and to patients that need them. Currently, the focus is around how treatments can be delivered in vivo, which means that the treatment is administered *inside* a fully developed living organism. The counterpart to in vivo is in vitro, which stands for when a process is taking place *outside* of an organism. Current clinical developments for both are taking place.

6.4.1 Chronic Pain Relief

Examples of chronic illnesses are heart disease, arthritis, osteoporosis, depression, stroke, high/low blood pressure, and diabetes. As per their namesake, chronic illnesses are incurable and have persisting symptoms that express themselves, sometimes to a very harmful effect, in individuals. Based on the source of the illness, synthetic mRNA is a highly viable avenue to pursue a treatment where the symptoms of a chronic illness are reduced or neutralized. A big category of chronic illnesses is those that cause pain due to wear and tear or damage to the body of an individual. There are currently several methods to address this issue: surgical replacement of the part, surgical repair of the part, or a medication that has an effect on pain or integrity of the problem area. In order to treat chronic pain, one novel therapeutic strategy introduced was the use of clustered regularly interspaced short palindromic repeats (CRISPR) to replace segments of non-coding RNA, which govern the expression of certain genes.[7] Chronic pain often results from an injury that causes inflammation or damage to the nerves in the area, which then trigger the natural mediators in the form of micro-RNA segments that signal neuropathic channels for pain reception.[8] Neuropathic channels of the body lead from and back to the central spinal cord and subsequently the brain, but after long periods of pain, the dorsal root ganglion that sits deep in the vertebrae of every spinal segment can have its neurons sensitized and become increasingly excitable.[8] This results in hypersensitivity (conditions like hyperalgesia) as a result of the constant signaling by the non-coding RNA strands.[8] The novel treatment proposed to this is to use a synthetic mRNA strand to reduce the sensitivity to pain by reducing the expression by the non-coding segments of RNA. This method of therapy is theoretically applicable to a wide array of chronic pain illnesses by way of regulating the pain response over long periods.[8] Furthermore, studies into tissue engineering using mRNA are starting to take place, which will be discussed in a later section.[9]

6.4.2 Deficiencies

Another type of illness that has a potential solution with mRNA technology are various kinds of deficiencies resulting from the body not generating the necessary hormones, biomolecules, or substrate to successfully trigger enzymes. One illness that falls in this category is type 2 diabetes, where the cells of the body can't take up the sugar put into the body because the cells have become resistant to insulin and the pancreas can't produce enough insulin to overcome the tolerance. From a study in Germany that ran a clinical trial on the drug AZD8601 with 42 men (ages 18 to 65) with type 2 diabetes, it was shown that the test groups for the drug had increased blood flow and cell permeability.[10] In addition to this, the blood vessels had grown in size and number, which is important for diabetic patients, who often have health complications as a result of constrictive blood vessels.[10] There were no concerning side effects, and the treatment effects were observed between 4 and 24 hours after administering the treatment.[10] What allowed for this duration of protein detention was, once again, a liposomal package that kept the synthesized genetic material safe from the body's immune system, as well as proteins that mimicked natural RNA identifiers.[10] Another study used mice to test the effectiveness of mRNA in being able to supplement deficiencies in organisms such as mice, and this study also references the use of a liposomal package to protect the synthetic mRNA from the immune system. In particular, the deficiency that needed to be supported was a lack of ornithine transcarbamylase (OTC), which is an enzyme that is important in the urea cycle (hydrolysis and expulsion of nitrogen from the body).[10] Allowing this deficiency to go untreated leads to high concentrations of ammonia in the blood, of which the toxicity can affect the nervous system. The results of the experiments showed that their treatment accounted for the OTC deficiency and that uptake of the mRNA by the liver (where the deficiency would be identified) was increased by about 200 percent in the first dosage alone over 10 days.[10] Using these data, the researchers also generated a model for humans which suggested that mRNA encoded for this particular deficiency would account for about 35 percent of the normal levels found in humans, most likely with the same delivery system using lipid nanoparticles.[10]

6.4.3 Genetic Illness

Seeing that mRNA is inherently genetic material that works as a command signal for much of the body's processes, it would also be able to rectify a problem which is rooted in a genetic cause. The DNA responsible for instructing RNA strands for certain protein synthesis may have errors that cause the naturally encoded RNA to create problems for the individual. This can be done one of two ways, either by targeting the affected facility of the "bad" mRNA strands or targeting the bad strands with synthetic mRNA that is intended to neutralize the production or lack thereof of biological molecules in an undesirable quantity.[11] One study involved the interference of naturally generated RNA that causes a disease known as acute intermittent porphyria, which is a metabolic disorder that can become toxic if left untreated and has a genetic root.[12] It is caused by mutation. The interfering strand is named RNA givosiran, a drug developed by Alnylam Pharmaceuticals.[12] In mice, the vectorization of the interference mRNA returned around 30 percent increase in liver function, which suggested clinical efficacy, but when applied to a human model (not a clinical trial), the transgene delivery suggested the effectiveness was insufficient in humans.[12]

6.5 IMMUNOTHERAPY

Immunotherapy is a type of biological therapy that aims to control the degree to which the immune system will function to fight numerous diseases. The response speed and efficacy of the immune system depend heavily on the novelty of a foreign invader to the body, as well as the information stored in memory cells regarding an invader to the body.[13] The immune system is composed of three main parts: physicochemical barriers (skin, hair, saliva, stomach acid), non-specific innate responses (broad trigger response of white blood cells to a plethora of pathogens), and specific adaptive responses where the body learns or remembers the specific pathogen and generates antibodies with the help of B-cells, which later store information for the next attack from the same pathogen.[13] mRNA immunotherapy is taking place in the world today through mRNA coronavirus vaccines which stimulate the immune system into a higher active state. Besides the nanostructures of liposomes, the enzyme known CRISPR-CAS13a plays an important role through its outlier function of targeting RNA exclusively instead of DNA.[14] Cas13a is also able to cleave and bind sites through an interference system which disrupts only the expression of a gene, instead of cutting out entire portions of the genomic sequence like Cas-9 does.[15] This would potentially make it a safer alternative, but it still requites a clinical trial period.

6.5.1 Herd Immunity Sans Retrovirus

The purpose of any kind of immunization treatment is to have as many people as possible retain the qualities of resilience against infection, leading to herd immunity. Herd immunity is when the majority of a community expresses immunity to a disease, making transmission more unlikely and protecting those who do not have total immunity as well.[16] One primary advantage of using a non-viral vector in immunotherapy is a higher transduction efficiency than if a retrovirus was used.[16] In addition to this, cell division is not needed for transduction to occur in a non-viral vector, since it becomes effective as soon as it transfects into the cytoplasm of immune cells.[16] This is the opposite with viral vectors, which need to transfect into the nucleus to transduct and have enough expression to trigger an immune response.[16] However, one big drawback of a non-viral vector for immunization is that the duration of expression is notably shorter than with viral templates that have a higher level of integration with the genome of the test individual (which is also a risk).[16] Generally, the benefits outweigh the drawbacks for non-viral vectorization through mRNA immunotherapy to achieve herd immunity, in that it is mostly safer, cheaper, and more effective in certain cases (propagation, etc.).

6.5.2 Sustainability

The sustainability of mRNA treatments for immunotherapy of a community is higher than that of a viral vector due to how quickly it can be adapted for a situation and used to combat emerging outbreaks.[17] This variability is a big advantage over using a retroviral solution that can generally only target one strain of infectious disease. This, combined with an efficacy rate of around 95 percent from the current major vaccine providers, suggests the longevity of this method of immunotherapy on the scale of global public health.[17]

6.5.3 Immuno-oncology

Immuno-oncology is an individual's way of fighting cancer. However, this is done by developing drugs and treatment options that make the most out of the patient's immune system. An individual's immune system plays a vital role in a normal person's body; however, it plays an even bigger role in a patient with cancer, as they are immunocompromised.[18] So, with immuno-oncology therapies, the patient benefits by being able to fight the cancer despite having a weak immune system.[18]

While many viral vectors are used in immuno-oncology, non-viral vectors are fairly new in the field, and hence, not much research has been published on non-viral vectors in this area. There are many up and coming studies in this field, but none which we had access to as students.

6.6 ELECTROPORATION

While viral vectors are a common method to treat diseases, non-viral vectors are becoming more and more common, since viral vectors tend to be a safety concern. Non-viral vectors, especially non-viral gene carriers, are popular because of the induction of transient gene expression in which polymers or liposomes with cationic lipids are kept for a few days until they are converted into a long, low-level expression.[19] One type of cell that non-viral gene therapy has been used on is natural killer cells, or NK cells.[19] A process known as electroporation is used to artificially inject nucleic materials into the NK cell. Electroporation is the induction of a temporary permeabilization of the cell membrane through the creation of an electric field so that the artificial nucleic substances can be injected into the desired cell. This process is used over viral vectors because with viral vectors, many problems could arise such as unwanted replication of the actual nucleic material, altering the individual's DNA. While electroporation can be a dangerous process, prior research has shown that lytic function, the major danger, has been restored and caused the patient no harm in the future.[19] Furthermore, studies have shown that electroporation of mRNA coding and anti-CD19 chimeric antigen receptors (CARs) have been successfully electroporated into blood-derived cells. Not only were these processes successful, but they were also efficient with an 81 percent efficiency rate.[19]

6.6.1 Cancer Treatment Using Electroporation

Electroporation is becoming a popular way of treating cancer. In one study, electroporation was useful and effective because the intratumoral injection of the drug bleomycin, which was administered, ended up having a higher uptake of the drug and it increased the number of cancer cells that were killed.[20] Hence, electroporation is proving to be an effective method of treating cancer due to the electric field, allowing a greater number of cancer cells to die. In this study, head and neck tumors were treated with a specific treatment known as the MedPulser, which allows for local electroporation therapy (EPT). Since EPT combined with bleomycin was effective in treating tumors in vitro, in mice, and in humans, this treatment was experimented on 10 patients with head and neck tumors through a phase I/II clinical trial.[20] The study revealed that five of the eight patients responded to the treatment completely, while three patients responded partially. A partial response in this study was defined as greater than or equal to 50 percent of a shrinkage in the tumor.[20] The remaining two patients had a partial treatment, which resulted in a local response. All of these results were confirmed with a biopsy and magnetic resonance imaging (MRI). All 10 patients were able to bear the treatment, and at the end of the treatment, none of them showed any significant adverse effects to the MedPulser.[20]

6.7 GENOME EDITING

Genome editing is also known gene editing, as it allows scientists to change an individual's DNA with the help of up-and-coming advanced technology. Genome editing is when genetic material is altered in some manner, including but not limited to the addition and removal of genetic material.[21] One specific genome editing system that has been developed is the CRISPR method.[21] The most recent study used CRISPR-Cas9, which stands for CRISPR-associated protein 9. CRISPR-Cas9 is a better alternative than the other genome editing programs because it uses advanced technology that is fast, cheap, and more accurate and efficient.[21]

6.7.1 CRISPR-Cas9

CRISPR-Cas9 was inspired by a bacterium that used genome editing. In this system, the bacteria use parts of the DNA from foreign viruses to create CRISPR arrays, which are the pieces that the bacteria remember from the virus.[21] Then, when the bacteria sense the virus again, they will produce RNA from the CRISPR arrays to attack the DNA from the virus. Lastly, the Cas9 part will come into play where the DNA of the virus is dissembled and destroyed.[21] This process is very similar to the lab in which genome editing is done. In the lab, scientists will make a tiny piece of RNA, which can then attach to the DNA of the target genome and the Cas9 enzyme.[21] This RNA is then able to identify the DNA of the genome, and Cas9 dissembles the DNA and allows for new genetic material to be added or existing genetic material to be removed.[21] Furthermore, this allows the scientist to construct the DNA to their will, allowing the perfect DNA structure to be created.

This research was done with DNA and CRISPR-Cas9; however, it can also be done with mRNA. CRISPR-Cas9 used with mRNA is shorter, as it can be detected in four to six hours after transfection since nuclear localization is not required.[22] Not only is this faster with mRNA, but it is also safer because there is a very slight chance of mutagenesis.[22] Additionally, since mRNA is shorter than DNA, there is a decreased chance of off-target effects, or the genome editing being in the wrong place. While this is a faster process than DNA, the Cas9 protein expression may not be noticed until 72 hours after transfection in vitro and 24 hours after injection in vivo.[22] While all of these are advantages to performing genome editing with mRNA over DNA, there are some consequences. The main challenge that has to be overcome is that special material is needed for CRISPR-Cas9 delivery in mRNA because of the difference in length in both compounds and the difference in the kinetics of expression.[22]

6.7.2 Successful Genome Editing Studies

Genome editing can be used in many different ways to get the outcome that scientists want in an organism. It is of great use when preventing or treating diseases in humans because genome editing gets rid of the part of the DNA that causes the disease to be there. Many of the genetic diseases that are faced by families every day would be eradicated with further use of genome editing. Additionally, fatal diseases such as cystic fibrosis can be treated using genome editing. For example, a case in the United Kingdom was successful in treating a one-year-old girl with leukemia.[23] The doctors used genome editing to help her fight leukemia and treated the young girl. However, they used another genome editing process known as transcription activator–like effector nucleases (TALENs), instead of CRISPR-Cas9.[23] While the doctors saved her life with this technology, many concerns were raised by society.

6.7.3 Germline Human Genome Editing

While the genome editing methods described earlier are examples of somatic gene therapies that change the DNA to treat or prevent diseases, there is also another type of genome editing method known as germline human genome editing. In this method, the genetic material of an embryo is altered.[24] This process changes the DNA of that individual, which would also cause their children's DNA to be altered.[24] Germline genome editing is restricted on humans in many places for a variety of reasons, including but not limited to the genome editing fixing one issue and causing another issue to arise.[24] Hence, this type of research is considered to be new and is done in petri dishes alone.

6.7.4 Consequences to Genome Editing

Many concerns arise when it comes to genome editing, despite all the advantages that it has to offer. The first problem that arises is an ecological imbalance when genetic material of bacteria, plants, and animals is edited. When gene editing is done on these organisms, gene drift occurs, leading to a higher off-target mutation possibility, which finally leads to an increase in the number of mutations in future generations.[25] Additionally, genetically modified organisms (GMOs) are hard to track by the federal government after leaving the lab.[25] This makes it hard for consumers to know if they are buying a product that is a GMO, and it also makes it difficult for researchers to keep track of the data to see if the GMO has caused any consequences or if it was a success.[25]

The overall theme with the concerns of genome editing seems to be that more research needs to be done before conducting genome editing on humans. If more research is conducted, then scientists can identify how to prevent the issues that society has addressed.

6.8 VACCINES

Vaccines are a form of delivery system that can be viral or non-viral. With non-viral vaccinations, the genetic material is delivered into the organism, which copies the virus and invokes an immune response.[26] Compared to viral vaccinations, non-viral vaccines are safer and faster since the live organism is not used inside the vaccine.[26] Since non-viral vaccines are fast and safer than viral vaccines, they can be administered to the public at a faster pace, which was seen during the coronavirus pandemic.[26]

There are two different vaccines, including DNA vaccines and RNA vaccines. For DNA vaccines, the DNA is transcribed into mRNA and then translated, which can cause many different problems, including mutagenesis and the possibility of the patient contracting a disease they did not previously have.[26] mRNA vaccines are an up-and-coming technology in which much research and development are being done. Recent studies have shown that mRNA vaccinations are used mostly in preventative and therapeutic measures.[26] Therapeutic vaccines are vaccinations that are used to treat patients who already have a certain disease. On the other hand, preventative vaccinations are vaccines that are administered to patients to protect them from contracting a certain disease.[27] Vaccinations made of mRNA are also used to avoid and handle the spread of infectious diseases such as the COVID-19 pandemic.[27]

6.8.1 COVID-19 Vaccination

During the start of the COVID-19 pandemic, scientists and researchers all around the world put their other research to the side and started working on a vaccine to control the spread of the virus. Many vaccinations were under development by late 2020 and early 2021. Many different technologies were used to create the vaccine, including virus-like particles, recombinant proteins, DNA, and mRNA.[28] In the United States two specific mRNA vaccinations have been administered to the public, including the BioNTech/FosunPharma/Pfizer vaccine and the Moderna/NIAID vaccine. The mRNA vaccines were approved and administered to the public at the pace they were not only because the world was facing a pandemic but also because mRNA vaccines proved to be faster and safer to produce and administer to individuals.[28] Both of the vaccines are administered by lipid nanoparticles (LNPs) through an intramuscular delivery method.[28] LNPs being delivered through a non-viral mRNA vector are advantageous for a number of reasons:

1. The LNP is able to adequately enclose and compress the mRNA.[28]
2. The LNP allows for the mRNA to get to the cytosol of the cell faster.[28]
3. The LNP protects the mRNA from being broken apart in the extracellular space by making the mRNA stronger.[28]
4. The LNP is made up of biocompatible materials that are safe for humans.[28]
5. The LNP is able to be produced and used on a large scale without any issues.[28]

6.9 REGENERATIVE MEDICINE

Regenerative medicine consists of repairing and restoring function to damaged cells by using stem cells to take over the function of the original cell to help the body function as it previously did.[29] A new and emerging field that is classified as regenerative medicine is through the use of stem cells. In particular, human mesenchymal stem cells (hMSCs) are used, which are adult stem cells that are located in different tissues.[30] They are specifically found in bone marrow, adipose tissue, and the umbilical cord of individuals.[30] These cells are special types of cells which can be placed near damaged tissue to repair the tissue and help in the healing process through an immune response.[30] Hence, hMSCs are undergoing major research, and they are being used to treat many different diseases with their unique abilities.[30] The most common active clinical trials range from autoimmune diseases to cancer. In MSCs, nucleic acid such as DNA and RNA are transfected using nanocarriers.[30] Nanocarriers are materials that use an electric charge to convert the nucleic acids into nanoparticles, which then use their charge and size to get inside the cell.[30] This is a similar process to electroporation; however, it is an alternative method which is being considered to be more advanced due to the nanotechnology that is used.

6.9.1 Non-Viral Delivery Methods of Regenerative Medicine

Non-viral delivery methods are preferred when working with MSCs due to the multiple advantages they have. More specifically, liposomes and cationic polymers are used when working with MSCs. Polyethyleneimine (PEI) is a cationic polymer, which is an agent that is used when creating MSC from different sources.[31] From the studies done so far, it has shown to be rather successful; however, more research has to be conducted to learn more in-depth information on the subject. It is more commonly used when working with DNA and is being experimented on with mRNA.[31] Furthermore, in a study conducted on mice, the MSCs were tested using non-viral delivery methods in a laboratory.[32] In this study, erythropoietin (EPO) was also used in order to develop red blood cells in bone marrow.[32] This study showed that non-viral gene delivery into MSCs is more efficient and safer than using viral gene delivery methods.

6.10 CONCLUSION

Genetic material is very important to an individual. Much research has been done with genetic material, especially with DNA. However, more research is currently being done on mRNA. mRNA is being used in more medicinal research using nanotechnology-based solutions, which has ample space to grow and develop into multiple revolutionary treatments for a diverse range of illnesses and diseases. The potential for future growth is expected to rise when observing the current trendlines and the current research with the development and approval of new drug applications due to the COVID-19 pandemic. Using non-viral vector–based mRNA medicine can be beneficial for not only public health crises but so much more in medicine with the help of various nanotechnologies.

6.10.1 Further COVID-19 Vaccination Research

While mRNA COVID-19 vaccines have had a very successful response in the United States, more research still needs to be done on possible adverse effects to the vaccinations, whether short term or long term. Additionally, the efficacy of mRNA treatments in regard to other viruses or illnesses should be considered. Alongside the appearance of new diseases, mutations in the preexisting ones should be acknowledged as well, potentially even the resurgence of certain strains.[28] Will the vaccine be effective long term? Will a booster shot be required? How long after? Will there be adverse effects to the vaccine long term? Science will never solve a problem without creating 10 more questions to ask, so much conclusive evidence can only be the subject of speculation.

REFERENCES

1. Try Stat+: The Story of mRNA: How a Once-dismissed Idea Became a Leading Technology in the Covid Vaccine Race. https://www.statnews.com/2020/11/10/the-story-of-mrna-how-a-once-dismissed-idea-became-a-leading-technology-in-the-covid-vaccine-race/.
2. Wolff JA, Malone RW, Williams P, et al. Direct Gene Transfer into Mouse Muscle in Vivo. *Science*. 1990; 247(4949):1465–1468.
3. Bayda, S, Adeel M, Tuccinardi T, Cordani M, Rizzolio F. The History of Nanoscience and Nanotechnology: From Chemical—Physical Applications to Nanomedicine. *Molecules*. 2019; 25(1):112.
4. Hoecke LV, Roose K. How mRNA Therapeutics are Entering the Monoclonal Antibody Field. *Journal of Translational Medicine*. 2019; 17(54):1804–1808.
5. Kose N, Fox JM, Sapparapu G, et al. A Lipid-Encapsulated mRNA Encoding a Potently Neutralizing Human Monoclonal Antibody Protects against Chikungunya Infection. *Science Immunology*. 2019; 4(35).
6. Kim YK. RNA Therapy: Current Status and Future Potential. *CMJ*. 2020; 56(2):87–93.
7. Genetic Engineering & Biotechnology News: CRISPR-Cas13 Developed as Combination Antiviral and Diagnostic System. https://www.genengnews.com/news/crispr-cas13-developed-as-combination-antiviral-and-diagnostic-system/.
8. Lutz BM, Bekker A, Tao YX. Noncoding RNAs: New Players in Chronic Pain. *Anesthesiology*. 2014; 121(2):409–417.
9. Patel S, Athirasala A, Menezes PP, et al. Messenger RNA Delivery for Tissue Engineering and Regenerative Medicine Applications. *Tissue Engineering Part A*. 2019; 25(1–2):91–112.
10. Science Business: Trial Shows RNA Therapy Safe for Diabetes. https://sciencebusiness.technewslit.com/?p=36037.
11. Berraondo P, Martini PGV, Avila MA, Fontanellas A. Messenger RNA Therapy for Rare Genetic Metabolic Diseases. *Gut*. 2019; 68(7):1323–1330.
12. Nature: Why Rare Genetic Diseases are a Logical Focus for RNA Therapies. https://www.nature.com/articles/d41586-019-03075-5.
13. News Medical Life Sciences: What are the Three Lines of Defense? https://www.news-medical.net/health/What-are-the-Three-Lines-of-Defense.aspx.
14. Zhang J, You Y. CRISPR-Cas13a System: A Novel Approach to Precision Oncology. *Cancer Biol Med*. 2020; 17(1):6–8.
15. Granados-Riveron, JT, Aquino-Jarquin G. CRISPR—Cas13 Precision Transcriptome Engineering in Cancer. *Cancer Research*. 2018; 78(15):4107–4113.
16. Eastern Michigan University: Risk-Benefit Analysis of the use of Viral Vectors in Gene Therapy. https://www.emich.edu/chhs/health-sciences/programs/clinical-research-administration/documents/theses/viral-vectors-in-gene-therapy.pdf.
17. Crommelin DJA, Anchordoquy TJ, Volkin DB, Jiskoot W, Mastrobattista E. Addressing the Cold Reality of mRNA Vaccine Stability. *J Pharm Sci*. 2021; 110(3):997–1001.
18. Cancer Care: Understanding the Role of Immuno-oncology in Treating Cancer. https://www.cancercare.org/publications/285-understanding_the_role_of_immuno-oncology_in_treating_cancer.
19. Matosevic S. Viral and Nonviral Engineering of Natural Killer Cells as Emerging Adoptive Cancer Immunotherapies. *J Immunol Res*. 2018; 4054815.

20. Hofmann GA, Dev SB, Dimmer S, Nanda GS. Electroporation Therapy: A New Approach for the Treatment of Head and Neck Cancer. *IEEE Trans Biomed Eng*. 1999; 46(6):752–759.
21. Medline Plus Trusted Health Information for You: What are Genome Editing and CRISPR-Cas9. https://medlineplus.gov/genetics/understanding/genomicresearch/genomeediting/#:~:text=Genome%20editing%20.
22. Rui Y, Wilson DR, Green JJ. Non-Viral Delivery to Enable Genome Editing. *Trends Biotechnol*. 2019; 37(3):281–293.
23. National Human Genome Research Institute: What is Genome Editing? https://www.genome.gov/about-genomics/policy-issues/what-is-Genome-Editing.
24. The Harvard Gazette: Perspectives on Gene Editing. https://news.harvard.edu/gazette/story/2019/01/perspectives-on-gene-editing/.
25. Yanoğlu FB, Elçin AE, Elçin YM. Bioethical Issues in Genome Editing by CRISPR-Cas9 Technology. *Turk J Biol*. 2020; 44(2):110–120.
26. Zhang C, Maruggi G, Shan H, Li J. Advances in mRNA Vaccines for Infectious Diseases. *Front Immunol*. 2019; 10:594.
27. Malaghan Instittue of Medical Research: Equipping our Immune System to Fight Disease-Preventive vs Therapeautic Vaccines. https://www.malaghan.org.nz/news/equipping-our-immune-system-to-fight-disease-preventive-vs-therapeutic-vaccines/#:~:text=The%20flu%20vaccine%2C%20as%20well,show%20signs%20of%20a%20disease
28. Park KS, Sun X, Aikins ME, Moon JJ. Non-Viral COVID-19 Vaccine Delivery Systems. *Adv Drug Deliv Rev*. 2021; 169:137–151.
29. Gómez-Aguado I, Rodríguez-Castejón J, Vicente-Pascual M, Rodríguez-Gascón A, Solinís MA, Pozo-Rodríguez A. Nanomedicines to Deliver mRNA: State of the Art and Future Perspectives. *Nanomaterials*. 2020; 10(2):364.
30. Hamann A, Nguyen A, Pannier AK. Nucleic Acid Delivery to Mesenchymal Stem Cells: A Review of Nonviral Methods and Applications. *Journal of Biological Engineering*. 2019; 13(9).
31. Ramos-Murillo AI, Rodríguez E, Beltrán K, Ricaurte C, et al. Efficient Non-Viral Gene Modification of Mesenchymal Stromal Cells from Umbilical Cord Wharton's Jelly with Polyethyleneimine. *Pharmaceutics*. 2020; 12(9):896.
32. Morshed M, Hasan A, Sharifi M, et al. Non-Viral Delivery Systems of DNA into Stem Cells: Promising and Multifarious Actions for Regenerative Medicine. *JDDST*. 2020; 60:101861.
33. Kyle P, Smita N, Kam L. Messenger RNA (mRNA) Nanoparticle Tumor Vaccination. *Nanoscale*. 2014; 6(14):7715–7729.
34. Chung YH, Beiss V, Fiering SN, Steinmetz NF. COVID-19 Vaccine Frontrunners and Their Nanotechnology Design. *ACS Nano*. 2020; 14(10):12522–12537.
35. Zhang X, Zhao W, Nguyen GN, et al. Functionalized Lipid-like Nanoparticles for in Vivo mRNA Delivery and Base Editing. *Science Advances* 2020, 6(34).
36. Pardi N, Hogan MJ, Porter FW, Weissman D. mRNA Vaccines—A New Era in Vaccinology. *Nature Reviews Drug Discovery*. 2018; 17(4):261–279.
37. Sturm G, Finotello F, Petitprez F, et al. Comprehensive Evaluation of Transcriptome-Based Cell-Type Quantification Methods for Immuno-Oncology. *Bioinformatics*. 2019; 35(14):i436–i445.
38. Dworkin MB, Dworkin-Rastl E. Functions of Maternal MRNA in Early Development. *Molecular Reproduction and Development*. 1990; 26(3):261–297.
39. Gurevich I, Tamir H, Arango V, Dwork A, Mann JJ, Schmauss C. Altered Editing of Serotonin 2C Receptor Pre-MRNA in the Prefrontal Cortex of Depressed Suicide Victims. *Neuron*. 2002; 34(3):349–356.
40. HHS Public Access Library. Sequence Variants in SLC16A11 Are a Common Risk Factor for Type 2 Diabetes in Mexico. *Nature*. 2013; 506(7486):97–101.

41. Urbina F, Morales-Pison S, Maldonado E. Enzymatic Protein Biopolymers as a Tool to Synthetize Eukaryotic Messenger Ribonucleic Acid (mRNA) with Uses in Vaccination, Immunotherapy and Nanotechnology. *Polymers*. 2020; 12(8):1633.
42. Van der Meel R. Nanotechnology for Organ-Tunable Gene Editing. *Nature Nanotechnology*. 2020; 15(4):253–255.
43. Tang Z, Zhang X, Shu Y, Guo M, Zhang H, Wei T. Insights from Nanotechnology in COVID-19 Treatment. *Nano Today*. 2021; 36:101019.
44. Milane L, Amiji M. Clinical Approval of Nanotechnology-Based SARS-CoV-2 MRNA Vaccines: Impact on Translational Nanomedicine. *Drug Delivery and Translational Research*. 2021.
45. Guo P. The Emerging Field of RNA Nanotechnology. *Nat Nanotechnol*. 2010; 5(12):833–842.
46. Chen YJ, Groves B, Muscat RA, Seelig G. DNA Nanotechnology from the Test Tube to the Cell. *Nature Nanotechnology*. 2015; 10(9):748–760.
47. Lin YX, Wang Y, Blake S, et al. RNA Nanotechnology-Mediated Cancer Immunotherapy. *Theranostics*. 2020; 10(1):281–299.
48. Islam MA, Reesor EK, Xu Y, Zope H, Zetter B, Shi J. Biomaterials for MRNA Delivery. *Biomaterials Science*. 2015; 3(12):1519–1533.
49. Cheng Q, Wei T, Farbiak L, Johnson LT, Dilliard SA, Siegwart C. Selective Organ Targeting (SORT) Nanoparticles for Tissue-Specific MRNA Delivery and CRISPR—Cas Gene Editing. *Nature Nanotechnology*. 2020; 15(4):313–320.
50. Wong DT. Salivary Diagnostics Powered by Nanotechnologies, Proteomics and Genomics. *JADA*. 2006; 137(3):313–321.
51. Lee K, Cui Y, Lee LP, Irudayarag J. Quantitative Imaging of Single MRNA Splice Variants in Living Cells. *Nat Nanotechnol*. 2014; 9(6):474–480.
52. Schatzlein AG. Non-Viral Vectors in Cancer Gene Therapy: Principles and Progress. *Anti-Cancer Drugs*. 2001; 12(4):275–304.
53. Kohn DB, Porteus MH, Scharenberg AM. Ethical and Regulatory Aspects of Genome Editing. *Blood*. 2016; 127(21):2553–2560.

7 RNA-Based Vaccines for Infectious Disease

Deepa Dehari, Aiswarya Chaudhuri, Sanjay Singh, and Ashish Kumar Agrawal

CONTENTS

7.1 INTRODUCTION

Vaccines have been produced to prevent and eradicate the transmission of contagious diseases since the 18th and 19th centuries [1]. They are the bedrock of worldwide social health initiatives and provide significant socioeconomic advantages [2]. Pre-exposure protection is provided by prophylactic immunization, which also aids in the production of herd immunity. Therapeutic vaccination, which is a type of immune responses, is used to fight infections [3]. The long-term interventional efficacy of presently licensed vaccines encourages more studies into novel vaccination programs. These initiatives are intended to improve therapeutic and preventive effectiveness, introducing new ideas, simplifying manufacturing techniques, and allowing for a quick response to evolving infective diseases [1, 4]. Synthesized sequences are being employed to convey antigenic peptides or proteins in situ in nucleic acid vaccines.

DOI: 10.1201/9781003186069-7

By triggering both humoral and cell-mediated responses, genomic immunization may enhance outstanding immune responses, and it has fabrication benefits over previous vaccines. Due to problems with RNA-based immunotherapy's stability and large manufacturing, early studies focused primarily on producing DNA candidates. DNA vaccines, on the other hand, have usually executed inadequately in human clinical trials, prompting growing attention in RNA vaccine development for communicable diseases. This transition has been inspired by the success of tumor immunotherapeutic studies to a certain point [5–6]. The safety spectrum of such nucleic acid vaccines is improved by the unique nature and cytoplasmic position of RNA in comparison with their more stabilized DNA counterparts that also necessitate nuclear delivery, target gene expression, and risk assimilation inside the host genetic material [7]. These characteristics have prompted considerable investment in RNA-based drug delivery in recent years. Traditional messenger RNA (mRNA) and self-amplifying RNA (saRNA) are the two kinds of artificial RNA vaccines available today [8]. So many preclinical and clinical trials have looked into the use of traditional mRNA techniques (also known as nonreplicating or nonamplifying mRNA) for infective illnesses and tumors. Vaccines based on in vitro transposed mRNAs encoding viral antigens were researched, while immunotherapy based on mRNAs encoding therapeutics, including antibodies or immunologic modulating agents, has been investigated [9]. The inclusion of chemically designed nucleotides, sequence standardization, and various purifying techniques enhance mRNA translation efficiency while reducing inherent immunogenic characteristics. Antigen expression, on the other hand, is dependent on the percentage of traditional mRNA transcripts delivered effectively during immunization. To achieve sufficient expression for safeguarding or immunomodulation, high amounts or multiple administrations may be required. This restriction is addressed by saRNA vaccines, which are genetically modified replicons obtained from self-replicating, single-stranded RNA viruses [8, 10]. They can be delivered as viral replicon particles (VRPs), with the saRNA assembled inside, or as a synthetically bioengineered saRNA obtained after in vitro transcription. Throughout manufacturing, envelope proteins are supplied in trans as defective helper constructs to produce replication-defective VRPs. Even after initial infection, the subsequent VRPs are unable to develop infective viral particles, and only the RNA can be amplified further. Positive-sense and negative-sense RNA viruses can both produce VRPs, but the latter is more complicated and requires reverse genetics to recover the VRPs [11].

The use of viral vectors for a vaccine design like gene therapy has several drawbacks. These include the vector's immunogenicity, which can induce an unwanted immune reaction and deter possible future booster injections with the same vector. A vaccine can also be rendered ineffective if the viral vector is already immune to it. Replication-competent alphavirus vectors, like live-attenuated vaccines, have the potential to reactivate the virus. To get around this, saRNA vaccines can be made and administered in the same way as mRNA vaccines. The Venezuelan equine encephalitis (VEE) virus, Sindbis virus (SINV), and Semliki forest virus (SFV) are all positive-sense alphavirus genomes that were utilized in the development of saRNA vaccines. The RNA-dependent RNA polymerase (RdRP) cluster encoded by the alphavirus replicase genes magnifies synthesized transcripts in situ. The immunogenic or therapeutic sequence is upregulated to a high extent as a distinct entity, and the immunogenic materials do not necessitate further proteolytic processing. Because of their self-replicative behavior, saRNA vaccines can acquire comparable antigen expression at lower doses than traditional mRNA vaccines [11–12].

The aim of this chapter is to introduce vaccine development history, the key benefits of saRNA over mRNA, and the immune response triggered by a saRNA-based vaccine. Further, it will cover preparation, purification, delivery, and pharmacokinetic aspects of saRNA-based vaccines. We have limited our discussion to the saRNA vaccine for infectious diseases, clinical translation, and their future prospects.

7.2 ADVANTAGES OF saRNA OVER mRNA

Because DNA or mRNA vaccines are convenient to produce and have better safety statuses than traditional vaccines, they may have a benefit over existing vaccines. In preclinical simulations, saRNA gains from alphavirus expression vectors have proven to be more effective than non-replicating mRNA and DNA in inducing humoral and cellular responses to a variety of antigens. This is primarily due to the fact that saRNA can produce significant levels of expression while also inducing powerful innate immune responses, thereby amplifying immunity. saRNA can be delivered as viral particles or DNA, but RNA transport is a safe, sustainable, and more straightforward option. Although saRNA can be transported as naked RNA, electroporation or crosslinking it with cationic lipids or polymers can improve in vivo transfection. Alphavirus saRNA could be used to immunize against a variety of human infectious agents, along with emerging ones such as SARS-CoV-2, for which an mRNA-based vaccine was recently approved. Figure 7.1 demonstrates advantages of saRNA over mRNA in intensifying the immune response [13–15].

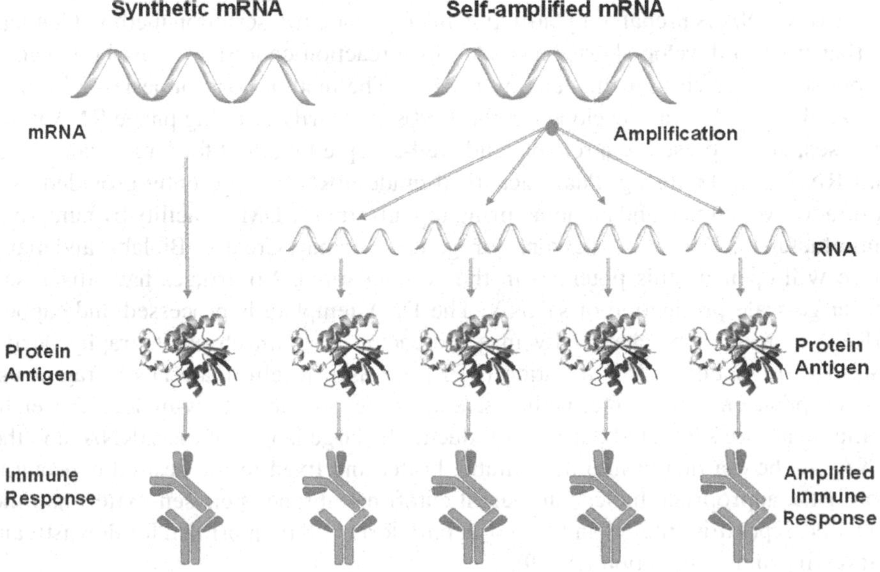

FIGURE 7.1 Advantages of saRNA over mRNA in intensifying the immune response.

7.3 saRNA VACCINE–INDUCED IMMUNE RESPONSE

saRNA only needs to be transcribed into the host cell cytoplasm, followed by its intracellular transportation. The mRNA simulates a viral infection during self-amplification and promotes an immunological response towards the expressed antigenic components of the virus. Non-viral delivery is a significant scientific area to be explored for saRNA vaccines [16].

A form of mRNA that has demonstrated extraordinary properties to provoke immune responses is saRNA. saRNA is obtained from the genes of many viruses such as alphaviruses and flaviviruses and has the ability of self-amplification, given the fact that it expresses a viral replicase (Rep), whereas the gene encoding for the virus structural proteins is replaced by the transgene of interest. Alphaviruses, such as VEEV, SFV, and SINV, provide the majority of saRNAs included in immunization research. An initial study demonstrated that substantial modification and alternative methodologies are essential for effective mRNA delivery as a vaccine candidate. Preliminary studies in animals suggested that saRNA-based non-viral delivery has the ability to generate a specific and potent immune response against viral infection. Figure 7.2 demonstrates the immunological response mediated by saRNA-based vaccines [13, 17].

7.4 PREPARATION OF saRNA-BASED VACCINES

A saRNA-based vaccine can be prepared by various methodologies. A widely accepted method is discussed next.

7.4.1 Cell-Free Synthesis Using an In Vitro Transcription Reaction

In vitro, saRNA is prepared by utilizing an enzymatic transcription method identical to that used to develop shorter mRNA, since reaction conditions must be tweaked to boost productivity for this lengthy mRNA. The method for synthesizing in vitro transcribed RNAs was developed in the 1990s, primarily utilizing phage RNA polymerases, and is presently a reliable and well-accepted method for large-scale artificial RNA manufacturing. Pharmaceutical-grade mRNA is presently provided as a contract development and manufacturing organization (CDMO) facility by numerous manufacturers: TriLink, Aldevron, Eurogentec, Biomay, Creative Biolabs, and many more will open up this potential in the coming years. No articles have discussed the large-scale production of saRNA. The DNA template is processed and capped mRNA is formed biochemically in a bioreactor. Column chromatography purification and tangential flow filtration (TFF) are used to eliminate DNA fragments, transcription enzymes, intermediates, and waste products. Low-molecular-weight components are separated during TFF due to the large length of the saRNA, and the RNA can be diafiltered into the suitable buffer and fixed to the desired concentration if the appropriate molecular weight cutoff membrane is chosen. After that, the RNA is aseptically filtered and stored in bulk form and then primed for downstream harvesting and formulation [18–19].

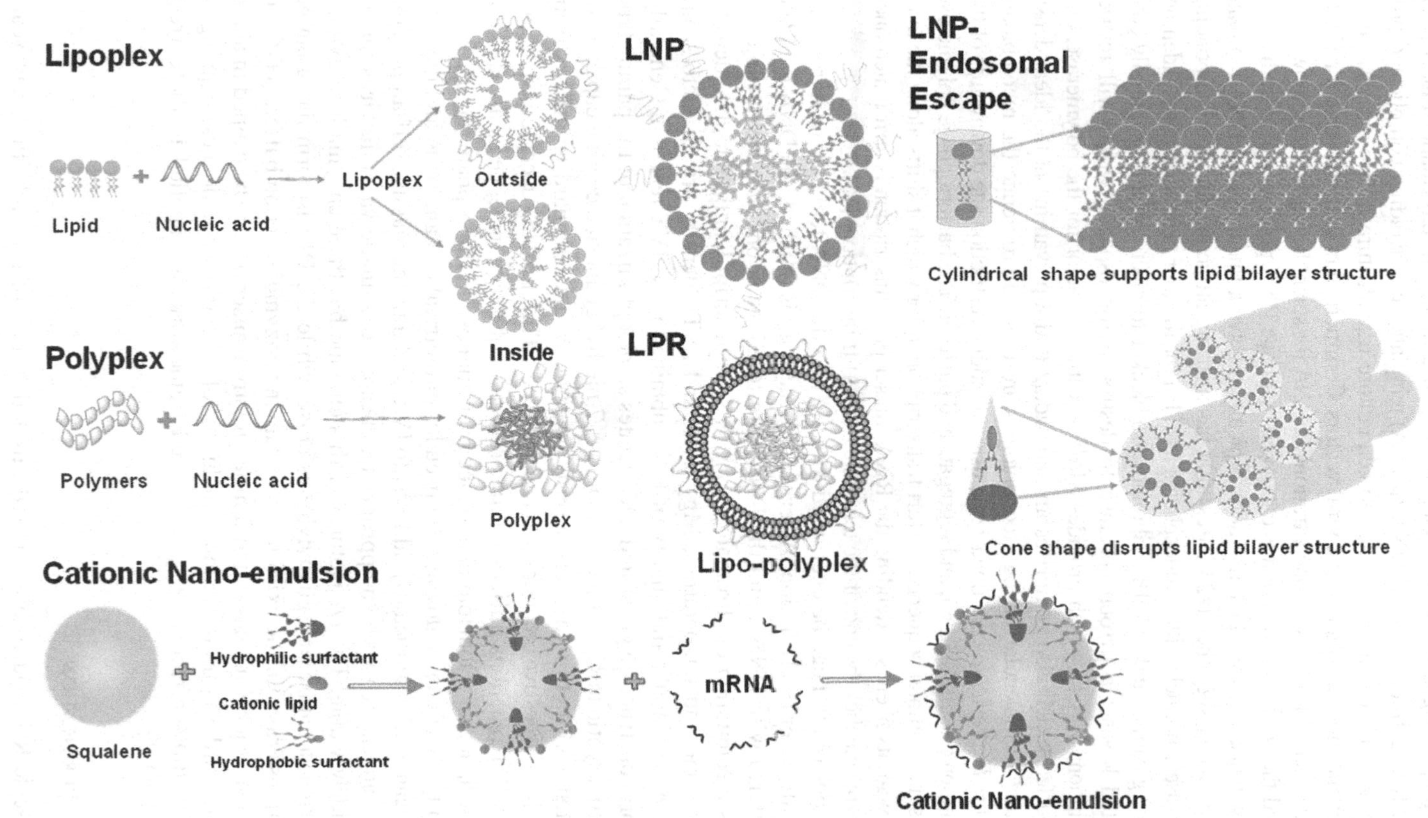

FIGURE 7.2 Schematic representation of immune response mediated by saRNA.

Self-amplifying mRNA is developed in vitro utilizing an enzymatic transcription process from a linear plasmid DNA (pDNA) template, thus avoiding complicated production and safety concerns related to cell culture manufacture of live viral vaccines, recombinant subunit proteins, and viral vectors. Commercial in vitro transcription (IVT) kits that generate milligram concentrations of RNA for scientific activities are now available, and the enzymatic reaction is catalyzed by phage RNA polymerase. In addition to the polymerase enzyme, IVT reactions typically involve a linear system DNA template with a promoter sequence (z23 bases) that has a strong attraction for its corresponding polymerase; ribonucleotide triphosphates (rNTPs) for the four necessary bases (adenine, cytosine, guanine, and uracil); a ribonuclease blocker to inactivate any potentially contaminated RNase; a pyrophosphatase to destroy pyrophosphate, which will restrict transcription; $MgCl_2$, which provides Mg^{2+} as with a cofactor for the polymerase; and a pH buffer, which also comprises an antioxidant and a polyamine at the ideal densities. Standard molecular biology technologies are used to proliferate the recombinant plasmid in *Escherichia coli*, linearize it using a unique restriction site downwards of the transcription cassette's 3' end, and segregate and purify it. The bacteriophage polymerase attaches the promoter sequence to start transcription, after which it shifts along the template toward its 5' ends, extending the RNA transcript. Transcription is terminated once the enzyme reaches the end of the template (run-off transcription) [15].

The poly(A) tail can be encrypted directly into the DNA template or introduced chemically after transcription. After the IVT activity is finished, the DNA template is splintered with DNase, and the RNA is restored using one of many techniques, such as precipitation or chromatography. RNA transcript length, template density, reaction time and temperature, Mg_2 level, and rNTP density are all factors that influence the amount and quality of RNA obtained in an IVT reaction. Generally, each form of structure generated necessitates some optimization of the parameters. Many eukaryotic mRNA molecules have 5' 7-methyl guanosine coating cap components that work both in triggering protein synthesis and safeguarding mRNA from intracellular digestive enzymes such as nucleases. The currently accepted technique used for IVT reactions utilizes the incorporation of a cap analogue as an activator of transcription at a fourfold abundance over guanosine triphosphate (GTP). There are two types of cap analogues: the pseudosymmetrical cap analogue and the anti-reverse cap. Both significantly add cost to IVT, and thus the massive self-amplifying mRNAs are capped with an appropriate, cheaper, enzymatic vaccinia virus that is now widely viable. The D1 isoform of this enzyme has three enzymatic activities: RNA triphosphatase and guanylyltransferase, while the D12 isoform has guanine methyltransferase. In the existence of a capping enzyme, reaction buffer, GTP, and the methyl donor S-adenosylmethionine, in vitro transcripts can be capped in about an hour. Unlike cotranscriptional inclusion of certain cap analogues, capping is generally 100% effective, and all capped frameworks are applied in the correct orientation [11].

7.4.2 Purification

Large-scale RNA purification is still an active area of research. In recent years there has been an increased interest in exploring methods for RNA manufacturing

[20–21]. An industrially feasible purification procedure must be customizable, implement good manufacturing practices, make it possible to eliminate all materials incorporated in the in vitro and capping reactions, and produce a sterilized finished bulk that meets numerous formulation and in vivo delivery specifications. Furthermore, organic reagents should be avoided in vaccine production processes due to prospective safety issues such as residual solvents, increased overall cost, environmental consequences, and prospective negative impacts on RNA stabilization and efficacy. Purification of DNA for biomedical applications has deep roots in comparison to RNA purification. Good manufacturing practice (GMP) manufacturing is presently on a gram-to-kilogram range, but the most frequently utilized procedures are vastly different from those essential for mRNA [22–23]. In *E. coli*, pDNA is manufactured by bacterial fermentation and accounts for around 2% (w/w) of the overall nucleic acid. Consequently, the pDNA should be purified away from bacterial cell waste products, which contain proteins, host DNA and RNA, and endotoxins. RNA is considered a waste product and is expelled with preferential precipitation utilizing Ca^{2+}, NH^{4+}, or Mg^{2+} ions or polyethylene glycol (PEG) [24]. Furthermore, there are three isoforms of pDNA (supercoiled, open circular, and linear), and the supercoiled species should be purified beyond a certain criterion. The downstream purifying method for pDNA is thus challenging and requires a variety of steps: cells lysis/disruption, solid/liquid segregation, abstraction, and purifying. Size-exclusion chromatography (SEC), reversed-phase chromatography, anion-exchange chromatography, hydrophobic interaction, and thiophilic adsorption chromatography are among the chromatographic methodologies used to purify pDNA [25–26].

As with DNA, mRNA has a negative-charge phosphodiester foundation, which can effectively be tailored to the purification of that molecule through any of the purification methods utilized for pDNA. But mRNA purification might be significantly easier than pDNA purification because of the well-understood comparatively low amount of the enzymatic transcription reaction materials needed that are not preceded by host cell trash [27–28]. The compliance demands for viral clearance and the procedure employs recombinant or animal-free industrial chemicals. The viruses, retroviruses, or prion proteins are therefore not contaminated. RNA may be easily precipitated, rinsed with alcohol, and put into a buffer for use in the immunization with LiCl for routine animal model work and in vivo immunization studies [29]. However, it would be incredibly difficult to incorporate such a procedure for the manufacturing of GMPs.

In the history of biophysical and structural analysis, large amounts (mg) of pure RNA were needed, and this has been accomplished by denatured polyacrylamide gel electrophoresis (PAGE) [30]. High capability and better resolution for separating short oligoribonucleotides are provided with column chromatography, but PAGE denaturation is usually the technique of purification for long (>30 mer), in vitro translated RNA [31–32]. Even so, the traditional PAGE gel is limited in its loading capability. The effectiveness of a high-performance liquid chromatography (HPLC) cleansing technique for mRNA gene therapeutic applications has been emphasized in numerous research studies [33]. The process includes its usefulness, and promising health concerns regarding organic solvent residues have been raised [34]. Major firms such as Asuragen in the Americas and CureVac GmbH in Europe are currently supplying pharmaceutical-grade mRNA. CureVac's current innovative work on the therapeutic manufacturing of smaller (z2 kb) mRNA that does not enhance the utilization of mRNA has demonstrated viability in human use in tumor vaccines at a huge scale. While the procedure is proprietary and unpublished, CureVac has shown that mRNAs have been cleared from the chromatographic purification by size and eliminate abortive (shorter) or aberrant (longer) transcripts generated during the enzyme reaction by trace quantities of impurities in the IVT reaction (proteins, DNAs) [11].

The self-amplifying mRNA vaccines of 10,000 bases are large mRNAs (MW z3 MDa). Due to the exclusion impacts of size and poor recovery, such molecules pose a number of extra difficulties, and no extensively feasible procedures remain. Chromatographic segregation of RNA premised on the HPLC reverse ion pairing or ion exchange resins is focused on the maximum loading of the substances [7]. It is efficient at purifying RNA molecules of around 400 to 5000 bases, so it is difficult to be useful as self-amplifying mRNA vaccination purifying methodologies. There is thus still a demand for advanced techniques for purifying RNA, especially among those who allow for the cost-effective and timely purifying of a significant quantity of RNAs at a greater output and therapeutic grade, while maintaining their stability, biochemical efficacy, and usability. At a substantial scale, chromatographic purification of RNA is complicated for numerous manufacturers and universities and is a popular field of research. An RNA method can be standard and separate from the encoded antigen in the vector and can produce significantly reduced times than that of recombinant protein manufacturing [11].

7.5 REFINING saRNA PHARMACOKINETICS

Many attempts have finally progressed into RNA manufacturing stability, translation, and drug kinetic model understanding and strengthening. Improving the 5' cap design monitoring the dimension of the poly(A) tail that includes modified nucleotides, standardization of the codon or sequence, and modifying the 5' and 3' UTRs (untranslated regions) are a few of the considerations. For lengthy saRNA transcripts, it is also essential to optimize the intrinsically and extrinsically immunologic qualities of synthesized RNA, antigen, and delivery. Several other researchers suggest that the incorporation of several pseudouridine-modified nucleotides during transcription showed improved translation and lowered RNA-related immunogenicity. Since saRNAs use host-cell factors in the replication of mRNA, adding altered nucleotides can be of minimal use, as they would be misplaced when amplified. Another feasible technique to enhance the translation of saRNA vaccines is by optimizing 5' and 3' UTRs, relying on the development of natural alphaviruses. The single-stranded genome of RNA can be transformed into a range of secondary structures that enable alphaviruses to circumvent normal host cellular functions and avoid immune reactions. It can also prove useful to revise the nsP1–4 gene sequence encryption. In order to recognize mutations in the nonstructural protein VEE which enhances the *in-situ* expressions of subgenomic RNAs in the in vitro transformation approach, the proficient cell interferon (IFN) was employed [12, 35–36].

7.5.1 Five-Prime Caps

Alteration of the synthesized 5' cap framework is a well-invested method of safeguarding in vitro translated RNAs against nuclease degradation. In situ translation of RNAs by only encapsulating transcripts of forwarding direction, the anti-reverse cap analogue, and new phosphorothioate derivatives have been shown to be better. Cap-1 structures are generated in combination with 2'-O-methyltransferases, which simulate biological eukaryotic mRNAs. The capping enzymes obtained from the Vaccinia virus have an increased capping efficiency. TriLink BioTechnologies has innovated the CleanCap platform to further enhance cotranscriptional capping. The new technologies can produce epitranscriptomic analogues of Cap 1, Cap 2, and Cap 1 including m6Am that will increase the stability of the RNA by preventing decapping of DCP2 encrypted metal enzymes. Interestingly, the Clean Cap Reagent AU has been specially designed with saRNA transcribers obtained from positive-sense alphaviruses to produce Cap 1 frameworks. Cap analogues can play a major rolc in the evasion of inborn immune reactions from cells, and Cap 0 RNAs can induce IFN reactions. Some alphaviruses thus circumvent the requirement for 2'-O-methylated caps, which indicates that the proper architecture of the 5' UTRs could ignore Cap 0 immunity [12, 37].

7.6 DELIVERY OF saRNA VACCINES

The effective non-viral delivery of nucleic acids to the cellular cytoplasm, in which an enclosed vaccine antigen amplifies and expresses can be a significant obstacle when realizing the total capability of self-amplifying mRNA vaccines. The non-virus supply of genes, such as the chemical supply by lipids, polymeric materials, emulsions, and other substances facilitating cell intake and physical delivery platform and devices, can be accomplished in many diverse ways. Many other investigated platforms for pDNA, antisense RNA, siRNA, and mRNA have been established. Transport of saRNA in vivo was found to be complicated, with multiple steps. Initially, RNA should reach the tissue at the same time it should prevent from deterioration and elimination mediated by RNase. If the target cell RNA needs to translocate to the cytosol via its cell membranes, use the host translation equipment and activate nonstructural protein translation. The hydrophilic nature and powerful net-negative RNA load hinder cell absorption considerably. In order to solve this obstacle, RNA can be compounded by electroporation or ballistic particle-media shipment with cationic liposomes or nanoparticles or physically shipped to enhance cellular absorption. Viruses have developed using advanced processes that manipulate or bypass cell signaling and traffic in host cells and transfer their genome to the relevant subcellular compartments. Various delivery aspects of saRNA-based vaccines are presented in Figure 7.3 [38–41].

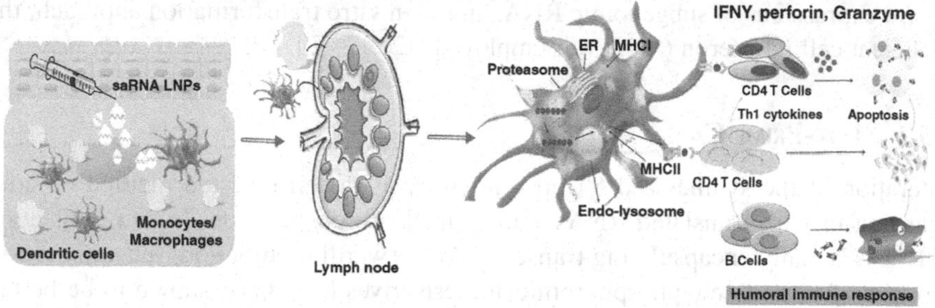

FIGURE 7.3 Delivery aspects of saRNA-based vaccines.

7.7 saRNA-BASED VACCINE DEVELOPMENT FOR INFECTIOUS DISEASE

7.7.1 HIV

Human immunodeficiency virus (HIV) is a virus that causes infection in humans. HIV-1 is the most common type of HIV. By damaging crucial cells that battle infectious agents, it diminishes a person's immune system and causes it to malfunction. HIV specifically harms and destroys CD4 cells, a type of immune cell known as a T cell. As HIV harms more CD4 cells, the body becomes more susceptible to a variety of diseases and cancers. HIV-1 infection can eventually lead to acute immunodeficiency syndrome (AIDS) [42–44]. Presently, there is no efficient treatment for HIV. It can, however, can be managed with the right medical care.

T-cell responses to HIV-1 need to focus on the most sensitive areas of the virus, the structurally invariant regions of HIV-1 proteins, which is a major element for vaccine success [45]. Individual CD8+ T cells and the population as a whole must exhibit a number of key characteristics for a T-cell vaccine to effectively control HIV-1 replication [46]. Immunization is prone to failure if any of these characteristics are inadequate. Incremental linear advances in clinical trials will be required to fine-tune the individual protective features of T cells [47]. The second-generation tHIVconsvX immunogens, on the other hand, direct CD8+ T cells to primarily preventive and retained epitopes [48].

Recently, Moyo and colleagues developed saRNA for delivering tHIVconsvX to the immunological system. They showed that saRNA vaccines triggered strongly precise, plurifunctional CD8+ and CD4+ T cells in BALB/c and crossbred mice that exhibited organized memory subgroups and were retained at significantly higher frequencies for at least 22 weeks after vaccination. It is one of the first comprehensive studies of T-cell responses evoked by mRNA vaccines. The integration of tHIVconsvX immunogens and the extremely customizable and easy-to-manufacture saRNA framework could offer a long-awaited ability to establish and optimize the activation of absolutely protective CD8+ T-cell parameters in human subjects [49].

Positive-strand RNA viruses' saRNA is an efficient vector for in situ expression of vaccine antigens, and it has the capability to become an innovative vaccine technology framework with world health systems. The saRNA vaccine concept is based on an artificial, non-viral delivery mechanism for saRNA. Bogers and colleagues reported on the safety and immunogenicity of an HIV-SAM™ vaccine in rhesus macaques encrypting a clade C envelope glycoprotein and delivered via a cationic nanoemulsion delivery method. The HIV saRNA immunization elicited stronger cellular immune reactions than saRNA assembled in a viral replicon particle or a recombinant HIV envelope protein developed with MF59 adjuvant, as well as anti-envelope adherence (together with anti-V1V2) and neutralizing antibody responses that outperformed the viral replicon particle vaccine. These findings are the first to show that HIV immunization with a comparatively low dose (50 μg) of prepared saRNA is both safe and immunogenic in animal models [50].

saRNA is a viable biotechnology therapeutics platform that has been utilized as a vaccine for both contagious illnesses and tumors. saRNA has been shown to stimulate protein expression for up to two months and to induce immune function at smaller concentrations than mRNA. Because saRNA is a large -ve charge molecule, it needs a shipping vehicle to enable optimal cellular uptake and safeguard from degeneration. Lipid nanoparticles (LNPs) have been popularly utilized in RNA preparations, with the present system being to encapsulate RNA inside the particle, along with the first Food and Drug Administration (FDA)–recommended small-interfering siRNA therapy. Blakney and colleagues prepared LNPs using cationic and ionizable lipids in which saRNA were encapsulated inside or attached to the particle surface. The nanoparticles formulated with positively charged lipids protected saRNA from RNAse degradation. Additionally, protective effects against RNAse degradation were retained even for surface decorated saRNA nanoparticles. Lastly, the study demonstrated that both formulations were able to produce the same extent of antibodies against HIV-1 Env gp140 as a model antigen. This study also demonstrated that saRNA either can be encapsulated or can be attached to the particle surface without affecting their intensity of immune response. In both back leg quadriceps muscles, female mice were administered C12–200, DDA, and DOTAP preparations with saRNA surface decoration (exterior) or encapsulated (interior) inside the nanoparticles. The mice were then visualized for luciferase expression on day 7 (Figure 7.4), which had initially been displayed to be the VEEV replicon's maximum luciferase expression [40].

7.7.1.1 Developmental Challenges for an HIV Vaccine

Efforts to develop an HIV vaccine have so far centered on stimulating antibodies that prohibit viral infection. Protein subunit vaccines, which use a recombinant viral protein as a target immunogen, have been the focus of most of the research in this field. The importance of tolerance mechanisms in restricting bnAb B-cell key ingredient advancement, external anergy, and the uncommon characteristic of bnAbs in neutralizing HIV are the principal obstacles to HIV bnAb vaccine innovation. Furthermore, because HIV evolves quickly and incorporates into host genes, elevated amounts of long-lasting antibodies to various bnAb Env epitopes should be available at the moment of infection to stop virus exit and offer additional sterilizing immunity. In order to stimulate defensive bnAb-mediated immunity, elevated titers of long-lasting neutralizing antibodies to numerous Env epitopes must be induced. It has been

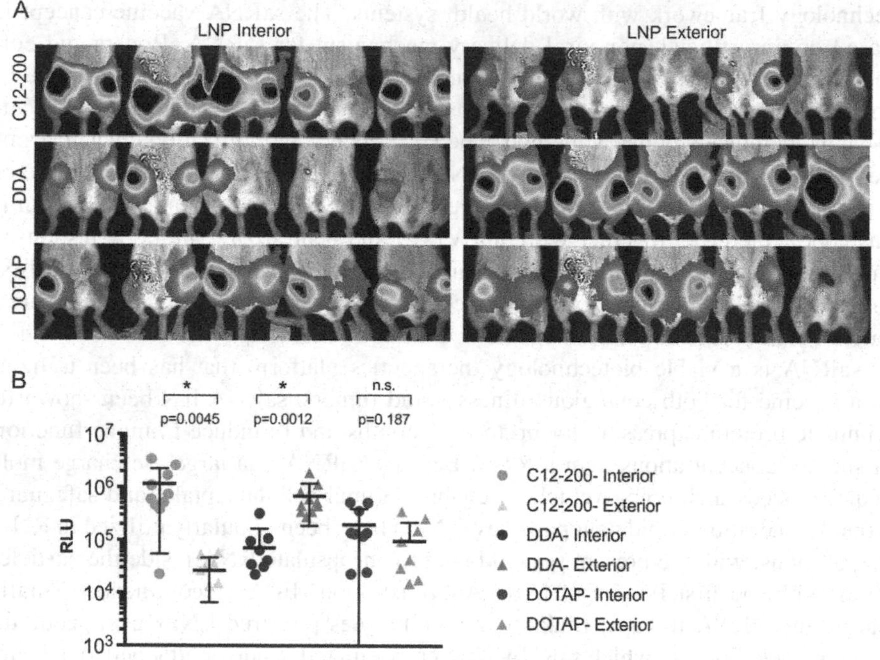

FIGURE 7.4 In vivo luciferase expression of saRNA complexed to the interior or exterior of LNPs. (A) In vivo imaging (IVIS) visualization of mice injected intramuscularly with 5 μg of fLuc saRNA per leg and imaged 7 days after injection. (B) Quantification of IVIS luciferase expression with a line at the mean ± standard deviation for n = 5 mice (n = 10 legs) per group. Units are expressed as relative light units (RLUs). Asterisk indicates significance applying an unpaired t-test with $*p < 0.05$ (p-values indicated); n.s., nonsignificant [40].

recommended that including a CD8+ T-cell triggering immunogen or framework in a bnAb vaccine could reduce the bnAb titers required for safeguarding [51].

7.7.2 Zika Virus

The Zika virus first appeared in the early 1900s, most likely in Uganda, and went unnoticed for decades. Scientists searching for the yellow fever virus at the Ugandan Viral Research Station did not discover Zika virus again until 1947, when sentinel rhesus macaque no. 776 developed a febrile sickness. Antibodies to the viral infection were found in 6 (6.1%) of the 99 Uganda people investigated from four distinct places. The significance of this evolving virus was uncertain and unpredictable at that time. Since there were no recognized illnesses or epidemics of significance in humans then, the response to Zika virus as a mystery made sense [52].

Zika virus is an evolving virus that poses a significant social health risk to humans. Although the majority of patients are symptomless or have mild, self-limiting symptoms, a limited proportion of individuals develop significant abnormalities, like congenital anomalies in the growing fetus of infected pregnant mothers and neurological dysfunction (e.g., Guillain-Barré syndrome). Zika virus is an arbovirus that corresponds to the Flaviviridae family of viruses, which also involves dengue, West Nile, and yellow fever viruses. The Zika virus has a single-stranded, +ve sense RNA genome that encrypts structural and non-structural proteins (capsid, precursor membrane [prM], and envelope [E]). The genetic code is transcribed into a single polypeptide, which is then sliced into specific proteins using proteolytic cleavage. The prM, E, and non-structural proteins are the most divergent from other flaviviruses in terms of pattern. East African, West African, and Asian Zika virus lineages have been identified [53–54].

Zika virus is responsible for an infant microcephalic pandemic and adult Guillain-Barre disorder [55]. Since no Zika virus immunology therapies or vaccinations are presently available, several global health organizations have made the development of safe and effective vaccines a top priority [56].

7.7.2.1 Immunological Responses to Zika Virus

Numerous cellular proteins have the ability to serve as entry receptors. Toll-like receptor 3, retinoic acid inducible gene-I, melanoma differentiation–associated gene 5 expression, secretion of type 1 and type 2 interferons, and overexpression of interferon triggered genes that facilitate antiviral responses are all characteristics of cellular illness with Zika virus. Glycosaminoglycans can help the Zika virus affix and enter the body. According to early findings, immune responses to Zika virus are analogous to those with other flaviviruses in that neutralizing antibodies (activity targeted at the E protein) are assumed to perform a key role in infection prevention. In reality, there is a lot of serological cross-reactivity with Zika virus as well as other flaviviruses, which has made it difficult to use screening procedures and seropositivity research in sectors in which other flavivirus antibodies are also visible. Monoinfection with Zika virus is less prevalent in some parts than coinfection with other flaviviruses [53, 57]. In mouse and rhesus monkey models of infection, a single dose of highly pure inactive virus vaccine or a plasmid DNA vaccine containing the prM and E proteins as immunogenic components provided full immunity against Zika virus. Additionally, in rhesus monkeys, a rhesus adenovirus (serotype 52) vaccine provided full immunity after just one dose. This DNA vaccine also triggered a protective immune response in animals that had their CD4+ or CD8+ T cells decimated prior to the viral threat, implying that humoral immune response is adequate to trigger clinical safety. These studies have started to look for a probable serological correspondence of E antibody levels and safeguards. It is still uncertain whether T cells are required for the commencement of Zika virus–specific B-cell responses [53, 58].

7.7.2.2 Zika Virus saRNA Vaccine Development

Luisi and colleagues have reported the advancement of Zika virus vaccine candidates utilizing the cationic nanoemulsion (CNE) self-amplifying RNA messenger technology platform, which provides a bedside mixture and is especially useful for quick response in a pandemic. It was observed that two vaccinations of the two different lead saRNA (CNE) vaccines in mice and non-human primates demonstrated the development of a potentially neutralizing antibody against the Zika virus. Further, the investigation suggested that mice and non-human primates were completely protected from the Zika virus. Hence, preclinical data revealed that the saRNA (CNE) vaccine is a suitable candidate for protecting against the Zika virus and the development of long-lasting protective immunity. Currently developed vaccines are able to provoke a protective immune response; the data are presented in Figure 7.5 [59].

7.7.3 SARS-CoV-2

Currently, the world is facing a pandemic caused by SARS-CoV-2 that triggered the fast-track development of a vaccine candidate. The widely accepted and trusted COVID-19 vaccine was developed by Moderna (USA-based pharmaceutical company) and Pfizer BioNtech (collaborated). Both vaccines have been approved by the FDA for vaccination and are premised on saRNA technology. The saRNA developed against SARS-CoV-2 has been found to have 95% efficacy. It was encapsulated inside the liposome core for effective delivery and to improve the stability profile of the vaccine [60–62].

In a study, McKay and colleagues designed an saRNA vaccine encrypting the SARS-CoV-2 spike protein, which was incorporated inside lipid-based nanoparticles. It was observed that a higher level of dose-dependent COVID-19–specific antibodies were present in mouse sera. It was also noted that viral neutralizing ability is directly proportional to the concentration of specific immunoglobulin G (IgG), which was in higher concentrations compared to that from patients who has recovered from COVID-19. Further, the study suggested that immunization with saRNA-loaded LNPs provoked a Thl-biased response in mice. Finally, when cells were re-stimulated with SARS-CoV-2 peptides, higher cell responses, as measured by IFN production, were noted. Quantitative analysis and neutralization of antibodies in SARS-CoV-2 saRNA immunized mice versus COVID-19–recovered individuals is presented in Figure 7.6. These findings shed light on vaccine development and immunogenicity testing, allowing for a quick transition to the health center [60].

7.7.4 Influenza (Flu)

The influenza virus is a pulmonary pathogenic virus responsible for 250,000 to 500,000 fatalities yearly globally, and immunization is the most inexpensive way to prevent and handle influenza incidence [63–64]. Currently approved inactivated influenza vaccines (IIVs) comprise the hemagglutinin (HA) viral surface protein and trigger strain-specific antibody responses that defend against serologically matched or closely linked virus infections. Due to the increased mutation rate in HA, periodic vaccines must be modified every year to fit the transmitted viruses. Seasonal vaccines fail to protect against newly evolving influenza virus infections or pandemic incidences. As a result, for the past two decades, researchers have been working on a "universal" influenza vaccine that can provide wider safeguards against all subgroups of influenza A virus. Adjuvants, such as MF59, improve the depth of immune response triggered by seasonal and pandemic influenza vaccines, but not enough to overcome the temporary vaccine strain that alters constraint [65–66].

In a study Magini and colleagues developed an LNP-encapsulated saRNA vector expressing influenza nucleoprotein that triggered excellent CD4 T helper cells

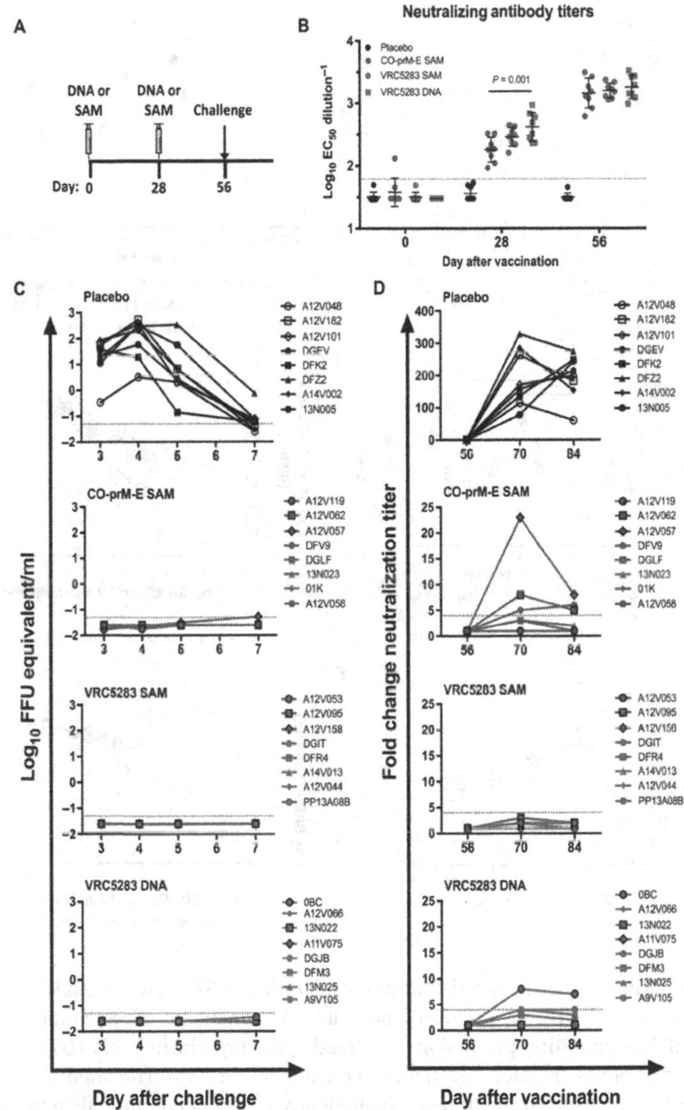

FIGURE 7.5 Zika virus saRTNA (SAM) (CNE) vaccines are immunogenic and protective in non-human primates. (A) Rhesus macaques (n = 8 per group) were immunized with the indicated vaccines at days 0 and 28 and subsequently challenged with 1000 FFU of Zika virus at day 56. (B) Neutralizing antibody activity was determined by Zika virus RVP assay at days 0, 28, and 56. Horizontal line and error bars represent the mean $\log_{10}$ reciprocal EC50 dilutions ± SD of eight animals per group, respectively. Statistical difference is shown between vaccines at each time point by two-way ANOVA with Tukey's multiple comparison posttest. Dotted line represents the LOC. Any replicates below the limit of detection were assigned a value of 0.5 LOC. (C) Viral loads were determined by qRT-PCR at days 3, 4, 5, and 7 after challenge. Each animal is depicted as a single line. Dotted line represents the LOC. Any replicates below the LOC were assigned a value of 0.5 LOC. (D) Post-challenge anamnestic antibody response. Fold change in EC_{50}-neutralizing antibody activity is shown relative to day 56. Each animal is depicted as a single line. Dotted line indicates a fold change of 4 [59].

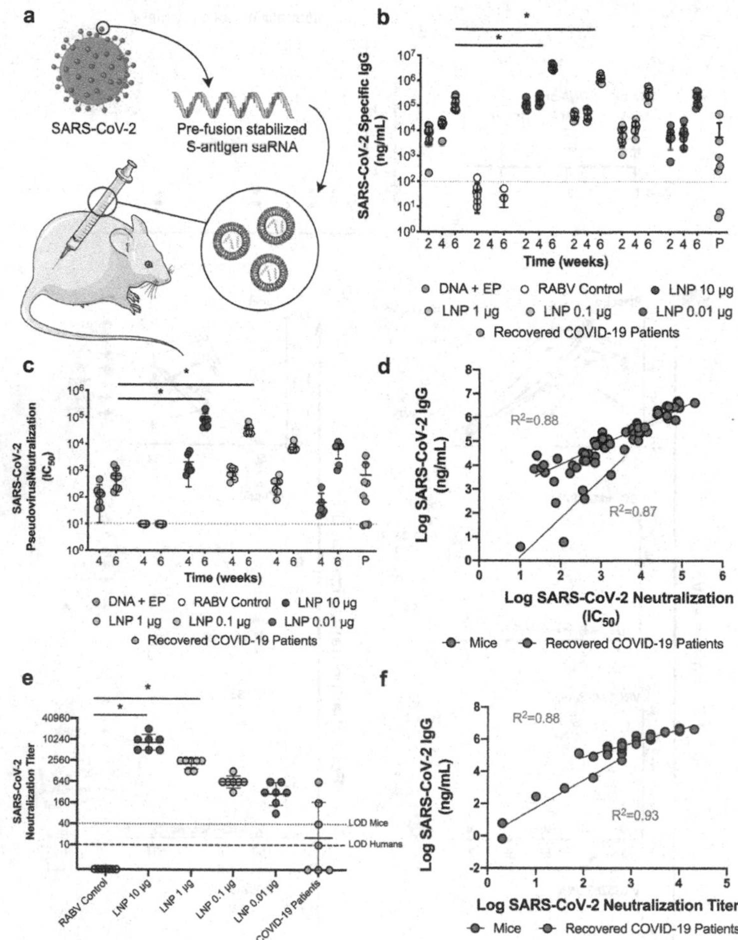

FIGURE 7.6 Antibody quantification and neutralization of SARS-CoV-2 saRNA vaccinated mice compared to COVID-19–recovered patients. (A) Schematic of vaccination of BALB/c mice with saRNA encoding pre-fusion stabilized spike protein in LNP. (B) SARS-CoV-2–specific IgG responses in mice vaccinated with doses of LNP-formulated saRNA ranging from 0.01 to 10 μg of saRNA with n = 7 biologically independent animals and COVID-19–recovered patients with n = 9 biologically independent samples. (C) SARS-CoV-2 pseudotyped virus neutralization of sera from BALB/c mice vaccinated with doses of LNP formulated saRNA ranging from 0.01 to 10 μg of saRNA with n = 7 biologically independent animals and COVID-19–recovered patients with n = 9 biologically independent samples. (D) Correlation between SARS-CoV-2–specific IgG and SARS-CoV-2 neutralization IC50 for vaccinated mice (n = 7 biologically independent animals) and recovered COVID-19 patients (n = 9 biologically independent samples). (E) SARS-CoV-2 viral neutralization of sera from BALB/c mice vaccinated with doses of LNP-formulated saRNA ranging from 0.01 to 10 μg of saRNA with n = 7 biologically independent animals. (F) Correlation between SARS-CoV-2–specific IgG and SARS-CoV-2 wild-type viral neutralization titers for vaccinated mice (n = 7 biologically independent animals). Electroporated pDNA (DNA + EP) was used as a positive control, while saRNA encoding the rabies glycoprotein (RABV) in pABOL was used as a negative control (RABV control). * indicates significance of $p < 0.05$ using a two-way ANOVA adjusted for multiple comparisons. Line and error bars indicated mean ± SD [60].

and CD8 cytotoxic cells, leading to a reduction in pulmonary viral load [67]. In another study Brazzoli and colleagues developed a cationic nanoemulsion loaded with saRNA expressed with influenza virus HA. It was noted that the developed nanosystem was able to inhibit viral replication in the upper respiratory tract in the animal infected with influenza virus [68].

saRNA vaccines have a number of advantages over mRNA vaccines in that they increase protein expression while lowering the dose needed. Even so, past delivery techniques were optimized for siRNA or mRNA, and because of structural dissimilarity between such RNAs, they do not always transport saRNA effectively, prompting the advancement of saRNA delivery technologies. Blakney and colleagues designed a linearly positively charged biologically reducible polymer called pABOL for saRNA transport. It was also demonstrated that an increase in molecular weight of the polymer promoted in vitro and in vivo delivery of saRNA. Further research shows that intramuscular (IM) and intradermal (ID) administration of pABOL improved protein activity and cellular absorption in vivo when contrasted to marketed accessible polymers and that IM administration provides full immunity from influenza. This polymer is expected to be strongly therapeutically transferable as a transport carrier for saRNA for both vaccines and therapeutics due to the robustness of polymer production and simplicity of formulation development. Figure 7.7 demonstrates cellular expression of saRNA after IM (mouse) or ID (human, mouse) administration with polyplex preparation [14].

To bridge the gap between pathogen evolution and vaccine certification, innovative vaccine technologies are required. RNA-based vaccines are an appealing choice for this position because they are harmless, manufactured without the use of cells, and can be developed quickly in response to a pathogen's rapid spread. Synthesized mRNA molecules encrypting only the antigen of concern are accessible, while saRNA is virally obtained and encrypts both the antigen of concern and proteins, allowing for RNA vaccine synthesis. Both technologies have been demonstrated to elicit immunity against infection, but it's unclear whether the method is the most effective. Vogel and colleagues contrasted the expression of influenza virus hemagglutinin by synthesized mRNA and saRNA. Both systems were prophylactic, but 1.25 mg saRNA provided comparable thresholds of safeguarding when contrasted to 80 mg mRNA (64-fold less material). They evaluated hemagglutinin from test varieties of influenza H1N1, H3N2 (X31), and B (Massachusetts) as saRNA vaccines after determining that saRNA was much more efficient than mRNA. All three variants safeguarded against challenge with infectious disease. When saRNA was coupled in a trivalent preparation, it provided protection against H1N1 and H3N2 in a systematic fashion. As a result, the researchers believe that saRNA is a viable technology for immunizations against infectious diseases [69].

7.8 TRANSLATING SARNA VACCINES TO CLINICAL PRACTICE (CLINICAL TRIALS)

Translation of saRNA-based vaccines to clinical practices requires deep understanding and thorough investigation of its safety and efficacy profile. Numerous preclinical and clinical studies have examined using an saRNA virus vector as a

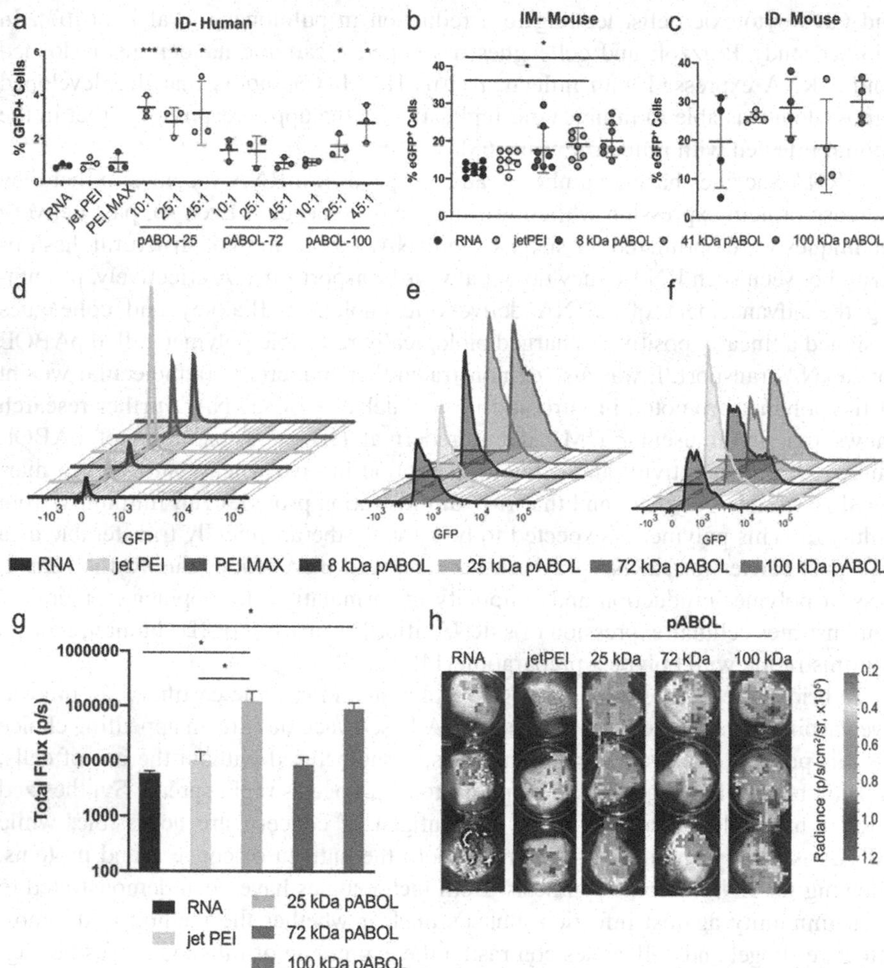

FIGURE 7.7 Cellular expression of saRNA after IM (mouse) or ID (human, mouse) injection with polyplex formulations. (A) Percentage of eGFP+ cells out of total live cells for each formulation after an intradermal injection of 2 μg of saRNA in human skin explants. Explants were analyzed 72 h after initial injection. jetPEI and PEI MAX were formulated at ratios of N/P = 8 and 1, respectively. pABOL formulations were prepared at ratios of 10:1, 25:1, and 45:1. Bars represent mean ± SD for n = 3, with *, **, and *** indicating significance of $p < 0.05$, 0.01, and 0.001 using an unpaired, two-tailed t-test, respectively. (B and C) Percentage of eGFP+ cells out of total live cells for each formulation after either IM (B) or ID (C) injection of 5 μg of saRNA in mice. Tissue was excised 7 d after initial injection. jetPEI was formulated at a ratio of N/P = 8, and pABOL formulations were prepared at a ratio of 45:1. Bars are mean ± SD for n = 8 (IM) and 4 (ID), with * indicating significance of $p < 0.05$ using an unpaired, two-tailed t-test. (D–F) Histograms of mean eGFP fluorescence intensity (MFI) for each formulation in human skin explants (D), IM injection in mice (E), and ID injection in mice (F). (G) fLuc expression of human skin explants after ID injection with 2 μg of saRNA. Explants were analyzed 72 h after initial injection. Bars represent mean ± SD for n = 3, with * indicating significance of $p < 0.05$ using an unpaired, two-tailed t-test. (H) Representative images corresponding to (G) [14].

promising vaccine candidate for prophylaxis and treatment of various infectious diseases [70].

In a phase 1 clinical study, 40 healthy volunteers were administered VEE particles intramuscularly expressed with cytomegalovirus (CMV) glycoprotein B. The vaccine was administered at both a lower dose (1×10^7 infectious units [IU]) and a higher dose (1×10^8 IU), and it was noted that each dose was tolerated by the volunteers. The further outcome suggested that the developed vaccine was safer and able to neutralize the immune response produced against the viral antigen, and hence was able to develop protective immunity [71].

In another phase 1 trial, healthy volunteers were subjected to subcutaneous administration of an increasing dose of VEE particles expressed with HIV-1 subtype C Gag protein. Physiological evaluation of the volunteers demonstrated that the vaccine was well tolerated and free from any severe allergic symptoms. Even though some of the volunteers reported five serious adverse events, upon evaluation, it was concluded that none of them was due to vaccination. It was also noted that even at the higher dose of vaccination, immune response was the poor and a low level of the antibodies was produced [72].

In the midst of the Ebola virus (EBOV) epidemic in 2014–2016, various vaccine research programs were launched, including the usage of saRNA virus vectors. In a phase 1 trial to evaluate the safety and immunogenic activity, vesicular stomatitis virus (VSV) particles displaying the glycoprotein of a Zaire EBOV strain (VSV-ZEBOV) were utilized to immunize 78 participants with one of three concentrations (3×10^6, 2×10^7, or 1×10^8 pfu). The vaccination precipitated some side effects, like pain at the site of injection, tiredness, muscle weakness, and headache, but the second vaccination had fewer side effects. The two heaviest injections had greater antibody titers toward ZEBOV glycoprotein than that of the smallest dose. Furthermore, after the second immunization, antibody titers were considerably greater but the effect faded after six months. Lastly, the immunization evoked anti-EBOV antibody responses, and the maximum dose must be investigated further before a decision on prophylaxis can be made [73–74].

7.9 CONCLUSION

The use of mRNA for immunization has now become feasible. In rats and large animal prototypes, combining such innovative techniques with saRNA has proven to be a very effective way to provoke both humoral and cellular immune responses that are superior to non-replicating mRNA. The possible explanation for this supremacy is that saRNA transfection simulates a viral infection in several aspects, provoking a slew of adjunctive stimuli that boost immune responses without causing toxic effects. One of the most appealing features of saRNA is its adaptability, as new vaccines can be made speedily by modifying the sequence coding for the antigen of relevance without affecting its yield. In reality, utilizing the identical techniques that are utilized to make mRNA, saRNA can be manufactured at a GMP level. This ease of manufacture and speed of development could enable the rapid manufacturing of sufficient vaccine doses to combat evolving viruses that are exacerbating worldwide crises, including Zika virus, Ebola virus and SARS-CoV-2.

7.10 FUTURE PROSPECTS OF saRNA VACCINES

This innovative vaccine platform is now in the early stages of development, and the effectiveness or tolerability of vaccines produced with it in humans has yet to be determined. Self-amplifying mRNA vaccines, like many other forms of nucleic acid vaccines, have the ability to integrate the positive characteristics of live attenuated vaccines while avoiding a few of the intrinsic possible safety constraints, according to clinical studies. Large-scale mRNA manufacturing was once thought to be an impossible challenge in terms of commercial viability, but that viewpoint has shifted, and the simplicity and scalability of manufacturing are now seen as one of the vaccine design's best attributes. In order to develop certified clinical therapeutics, the stability problem of mRNA should be resolved, and this will be a significant aspect of future research. Clinical trials of simple traditional mRNA tumor vaccines have helped to break down some of these obstacles. Outside of the vaccine sector, there has been a lot of interest in improving the non-viral transport of smaller nucleic acids (e.g., siRNA) into the cytosol across the last 10 years. This has given us a better understanding of the prerequisites for cytosolic RNA transport, which is less difficult than nuclear pDNA transport. Each of these modifications has prompted breakthroughs in vector architecture non-viral shipment and large-scale manufacturing of saRNA, allowing the platform to advance rapidly. Whereas saRNA vaccines have clinical capability, their potency and immunogenicity in larger species of mammals such as non-human primates could be the main indicator of human success. The saRNA vector has been evaluated in humans and found to be antigenically utilizing viral transportation.

REFERENCES

1. Greenwood B. The contribution of vaccination to global health: Past, present and future. *Philos Trans R Soc Lond B Biol Sci.* 2014;369(1645):20130433. https://doi.org/10.1098/rstb.2013.0433
2. Riedel S. Edward Jenner and the history of smallpox and vaccination. *Proc (Bayl Univ Med Cent).* 2005;18(1):21–25. https://doi.org/10.1080/08998280.2005.11928028
3. Goldenthal KL, Midthun K, Zoon KC. Control of viral infections and diseases. In: Baron S, editor. *Medical Microbiology.* Galveston, TX: University of Texas Medical Branch at Galveston Copyright © 1996, The University of Texas Medical Branch at Galveston. 1996.
4. Mehata AK, Dehari D. Bradford assay as a high-throughput bioanalytical screening method for conforming pathophysiological state of the animal. *Journal of Drug Delivery Therapeutics.* 2020;10(1-s):105–110. https://doi.org/10.22270/jddt.v10i1-s.3921
5. Hobernik D, Bros M. DNA vaccines-how far from clinical use? *Int J Mol Sci.* 2018;19(11). https://doi.org/10.3390/ijms19113605
6. Zhang C, Maruggi G, Shan H, Li J. Advances in mRNA vaccines for infectious diseases. *Front Immunol.* 2019;10:594. https://doi.org/10.3389/fimmu.2019.00594
7. Maruggi G, Zhang C, Li J, Ulmer JB, Yu D. mRNA as a transformative technology for vaccine development to control infectious diseases. *Mol Ther.* 2019;27(4):757–772. https://doi.org/10.1016/j.ymthe.2019.01.020
8. Xu S, Yang K, Li R, Zhang L. mRNA vaccine era-mechanisms, drug platform and clinical prospection. *Int J Mol Sci.* 2020;21(18). https://doi.org/10.3390/ijms21186582
9. Pascolo S. Messenger RNA-based vaccines. *Expert Opin Biol Ther.* 2004;4(8):1285–1294. https://doi.org/10.1517/14712598.4.8.1285

10. Tombácz I, Weissman D, Pardi N. Vaccination with messenger RNA: A promising alternative to DNA vaccination. *Methods Mol Biol.* 2021;2197:13–31. https://doi.org/10.1007/978-1-0716-0872-2_2
11. Brito LA, Kommareddy S, Maione D, Uematsu Y, Giovani C, Scorza FB, et al. Self-amplifying mRNA vaccines. *Advances in genetics: Elsevier.* 2015; 179–233. https://doi.org/10.1016/bs.adgen.2014.10.005
12. Bloom K, van den Berg F, Arbuthnot P. Self-amplifying RNA vaccines for infectious diseases. *Gene Ther.* 2020:1–13. https://doi.org/10.1038/s41434-020-00204-y
13. Ballesteros-Briones MC, Silva-Pilipich N, Herrador-Cañete G, Vanrell L, Smerdou C. A new generation of vaccines based on alphavirus self-amplifying RNA. *Curr Opin Virol.* 2020;44:145–153. https://doi.org/10.1016/j.coviro.2020.08.003
14. Blakney AK, Zhu Y, McKay PF, Bouton CR, Yeow J, Tang J, et al. Big is beautiful: Enhanced saRNA delivery and immunogenicity by a higher molecular weight, bioreducible, cationic polymer. *ACS Nano.* 2020;14(5):5711–5727. https://doi.org/10.1021/acsnano.0c00326
15. Blakney AK, Ip S, Geall AJ. An update on self-amplifying mRNA vaccine development. *Vaccines (Basel).* 2021;9(2). https://doi.org/10.3390/vaccines9020097
16. Beissert T, Perkovic M, Vogel A, Erbar S, Walzer KC, Hempel T, et al. A trans-amplifying RNA vaccine strategy for induction of potent protective immunity. *Mol Ther.* 2020;28(1):119–128. https://doi.org/10.1016/j.ymthe.2019.09.009
17. Blakney AK, McKay PF, Christensen D, Yus BI, Aldon Y, Follmann F, et al. Effects of cationic adjuvant formulation particle type, fluidity and immunomodulators on delivery and immunogenicity of saRNA. *J Control Release.* 2019;304:65–74. https://doi.org/10.1016/j.jconrel.2019.04.043
18. Stech M, Nikolaeva O, Thoring L, Stöcklein WFM, Wüstenhagen DA, Hust M, et al. Cell-free synthesis of functional antibodies using a coupled in vitro transcription-translation system based on CHO cell lysates. *Sci Rep.* 2017;7(1):12030. https://doi.org/10.1038/s41598-017-12364-w
19. Schlake T, Thess A, Fotin-Mleczek M, Kallen KJ. Developing mRNA-vaccine technologies. *RNA Biol.* 2012;9(11):1319–1330. https://doi.org/10.4161/rna.22269
20. Baronti L, Karlsson H, Marušič M, Petzold K. A guide to large-scale RNA sample preparation. *Anal Bioanal Chem.* 2018;410(14):3239–3252. https://doi.org/10.1007/s00216-018-0943-8
21. Katayama S, Skoog T, Söderhäll C, Einarsdottir E, Krjutškov K, Kere J. Guide for library design and bias correction for large-scale transcriptome studies using highly multiplexed RNAseq methods. *BMC Bioinformatics.* 2019;20(1):418. https://doi.org/10.1186/s12859-019-3017-9
22. Plotkin S, Robinson JM, Cunningham G, Iqbal R, Larsen S. The complexity and cost of vaccine manufacturing—An overview. *Vaccine.* 2017;35(33):4064–4071. https://doi.org/10.1016/j.vaccine.2017.06.003
23. Kis Z, Shattock R, Shah N, Kontoravdi C. Emerging technologies for low-cost, rapid vaccine manufacture. *Biotechnol J.* 2019;14(1):e1800376. https://doi.org/10.1002/biot.201800376
24. Tan SC, Yiap BC. DNA, RNA, and protein extraction: The past and the present. *J Biomed Biotechnol.* 2009;2009:574398. https://doi.org/10.1155/2009/574398
25. Li H, Bo H, Wang J, Shao H, Huang S. Separation of supercoiled from open circular forms of plasmid DNA, and biological activity detection. *Cytotechnology.* 2011;63(1):7–12. https://doi.org/10.1007/s10616-010-9322-9
26. Bo H, Wang J, Chen Q, Shen H, Wu F, Shao H, et al. Using a single hydrophobic-interaction chromatography to purify pharmaceutical-grade supercoiled plasmid DNA from other isoforms. *Pharm Biol.* 2013;51(1):42–48. https://doi.org/10.3109/13880209.2012.703678

27. Berensmeier S. Magnetic particles for the separation and purification of nucleic acids. *Appl Microbiol Biotechnol.* 2006;73(3):495–504. https://doi.org/10.1007/s00253-006-0675-0
28. Ali N, Rampazzo RCP, Costa ADT, Krieger MA. Current nucleic acid extraction methods and their implications to point-of-care diagnostics. *Biomed Res Int.* 2017;2017:9306564. https://doi.org/10.1155/2017/9306564
29. Klenner J, Kohl C, Dabrowski PW, Nitsche A. Comparing viral metagenomic extraction methods. *Curr Issues Mol Biol.* 2017;24:59–70. https://doi.org/10.21775/cimb.024.059
30. Steger G, Riesner D. Viroid research and its significance for RNA technology and basic biochemistry. *Nucleic Acids Res.* 2018;46(20):10563–10576. https://doi.org/10.1093/nar/gky903
31. Kim I, McKenna SA, Viani Puglisi E, Puglisi JD. Rapid purification of RNAs using fast performance liquid chromatography (FPLC). *RNA.* 2007;13(2):289–294. https://doi.org/10.1261/rna.342607
32. Easton LE, Shibata Y, Lukavsky PJ. Rapid, nondenaturing RNA purification using weak anion-exchange fast performance liquid chromatography. *RNA.* 2010;16(3):47–653. https://doi.org/10.1261/rna.1862210
33. Karikó K, Muramatsu H, Ludwig J, Weissman D. Generating the optimal mRNA for therapy: HPLC purification eliminates immune activation and improves translation of nucleoside-modified, protein-encoding mRNA. *Nucleic Acids Res.* 2011;39(21):e142. https://doi.org/10.1093/nar/gkr695
34. Wadhwa A, Aljabbari A, Lokras A, Foged C, Thakur A. Opportunities and challenges in the delivery of mRNA-based vaccines. *Pharmaceutics.* 2020;12(2). https://doi.org/10.3390/pharmaceutics12020102
35. Kwok A, Raulf N, Habib N. Developing small activating RNA as a therapeutic: Current challenges and promises. *Ther Deliv.* 2019;10(3):151–164. https://doi.org/10.4155/tde-2018-0061
36. Kaczmarek JC, Kowalski PS, Anderson DG. Advances in the delivery of RNA therapeutics: From concept to clinical reality. *Genome Med.* 2017;9(1):60. https://doi.org/10.1186/s13073-017-0450-0
37. Warminski M, Kowalska J, Nowak E, Kubacka D, Tibble R, Kasprzyk R, et al. Structural insights into the interaction of clinically relevant phosphorothioate mRNA cap analogs with translation initiation factor 4E reveal stabilization via electrostatic thio-effect. *ACS Chem Biol.* 2021;16(2):334–343. https://doi.org/10.1021/acschembio.0c00864
38. Biddlecome A, Habte HH, McGrath KM, Sambanthamoorthy S, Wurm M, Sykora MM, et al. Delivery of self-amplifying RNA vaccines in in vitro reconstituted virus-like particles. *PLoS One.* 2019;14(6):e0215031. https://doi.org/10.1371/journal.pone.0215031
39. Geall AJ, Verma A, Otten GR, Shaw CA, Hekele A, Banerjee K, et al. Nonviral delivery of self-amplifying RNA vaccines. *Proc Natl Acad Sci U S A.* 2012;109(36):14604–14609. https://doi.org/10.1073/pnas.1209367109
40. Blakney AK, McKay PF, Yus BI, Aldon Y, Shattock RJ. Inside out: Optimization of lipid nanoparticle formulations for exterior complexation and in vivo delivery of saRNA. *Gene Ther.* 2019;26(9):363–372. https://doi.org/10.1038/s41434-019-0095-2
41. Beissert T, Koste L, Perkovic M, Walzer KC, Erbar S, Selmi A, et al. Improvement of in vivo expression of genes delivered by self-amplifying RNA using vaccinia virus immune evasion proteins. *Hum Gene Ther.* 2017;28(12):1138–1146. https://doi.org/10.1089/hum.2017.121
42. Levy JA. Pathogenesis of human immunodeficiency virus infection. *Microbiol Rev.* 1993;57(1):183–289.
43. Lucas S, Nelson AM. HIV and the spectrum of human disease. *J Pathol.* 2015;235(2):229–241. https://doi.org/10.1002/path.4449
44. Ferguson MR, Rojo DR, von Lindern JJ, O'Brien WA. HIV-1 replication cycle. *Clin Lab Med.* 2002;22(3):611–635. https://doi.org/10.1016/s0272-2712(02)00015-x

45. Lassen KG, Hebbeler AM, Bhattacharyya D, Lobritz MA, Greene WC. A flexible model of HIV-1 latency permitting evaluation of many primary CD4 T-cell reservoirs. *PLoS One*. 2012;7(1):e30176. https://doi.org/10.1371/journal.pone.0030176
46. Kuse N, Sun X, Akahoshi T, Lissina A, Yamamoto T, Appay V, et al. Priming of HIV-1-specific CD8(+) T cells with strong functional properties from naïve T cells. *EBioMedicine*. 2019;42:109–119. https://doi.org/10.1016/j.ebiom.2019.03.078
47. Mehata AK, Viswanadh MK, Priya V, Muthu MS. Dendritic cell-targeted theranostic nanomedicine: Advanced cancer nanotechnology for diagnosis and therapy. *Nanomedicine (Lond)*. 2020;15(10):947–949. https://doi.org/10.2217/nnm-2020-0032
48. Zou C, Murakoshi H, Kuse N, Akahoshi T, Chikata T, Gatanaga H, et al. Effective suppression of HIV-1 replication by cytotoxic T lymphocytes specific for pol epitopes in conserved mosaic vaccine immunogens. *J Virol*. 2019;93(7). https://doi.org/10.1128/jvi.02142-18
49. Moyo N, Vogel AB, Buus S, Erbar S, Wee EG, Sahin U, et al. Efficient induction of T cells against conserved HIV-1 regions by mosaic vaccines delivered as self-amplifying mRNA. *Mol Ther Methods Clin Dev*. 2019;12:32–46. https://doi.org/10.1016/j.omtm.2018.10.010
50. Bogers WM, Oostermeijer H, Mooij P, Koopman G, Verschoor EJ, Davis D, et al. Potent immune responses in rhesus macaques induced by nonviral delivery of a self-amplifying RNA vaccine expressing HIV type 1 envelope with a cationic nanoemulsion. *J Infect Dis*. 2015;211(6):947–955. https://doi.org/10.1093/infdis/jiu522
51. Mu Z, Haynes BF, Cain DW. HIV mRNA vaccines-progress and future paths. *Vaccines (Basel)*. 2021;9(2). https://doi.org/10.3390/vaccines9020134
52. Weinbren MP, Williams MC. Zika virus: Further isolations in the Zika area, and some studies on the strains isolated. *Trans R Soc Trop Med Hyg*. 1958;52(3):263–268. https://doi.org/10.1016/0035-9203(58)90085-3
53. Poland GA, Kennedy RB, Ovsyannikova IG, Palacios R, Ho PL, Kalil J. Development of vaccines against Zika virus. *Lancet Infect Dis*. 2018;18(7):e211–e219. https://doi.org/10.1016/s1473-3099(18)30063-x
54. Gatherer D, Kohl A. Zika virus: A previously slow pandemic spreads rapidly through the Americas. *J Gen Virol*. 2016;97(2):269–273. https://doi.org/10.1099/jgv.0.000381
55. Musso D, Gubler DJ. Zika virus. *Clin Microbiol Rev*. 2016;29(3):487–524. https://doi.org/10.1128/cmr.00072-15
56. Morabito KM, Graham BS. Zika virus vaccine development. *J Infect Dis*. 2017;216(suppl_10):S957–s963. https://doi.org/10.1093/infdis/jix464
57. Ngono AE, Shresta S. Immune response to dengue and zika. *Annu Rev Immunol*. 2018;36:279–308. https://doi.org/10.1146/annurev-immunol-042617-053142
58. Abbink P, Larocca RA, De La Barrera RA, Bricault CA, Moseley ET, Boyd M, et al. Protective efficacy of multiple vaccine platforms against Zika virus challenge in rhesus monkeys. *Science*. 2016;353(6304):1129–1132. https://doi.org/10.1126/science.aah6157
59. Luisi K, Morabito KM, Burgomaster KE, Sharma M, Kong WP, Foreman BM, et al. Development of a potent Zika virus vaccine using self-amplifying messenger RNA. *Sci Adv*. 2020;6(32):eaba5068. https://doi.org/10.1126/sciadv.aba5068
60. McKay PF, Hu K, Blakney AK, Samnuan K, Brown JC, Penn R, et al. Self-amplifying RNA SARS-CoV-2 lipid nanoparticle vaccine candidate induces high neutralizing antibody titers in mice. *Nat Commun*. 2020;11(1):3523. https://doi.org/10.1038/s41467-020-17409-9
61. Mehata AK, Dehari D, Mehta AK, Miya A. Boosting innate immunity during SARS-CoV-2 clearance. *Coronaviruses*. 2021;2(1). https://doi.org/10.2174/2666796701999201222113659
62. Baden LR, El Sahly HM, Essink B, Kotloff K, Frey S, Novak R, et al. Efficacy and safety of the mRNA-1273 SARS-CoV-2 vaccine. *N Engl J Med*. 2021;384(5):403–416. https://doi.org/10.1056/NEJMoa2035389

63. Peteranderl C, Herold S, Schmoldt C. Human influenza virus infections. *Semin Respir Crit Care Med.* 2016;37(4):487–500. https://doi.org/10.1055/s-0036-1584801
64. Wolff GG. Influenza vaccination and respiratory virus interference among Department of Defense personnel during the 2017–2018 influenza season. *Vaccine.* 2020;38(2): 350–354. https://doi.org/10.1016/j.vaccine.2019.10.005
65. Soema PC, Kompier R, Amorij JP, Kersten GF. Current and next generation influenza vaccines: Formulation and production strategies. *Eur J Pharm Biopharm.* 2015;94: 251–263. https://doi.org/10.1016/j.ejpb.2015.05.023
66. de Jong JC, Beyer WE, Palache AM, Rimmelzwaan GF, Osterhaus AD. Mismatch between the 1997/1998 influenza vaccine and the major epidemic A(H3N2) virus strain as the cause of an inadequate vaccine-induced antibody response to this strain in the elderly. *J Med Virol.* 2000;61(1):94–99.
67. Magini D, Giovani C, Mangiavacchi S, Maccari S, Cecchi R, Ulmer JB, et al. Self-amplifying mRNA vaccines expressing multiple conserved influenza antigens confer protection against homologous and heterosubtypic viral challenge. *PLoS One.* 2016;11(8):e0161193. https://doi.org/10.1371/journal.pone.0161193
68. Brazzoli M, Magini D, Bonci A, Buccato S, Giovani C, Kratzer R, et al. Induction of broad-based immunity and protective efficacy by self-amplifying mRNA vaccines encoding influenza virus hemagglutinin. *J Virol.* 2016;90(1):332–344. https://doi.org/10.1128/jvi.01786-15
69. Vogel AB, Lambert L, Kinnear E, Busse D, Erbar S, Reuter KC, et al. Self-amplifying RNA vaccines give equivalent protection against influenza to mRNA vaccines but at much lower doses. *Mol Ther.* 2018;26(2):446–455. https://doi.org/10.1016/j.ymthe.2017.11.017
70. Sandbrink JB, Shattock RJ. RNA vaccines: A suitable platform for tackling emerging pandemics? *Front Immunol.* 2020;11:608460. https://doi.org/10.3389/fimmu.2020.608460
71. Bernstein DI, Reap EA, Katen K, Watson A, Smith K, Norberg P, et al. Randomized, double-blind, Phase 1 trial of an alphavirus replicon vaccine for cytomegalovirus in CMV seronegative adult volunteers. *Vaccine.* 2009;28(2):484–493. https://doi.org/10.1016/j.vaccine.2009.09.135
72. Wecker M, Gilbert P, Russell N, Hural J, Allen M, Pensiero M, et al. Phase I safety and immunogenicity evaluations of an alphavirus replicon HIV-1 subtype C gag vaccine in healthy HIV-1-uninfected adults. *Clin Vaccine Immunol.* 2012;19(10):1651–1660. https://doi.org/10.1128/cvi.00258-12
73. Lundstrom K. Self-amplifying RNA viruses as RNA vaccines. *Int J Mol Sci.* 2020;21(14). https://doi.org/10.3390/ijms21145130
74. Regules JA, Beigel JH, Paolino KM, Voell J, Castellano AR, Hu Z, et al. A recombinant vesicular stomatitis virus Ebola vaccine. *N Engl J Med.* 2017;376(4):330–341. https://doi.org/10.1056/NEJMoa1414216

8 Conditional Replication of Oncolytic Virus Based on Detection of Oncogenic mRNA

Rakesh Sharma, Arvind Trivedi and Robert Moffatt

CONTENTS

8.1 INTRODUCTION

Oncolytic viruses are replicating microorganisms that have been selected or engineered to grow inside tumor cells. Oncolytic viruses specifically target cancer cells because they are able to exploit the very same cellular defects that promote tumor growth. These oncolytic viruses initially were viewed with skepticism for virus therapies. Virus therapy concept emerged based on tumor-specific mutations, including genetically engineered for specific signaling pathways or transcription activation programs and restricted virus entry in tumor cells (antigens overexpressed on the tumor cell surface) to kill tumor cells by oncolytic virus by cellular translational and transcriptional machinery, were discovered ultimately to induce cell necrosis or apoptosis. In the last decade, patients were treated in the first bona fide clinical trials of

DOI: 10.1201/9781003186069-8

oncolytic virus therapy after a few valid phase I or II clinical trials and a single published ONYX-015 phase III incomplete trial. So clinical experience is limited to optimize the efficacy of certain oncolytic viruses: vaccinia virus, adenovirus, reovirus, Newcastle disease virus (NDV), coxsackie virus and herpes simplex virus (HSV).

8.2 HISTORICAL PERSPECTIVE

From the 1950s to 1970s, years before the advent of the World Wide Web, the clinical concept of "viral" or "virulence" was used for pathogenic viruses to treat and cure cancer. These viruses continue to provide hope as a useful tool for virus therapies. The foundation of virus therapy by "good viruses" was laid in 1904 by Dr. George Dock at the University of Michigan for his famous experiment on a 42-year-old woman with acute leukemia who experienced a temporary remission after a presumed infection with influenza in 1896 (1). However, the relationship between the influenza virus and the infectious syndrome it caused was not established at that time. Similarly, in 1912, a cervical cancer patient bitten by a dog developed extensive tumor necrosis. Later, administration of a live attenuated rabies virus improved postexposure prophylaxis (2). In addition, spontaneous clinical remissions were observed in Hodgkin lymphoma (3) and Burkitt's lymphoma (4) after natural infections with measles virus. Many more spontaneous remissions and regressions of tumors occurred and were reported on in the setting of naturally acquired viral infections (5), possibly due to stimulation of an antitumor immune response and/or direct oncolysis (6). Such anecdotal observations prompted hundreds of clinical trials initiated in the 1950s and 1970s to develop a treatment for cancer by administration of different wild-type viruses such as hepatitis, West Nile, yellow fever, dengue fever, Uganda and adenoviruses to establish their potential to provide a cure (5). They all used wild-type viruses because these clinical trials laid the foundation of modern molecular biology techniques to modify their viral genomes. These early trials were not performed as per current clinical standards because interpreting the data still is difficult due to a lack of stringent quality control and testing. Moreover, in some cases patients were inoculated with viruses from previous patients or the same patients received multiple injections of different viruses (e.g., West Nile, Newcastle, vaccinia) (7–8). The consequences of such haphazard and uncoordinated administration in terms of safety were predictably disastrous with a high risk of encephalitis spread from West Nile, Uganda, dengue, and yellow fever (9).

On the other hand, adenovirus (or adenoidal-pharyngeal-conjunctival virus) emerged to prominence in cervical cancer clinical trials based on demonstration of safe delivery of adenovirus with mild flu-like symptoms as the main adverse event, with apparent efficacy in the form of marked tumor necrosis or liquefaction of tumors (10). However, the enthusiasm for oncolytic adenoviruses was short, as the antitumor responses only lasted a period of months and did not translate into an overall long-term survival benefit (11–13). In addition, extensive necrosis developed within the treated tumors (14). Subsequently, alternative options of promising new chemotherapy agents were introduced in the late 1970s. Moreover, during World-War periods, oncolytic virus therapy was not option to treat cancer (15). Major attention was focused on the discovery and use of clinically active chemical molecules that demonstrated an exciting therapeutic potential of new combination chemotherapy regimens at the bedside. Chemotherapy promised to revolutionize the treatment of cancer. In the optimism for combination chemotherapies to control viruses, old methods of virus therapies were forgotten. In the late 1970s, the utility of "virus therapy" suddenly again surfaced in the anticancer therapy scene as the potential answer to cancer but then in the 1980s, faded away again. After the mid-1980s, joint efforts between molecular biology and virus therapy emerged as a potential tool for the development of adeno and retroviral vectors for transgene delivery in different dreaded diseases, including cancer (16). However, the scientific community was not convinced for long time for possible use of oncolytic virus therapy.

After the success of gene transfer experiments, by and large, the potential of gene therapy and virus therapy for clinical use was poorly demonstrated. A major setback was a lack of understanding of how gene transfer vectors interacted with the host in the absence of suitable animal gene therapy models until the early 2000s (17). With time, viruses were investigated to modify them by recombinant DNA technology, as "designer viruses" means the addition of genes to code them for immune-stimulatory products or tumor-specific inflammation as multimodal therapeutic oncolytic viruses. These oncolytic viruses self-replicate within the cancer cell and have unique pharmacokinetic properties to target tumors and replicate to kill tumor cells. This arsenal of oncolytic viruses are under development with ever-expanding creative strategies for achieving tumor-specific replication. However, the complexities of tumor biology and the heterogeneity of human tissues again proved to be a setback with the demand of applying more than one kind of virus, or multitargeting strategy, to treat all cancers. In the 2000s the worldwide rights of genetically engineered adenovirus dl1520 (ONYX-015) were sold to the Chinese company Shanghai Sunway Biotech for conducting multiple phase I and phase II trials. After phase II trials on ONYX-015, Shanghai Sunway Biotech halted the phase III trials. This gave the impression that ONYX-015 was an ineffective therapeutic strategy in the absence of phase III data on the primary overall survival (OS) endpoint (18). In dubious attempts, the Chinese State Food and Drug Administration abandoned or secretly used ONYX-015 phase III results but developed successful H101 (Oncorine) phase III data, an oncolytic adenovirus similar to ONYX-015 and approved H101 for use in combination with chemotherapy for the treatment of late-stage refractory nasopharyngeal cancer in late 2005 (19). Since then, Warner Lambert, in partnership with Pfizer, revived their ONYX-015 phase III trials using old phase I and II clinical trial data for development of a virus therapy. Within five years, Onyx, in partnership with Bayer, developed the tyrosine kinase inhibitor sorafenib (Nexavar), which was subsequently approved for hepatocellular carcinoma (HCC) in 2005 (20). These results of the ONYX-015 trials led to the term "virus therapy" (21). In parallel, regulatory approval was given to Chinese H101 (Oncorine), a closely related adenovirus developed by Shanghai Sunway Biotech, for the treatment of head and neck cancers in China. Still, it was hard to convince the scientific community and governments of the possibility of "virus therapy" without regulatory guidelines (22).

Recently, development of effective immunotherapeutic agents for synergistic and rational combinations of checkpoint inhibitors, radiotherapy, and adoptive "cell therapy" has taken place. Simultaneously, oncolytic viruses caught the attention of the scientific community for "induced cellular immune response of oncolytic viruses". Soon, oncolytic viruses were believed to enhance anticancer efficacy because they could be "armed" with additional therapeutic genes (gene therapy) to drive a systemic antitumor immune response. With this approach, several viruses, including herpes virus, reovirus, polio virus, rhabdovirus, parvovirus, and vaccinia, have been successfully entered in clinical trials to favor gene therapy (23–24).

This chapter reviews the biology of recently used oncolytic adenoviruses, HSV and others with data from current clinical trials and finally explores future directions in combination with immunotherapy. Non-adenoviral oncolytics have also undergone extensive clinical development and entered late-phase clinical trials (25). Most notably are herpes virus (talimogene laherparepvec, previously called Oncovex) (26–31), vaccinia (pexa-vec, previously known as JX-594) (32–36) and reovirus (Reolysin), (37–46). Moreover, other viruses are also emerging as potential therapeutics. The specific roles of proteins in gene transfer and gene therapy are highlighted in killing tumors.

8.3 HOW DO ONCOLYTIC VIRUSES WORK?

The ideal criteria for a successful oncolytic virus is: (1) it is easily produced, easily manipulated, and selectively lytic to cancer cells; (2) it is systemically deliverable; and (3) it can be safely administered with low intrinsic pathogenicity. Over years, these criteria were met by the adenoviridae oncolytic virus. By contrast, vaccinia and HSV, with large double-stranded DNA (dsDNA) genomes that encode hundreds of proteins, require multiple deletions for safety and specificity, while retroviruses pose the theoretical risk of insertional mutagenesis (i.e., insertion of viral genomes into the host genome) (25). For interested readers, the following is a brief summary of oncolytic viruses used in oncolytic therapy (26–46). Adenovirus is a non-enveloped virus with a double-stranded, linear DNA genome that forms particles 70–90 nm in size. There are multiple engineered versions in clinical trials, including ONYX-015 and H101. Reovirus is a non-enveloped virus with a double-stranded, segmented RNA genome that forms particles 60–90 nm in size. The type III Dearing strain is in clinical trials for the treatment of patients with cancer. NDV is an enveloped virus with a single-stranded, negative-sense RNA genome that forms pleiomorphic particles ranging from 150 to 300 nm in size. Its PV701 strain is in clinical development. Poxvirus contains a double-stranded, linear DNA genome and forms particles 200 nm in diameter and 300 nm in length. HSV is an enveloped virus with a double-stranded, linear DNA genome that forms particles 150–200 nm in size. Many engineered versions of HSV strains G207, 1716 and NV 1020 are in clinical development. Picornaviruses are a family of non-enveloped viruses with single-stranded, positive-sense RNA genomes that form particles that range from 18 to 30 nm in size. The coxsackie viruses and engineered versions of poliovirus are used in oncolytic therapy. Myxoma, vesicular stomatitis and vaccinia viruses are family members that are under therapeutic development in mouse models.

8.4 BIOLOGY OF HUMAN ADENOVIRUS GENES AND TUMOR KILLING

Adenovirus biology offers the basis of a rational design of conditionally replicative adenoviruses. In humans, more than 50 different serotypes of adenovirus are known (47). On the basis of sequence homology and their ability to agglutinate red blood cells (48), these serotypes are divided into six species or subgroups, most of which are responsible for benign respiratory tract and gastrointestinal infections (49). The two most commonly described and developed for oncolytic therapy. The 2 and 5 (group C), species are non-oncogenic since the viruses replicate episomally (i.e., extrachromosomally) without host genome insertion (50, 51). Adenoviridae are a family of icosahedral, non-enveloped viruses, as they possess a protein capsid instead of a lipid membrane. These viruses have an approximately 30–40 kb linear dsDNA genome (51). The capsid protein, having a hexon, penton base and fiber, is principally responsible for host-receptor binding primarily through the coxsackie and adenovirus receptor (CAR) and virus internalization (see Figure 8.1) (32, 52). These capsid proteins disassemble inside the cell and result in the subsequent nuclear import of the viral genome (53) for commencement of viral transcription.

Depending on the type of virus, replication and viral gene expression can take place entirely in the cell cytoplasm (such as for vesicular stomatitis virus) or in the nucleus and cytoplasm (such as for adenovirus). In either case, the virus is largely dependent on cellular machinery for viral gene expression and synthesis of viral proteins. Viral gene expression and replication lead to the activation of cellular antiviral defenses, such as apoptosis, that are operational in normal cells but are often inactivated in tumor cells. Expression of viral proteins will eventually lead to immune-mediated lysis of infected cells by CD8+ T cells, which recognize viral peptide epitopes that are presented by major histocompatability complex (MHC) class I molecules on the surface of the infected cell. Alternatively, cells might be lysed owing to an overwhelming amount of budding and release of progeny virions from the cell surface, or by the activation of apoptosis during the course of viral replication and gene expression.

The well-studied modified oncolytic virus ONYX-015 by McCormick originally postulated the adenovirus cycle as an option of a p53-selective cancer therapy (32). In fact, ONYX-015 does not have E1B-55 K gene product to degrade normal cell p53, but suitably replicates only in the cancer cell (which lacks p53), so it destroys cancer cells. Because of this tumor-killing action, adenovirus genes play a significant role in the virus replication cycle. The adenovirus replicative cycle is divided into two phases: early (E1–E4) and late (L1–L5), as shown in Table 8.1 (32). The first expressed viral transcription unit E1A contains four highly conserved regions (CR1–CR4) (54). The two major E1A messenger RNA (mRNA) gene products (size 12S and 13S) promote epigenetic alterations through their interaction with chromatin remodeling protein p400 and histone acetyltransferases (HATs) p300/CBP protein (55). The second viral transcription unit E2F dissociates from its E2F-retinoblastoma (Rb) complex to activate E2F-mediated transcription of the other adenovirus early transcription units (E1B, E2, E3 and E4) involved in DNA synthesis and S-phase induction (56).

E2F, the host cell transcription factor, activates the transcription of the adenovirus E2 gene to induce p53-dependent apoptosis (57). Alternatively, if the E2F transcription factor avoids its induction of p53-dependent apoptosis, adenoviruses can produce a 55K-size E1b protein which binds to p53 (58). This E1b-p53 complex enters

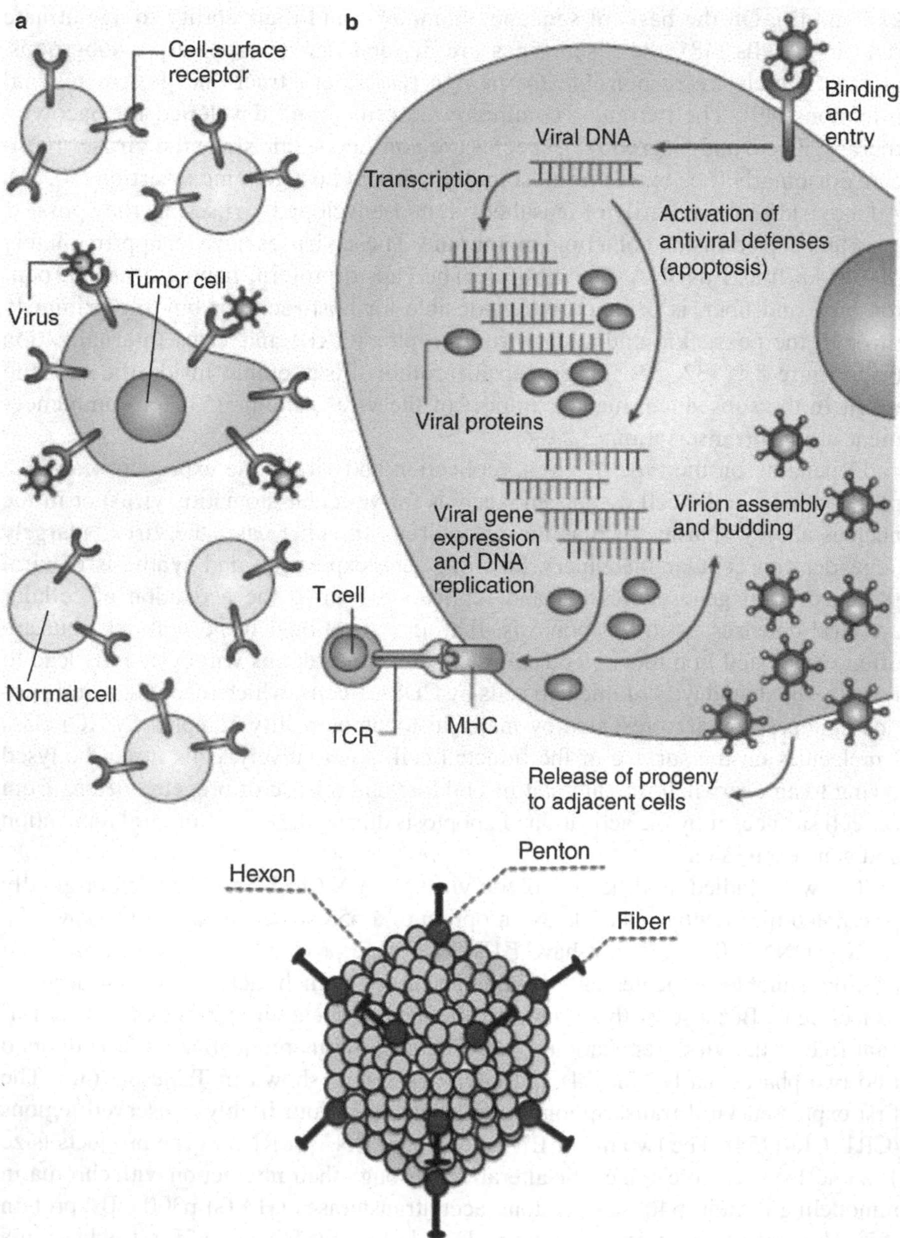

FIGURE 8.1 In general, adenovirus has major capsid proteins (fiber, penton, and hexon) for binding to the host cell. As shown in the upper right, adenoviruses interact with specific cell-surface receptors. Panel a shows proteins overexpressed by tumor cells (dark gray) compared with normal cells (shown in light gray). The virus will probably infect the tumor cell. Panel b shows that following binding to the cell surface receptor, the virus is internalized by endocytosis or membrane fusion, and its genome is released into the cell. (Modified from Ref. (32), fig. 1).

TABLE 8.1
Functions of Adenovirus Genes

E = Early transcription phase (before replication, <8 hours)
L = Late transcription phase (after replication, >12 hours)

Gene	Function
E1A	Modifies the function of key host and viral regulatory proteins such as retinoblastoma (Rb) and the chromatin remodeling protein p400
E2	Encodes the proteins for viral DNA replication
E3	Modulates host defense mechanisms
E4, E1B	Progression to late phase
L1–L5	Capsid proteins

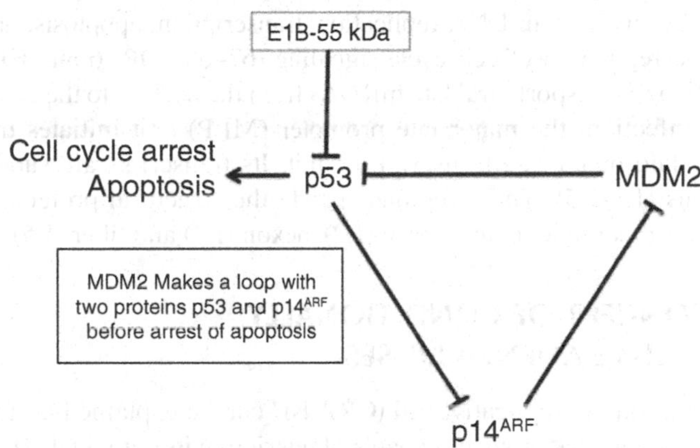

FIGURE 8.2 The p53-MDM2-p14^{ARF} feedback loop. MDM2 negatively regulates p53 by promoting p53 degradation. p14^{ARF} (p19^{ARF} in the mouse) binds to and sequesters MDM2, thereby preventing MDM2 from targeting p53 for degradation, while p53 negatively regulates p14^{ARF} expression. E1B-55kDa binds to and degrades p53. The removal of this gene in the ONYX-015 virus did not necessarily relieve p53 inhibition due to the presence of the other two components of the feedback loop in the tumor: MDM2 and p14^{ARF}. (Reproduced from Ref. (32)).

the cytoplasm for degradation, thus keeping the host cell alive long enough for progressive infection (59).

The ONYX-015 virus was postulated to act based on the E1B-55k-deleted mechanism (32, 60). However, McCormick (61) and others later reported that ONYX-015 replicates efficiently in p53 lacking cancer tumor cells (60, 62–63). Possibly, p53 tumors inhibit the p53 activity through other mechanisms such as overexpression of the endogenous p53 inhibitor, MDM2 or the loss of p14^{ARF}, which downregulates MDM2 (see Figure 8.2).

The E1B transcription unit is transcribed shortly after E1A and encodes the 55K protein (58). This protein inhibits the function of p53 as well as a 19K protein, a homolog of cellular Bcl-2, which prevents bax- and bak-mediated mitochondrial apoptosis. The E2 gene encodes three proteins required for replication of the viral genome: DNA polymerase, pre-terminal protein and the 72-kDa single-stranded DNA-binding protein (64).

The E3 transcription unit encodes the glycoproteins that function to subvert the immune response. These glycoproteins are 19 kDa in size. These glycoproteins downregulate the class I MHC-mediated antigen, which is required for cytotoxic T lymphocytes to prevent the T-cell recognition of infected host cells (65). Three other proteins, 10.4K, 14.5K and 14.7K (66), protect host cells from the lytic effects of tumor necrosis factor-α (TNF-α). Because the E3 transcription unit is nonessential, it is often deleted to allow for insertion of foreign DNA (approximately 3.3 kb).

The E4 transcription unit produces transcripts for six viral proteins named after their open reading frames: ORF1, ORF2, ORF3, ORF4, ORF6 and ORF6/7. These viral proteins are involved in DNA replication, transcription, apoptosis, host cell protein shutoff and regulation of cell cycle signaling (67–68). ORF6 and E1b-55K both inhibit p53 action to transport viral late mRNAs from the nucleus to the cytoplasm (69).

Late after infection, the major late promoter (MLP) unit initiates transcription from the so-called major late transcription unit. Its transcripts are subdivided into five late regions (L1–L5). These regions encode the structural proteins needed for progeny virus, for example, penton base (L2), hexon (L3) and fiber (L5) (32, 70).

8.5 THE CONCEPT OF CONDITIONALLY REPLICATIVE ADENOVIRUSES

The term "conditionally replicative Ad (CRAds)" can be explained as a replication-efficient and competent adenovirus capable of restricting its cytocidal effect on tumor cells while sparing normal cells. It means "Do Harm But Save the Base"—in other words, engineering a virus to only recognize the tumor cell surface and restrict replication of a potent oncolytic virus to malignant cells. In normal tissues, the promoter is inactive, so no viral transcription results and no infection. It is accomplished by microRNAs (miRNAs), smart regulators of gene expression in humans. The human genome encodes hundreds of miRNAs. More than 10% of human genes are under miRNA regulation. In human, miRNAs are expressed in tissue and differentiation state-specific patterns differentially expressed or deleted in common human cancers. Conceptually, after transcription and processing, miRNAs are incorporated into a protein complex RNA-induced silencing complex (RISC) to suppress the target gene expression via translational inhibition or mRNA degradation. The endogenous miRNA acts as a versatile and efficient system for the experimental targeting of gene expression in several tissues, cell types, cell lineages and differentiation states.

Many examples of conditionally replicating viruses are cited in the literature. The studies reported the introduction of a target site for the expressed let-7 miRNA into the positive-strand RNA genome of poliovirus and vesicular stomatitis virus to suppress animal virus replication by cellular RNA interference machinery (71). The let-7 target-modified vesicular stomatitis virus replication in these cells is a good choice for oncolytic virus therapy. CRAds HSV 1 and 2 strains have emerged as a possible modality for the treatment of cancer. Two types of approaches are used to achieve tumor-selective viral replication: (1) introduce loss-of-function mutations into the viral regulatory protein E1A or E1B that compromise viral replication in normal but not in transformed cells that typically have defects in the Rb/p16 and p53/p14ARF signaling pathways and (2) use heterologous regulatory elements to achieve cancer cell–specific expression of E1A. The cell sequencing selects first one or more target mRNA transcripts. Multi-sample sequencing subsequently identifies truncal mutations in the primary tumors or multiple regions of all the metastases. The large portion of one or more metastases in natural cancer cells lose targeted mutations and metastasize from the primary tumor cells or another metastasis. HSV type 1 and type 2 act as ideal vectors for oncolytic virus treatment. Extra DNA can be added or deleted to the HSV 1/2 genome without affecting its replication. This unique property of viral genes permits the ability to target relevant mutations. Interestingly, viral genes offer many conceivable therapeutic genetic elements (72). Other examples are (1) prostate-specific antigen (PSA) gene enhancer element upstream of the E1A gene to restrict viral replication to prostate cancer cells; (2) regulatory elements from prostaglandin-endoperoxide synthase-2; and (3) fibroblast growth factor-2 to favor the stability and translation, respectively, of E1A mRNA in certain types of cancer cells. Currently, cancer- and tissue-specific targeting of adenoviral replication is needed. In humans and non-human primates, systemic administration of replication-competent as well as replication-deficient adenoviruses are used as oncolytic adenoviruses. The most cited adenoviral biology classifies two broad types of replication-competent oncolytic adenoviruses. In infected cells, two types of CRAds infect. The first type of CRAd involved a modification of a viral gene sequence important for efficient viral replication in normal cells but dispensable or expendable in tumor cells (73). In the second type of CRAd, tissue/tumor-specific promoters were inserted to restrict viral replication to deregulate the tumors with their ability to activate these promoters. Examples include the human telomerase reverse transcriptase (hTERT)–regulated adenovirus active in multiple tumor types, and PSA-regulated adenovirus CG7870 developed for the treatment of prostate carcinoma (74). These approaches both act after the step of viral entry into the cell: the virus is not modified to selectively enter cancerous cells rather than normal cells, but is modified so it cannot carry out a productive infection to release progeny except in cancerous cells. Modifications to the fiber protein leading to selective entry into cancer cells have also been described and have made it into clinical trials (75, 76), but are generally used in combination with one of the previously mentioned types of modifications to confer additional specificity. Later, the absence of adenovirus gene sequence Elb-55k was identified as unique in CRAds for conditional replication to kill p53 depleted cells or tumor cells.

8.6 CLINICAL USE OF CONDITIONALLY REPLICATIVE ADENOVIRUSES

The first engineered adenovirus, ONYX-015, was a success in the CRAd clinical trials. It has been closely followed by other Elb-55k gene–lacking viruses with similar efficacy and toxicity profiles. This class of viruses was designed with deletion of the

800 bp Elb-55k gene. The difference with the absent Elb-55k was a unique modification in ONYX-015 to carry therapeutic transgenes. In theory, lacking a functional E1B-55 kDa for p53 degradation, the ONYX-015 adenovirus should replicate in cells with wild-type p53 but not in tumor cells where p53 was mutated or defective. In fact, ONYX-015 replication was p53-indcpendent due to the complexity of the p53-MDM2-p14ARF feedback loop, as shown in Figure 8.2.

In fact, O'Shea and colleagues demonstrated the mechanism of tumor selectivity related to the presence of the protein Y-box binding factor 1 (YB-1) expressed in cancer cells but not found in normal tissue. In cancer cells, the multifunctional E1B-55 kDa protein mediates the export of late adenoviral mRNA in normal cells as well as p53 inhibition (77). The YB-1 protein substitutes for the mRNA export function of E1B-55K only in tumors leading to cancer cell–restricted ONYX-015 replication. In retrospect, this proposed mechanism of action helps to explain the ONYX-015 clinical trial data and suggests future strategies to optimize and improve therapeutic outcomes. Moreover, other CRAd mechanisms of tumor selectivity are also proposed based on specific proteins. Major antitumor mechanisms are vectors targeting tumor antigens, engineered vectors binding tumor antigens, targeting vectors to the tumor microenviroment, vectors replicating only in tumor cells, vectors made from non-pathogenic viruses, cloaking (covering) strategies to evade the adaptive immune response and immune suppression. On the one hand, these defense mechanisms pose an impediment to the delivery and/or spread of oncolytic viruses. On the other hand, viral stimulation of the adaptive immune system seems to activate anti-tumor immune surveillance systems, increasing the effectiveness of oncolytic virus therapy (32).

8.7 SPECIFIC PROTEINS IN ONCOLYTIC VIRUS GENE THERAPY

Two cellular receptors: CD46, a member of the complement-regulatory protein family and SLAM (signaling lymphocytic-activation molecule) proteins, were reported to target the measles H-protein with carboxy-terminal extensions of epidermal growth factor (EGF), insulin-like growth factor 1 (IGF1), single-chain antibodies (scFvs) against tumor antigens such as carcinoembryonic antigen (CEA), CD20 and CD38 to mediate transient immunosuppression (78). The fusion (F)-protein of the measles virus was activated by a protease matrix metalloproteinase 2 (MMP2)–rich cancer microenvironment. The α2β1 integrin is often overexpressed on ovarian cancer cells. Coxsackievirus A21 binds to intercellular adhesion molecule 1 (ICAM1), which is abundant on the melanoma cell surface (79). A recombinant poliovirus, PV1(RIPO), binds to the receptor CD155 protein overexpressed on various tumor cell types (80). In oncolytic therapeutics, antiviral interferon proteins suppress the replication in interferon-responsive normal tissues but stimulate replication in tumor cells. So, tumor-selective oncolytic activity could be achieved by deleting or attenuating these anti-interferon-gene (ISG) products. In vesicular stomatitis virus (VSV), the M-protein binds to nuclear RAE1 mRNA export factor to block ISGs in the infected cells. VSV M-protein mutants that have lost this activity to induce the interferon response and limit the growth of VSV in normal tissues. The M-protein mutant vesicular stomatitis viruses can replicate and kill tumor cells that do not respond to interferon (81). The V-protein of NDV virus facilitates transcription in mammalian cells by binding to

STAT proteins in interferon signaling. Influenza virus encodes non-structural protein 1 (NS1) to inhibit responses to interferon by various mechanisms (32, 82) The protein kinase antagonist HSV gene product ICP34.5 is deleted in the oncolytic virus G207. This oncolytic virus replicates in tumor cells and kills them. The oncolytic activity of VSV in p53-deficient tumor cells was due to the loss of innate immunity (83). The protein kinase enzyme in the EGF receptor (EGFR)–RAS signaling pathway reduces innate immunity of the deleted vaccinia *E3L* gene product, which functions as a PKR antagonist and an anti-apoptotic factor to target cancer cells.

8.8 RESULTS FROM CLINICAL TRIALS WITH ONCOLYTIC VIRUSES

The lack of mRNA export function of E1B-55K with no p53 destruction in a cellular process in tumor cells provides oncolytic activity in ONYX-015 as tested in a phase III study (19, 61). In this trial, an *E1B-55K*–deleted adenovirus, H101, was given by intratumoral injection to patients who received cisplatin-based chemotherapy (19). In studies of patients with squamous cell cancer of the head and neck or of the esophagus, the response rate was significantly higher (78%) in patients who received the combination of viral therapy and chemotherapy than in patients who were treated with chemotherapy alone (39%) (61). A small number of patients treated with the oncolytic virus also had some regression of metastases. Oncolytic intravenous application of oncolytic reovirus, vaccinia virus and NDV vectors is underway for to determine the clinical potential of its therapeutic safety and efficacy. A brief summary is given on clinical use of oncolytic viruses in Table 8.2.

TABLE 8.2
Current Status of Oncolytic Viruses in Treatment of Cancer Clinical Trials in Phase I, II and III Stages

Virus	Mechanism of Tumor Targeting	Phase of Development	Results	Ref.
Adenovirus	Targets to tumor antigens; conditionally replicating	Phase III conducted	H101 – E1B-deleted vector is tested with cisplatin by intratumoral injection in patients with squamous head and neck carcinoma; greater response in patients given virus therapy with chemotherapy than chemotherapy alone	47
Reovirus	Selectively infects RAS-transformed cells	Phase I conducted	Currently in trials to compare intratumoral administration with cutaneous and IV administration in melanoma and malignant glioma patients	37–46, 61

(*Continued*)

TABLE 8.2 (Continued)

Virus	Mechanism of Tumor Targeting	Phase of Development	Results	Ref.
Herpes simplex virus	Only replicates in tumor cells	Phase I conducted, Additional trials planned	G207 and HSV1716 vectors were found to be well-tolerated when given by intratumoral injection in glioma patients	26–31
Newcastle disease virus	Selectively replicates in interferon-defective cells	Phase I conducted	PV701 vector was found to be well-tolerated when given intravenously; some patients had anti-tumor responses	34
Vaccinia virus	Gains access to tumor by vascular leakiness	Phase I conducted, phase II planned	JX-594 vector was found to be well-tolerated in phase I clinical trial when given by intratumoral injection into melanomas; trials are planned for intravenous delivery	32–36
Coxsackievirus	Selectively infects tumor cells that overexpress DAF	Phase I conducted	Coxsackievirus A21 vector was found to be well-tolerated when administered by intratumoral injection in patients with melanoma	52
Measles virus	Virus re-targeting tumor antigens; overexpression of virus receptor (CD46) on some tumor cells	Phase I conducted	Was found to be well-tolerated when administered via intraperitoneal injection in patients with ovarian cancer	78,79
Vesicular stomatitis virus	Selective replication in interferon-defective cells	Tested in preclinical (mouse) models	Shown to have antitumor effects in xenografts and metastatic tumors	71
Influenza virus	Non-structural protein 1-deleted virus replicates in interferon-ve cells	Tested in preclinical (mouse) models	Shown to selectively replicate in tumor cells	82
Retroviruses	Tumor-specific promoter expression only in cancer cells	Tested in preclinical (mouse) models	Replicates specifically in tumor cells; potential to include suicide genes in vector	884
Myxoma virus	Replicates specifically in tumor cells	In vitro cells	Replicates in signal transducer and activator of transcription 1 (STAT1) or interferon-deficient cells	26-46

8.9 RESULTS FROM CLINICAL TRIALS WITH ADENOVIRUS ONYX-015 (DL1520)

The advent of viral therapy showed concerns about its safety when retroviral integration causing activation of the proto-oncogene LMO2 led to leukemia in patients treated for severe combined immunodeficiency (SCID). In fact, a significant adverse effect was the death of a patient with ornithine transcarbamylase deficiency treated with adenoviral gene therapy became concern (79, 84). Such fatal adverse events were less in cancer patients treated with adenoviruses. In cancer, a lack of chromosomal integration (more selective killing of infected cells) mitigates the risks of chromosomal integration harm. In phase I and II trials, ONYX-015 was safe and well tolerated; even at the highest dose of 3×10^{11} plaque forming units (PFU), no dose-limiting toxicities were reached by intravenous, intratumoral or hepatic artery administration. The most common reported adverse effect was short-lived flulike symptoms (82, 85). However, the clinical evaluation of ONYX-015 efficacy was more complex because of the induced tumor swelling effect. The RECIST response rates as a single event were also low in its trials that predated the development of immune-related response criteria for pseudo-progressive changes. Pseudo-progression is a therapy-mediated tumor swelling. It can transiently occur before the tumor regression (conditionally replicative adenovirus action). Pseudo-progression is also a common event after several therapies: (1) use of checkpoint inhibitors ipilimumab and nivolumab (84, 86); (2) use of whole-brain radiotherapy (WBRT) (85, 87); (3) use of imatinib in gastrointestinal stromal tumor (GIST) (86, 88); (4) use of a phase II pan-epigenetic inhibitor; and (5) use of RRx-001 (87, 89). However, the kinetic responses to these agents are typically slower than with standard chemotherapy.

Similarly, Reid and colleagues reported a pattern of acute tumor enlargement followed by regression of tumor size after intrahepatic injection of ONYX-015 in combination with 5-FU/leucovorin for hepatic colorectal metastases in 11 of 24 patients (46%) (88, 90), suggestive of an ipilimumab-like pseudo-progression and predictive for improved survival (see Figure 8.3) A phase II trial of talimogene laherparepvec (then called Oncovex), an attenuated herpesvirus that expresses granulocyte macrophage colony-stimulating factor (GM-CSF), showed delayed responses occurring up to 10 months after starting treatment and often preceded by apparent tumor progression (29). These trials suggest that pseudo-progression may be a common theme in oncolytic virus therapy.

8.10 ROLE OF E1B-55K GENE AND PROTEINS IN TUMOR KILLING

The ONYX-015 agent was further improved by viral genetic modification. An E1b-55k is a multifunctional protein with pleiotropic properties, including mRNA transport, and its deletion alters the replication. E1b-55k renders the virus YB-1-dependent replication efficiency and lytic activity in tumors expressing YB-1. However, with an intact E1b-55k gene, tumors remain fully permissive and susceptible (CRAd effect) to adenovirus infection. For example, adenovirus 5 mutants dl922–947 and D24 retain E1b-55k and carry a mutation in the conserved region 2 (CR-2) of the E1A gene. Such presence of E1b-55k abolishes the binding of E1A to the Rb protein

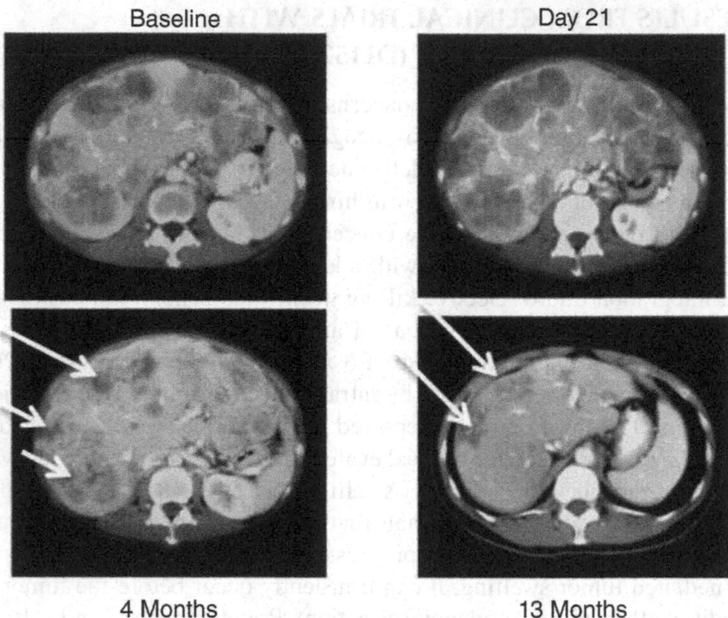

FIGURE 8.3 Computed tomography (CT) scans of a patient receiving ONYX-015 show virus therapy effect as liver lobe enlargement at baseline, pseudoregression after day 21, 4 months and 13 months in the panels. The baseline CT scan of this patient demonstrates extensive disease in all lobes of the liver. ONYX-015 in combination with 5-FU/leucovorin showed improvement of the tumor masses *(white arrows)* after 4 months and completely resolved masses *(white arrows)* after 13 months. (Modified from Refs. (88, 90)).

and prevents release of the E2F transcription factor. Restricted E1A and Rb protein and no E2F release have demonstrated significantly greater potency of the E1b-55k gene compared to ONYX-015 both in vitro and in vivo (91). ONYX-015 has cancer-selective replication due to the E1B-55k deletion. Without deletion, perhaps ONYX-015 does not carry a therapeutic "cargo" transgene. Other adenoviruses with various cargo transgenes have been tested in clinical trials with varying degrees of success based on responses to virally delivered cytokines and other immunologic factors in play (92). The viral transgene packaging system exhibits an innate host response even without viral replication or even cellular expression of foreign proteins. Moreover, several replicating viruses stimulate the same innate and adaptive immune response as a natural viral infection.

Systemically administered interleukin-2 can induce durable disease control in about 10% of treated patients. Interestingly, a replication-defective adenovirus exhibited the interleukin-2 gene–induced responses in some tumor locations directly injected with the adenovirus but not in distant metastases (93). In the replication-defective adenovirus TNFerade, TNF alpha cytokine was driven by a radiation-inducible promoter to achieve high local TNF levels without detectable levels in the blood and the associated toxicities of systemic TNF (94). Early phase trials of TNFerade gave

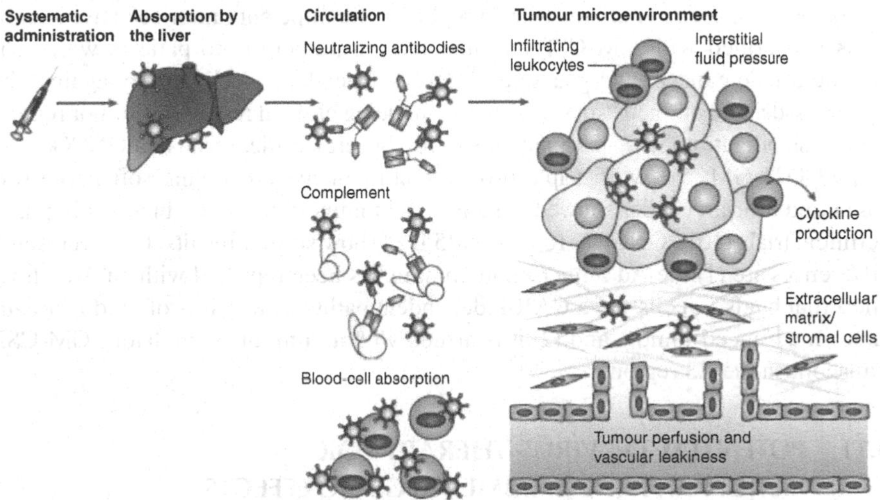

FIGURE 8.4 Delivery of oncolytic viruses to tumors in vivo is given to a patient by intravenous injection. Many barriers prevent oncolytic viruses from reaching the tumor and treating cancer cells. Within minutes, most of the initial virus inoculum is absorbed by the liver; the rest is absorbed or neutralized by blood cells through the complement cascade or by neutralizing antibodies (preexisting immunity). For oncolytic virus therapy, a virus gets access to the tumor, leaving the circulation, and traverses or leaks through the vascular endothelium against a gradient of interstitial fluid pressure. Resident or infiltrating leukocytes also the limit cell–cell spread of the virus (antiviral activity) or indirectly by the release of soluble inflammatory mediators, including interferons and other cytokines. (Modified from Ref. (32)).

encouraging results with melanoma (95). A phase III trial recently found no survival benefit in patients with pancreatic cancer (96). So, it was not established whether the radiation-inducible promoter present in that non-replicating oncolytic virus actually led to significant TNF expression in patients. CD154 has shown promise—in a phase I/IIa trial of patients with urothelial carcinoma of the bladder, intravesicular adenovirus carrying CD154 led to the absence of tumors on cystectomy in three out of five patients with high-risk cancer with plans for cystectomy and to tumor shrinkage in one out of three patients who had stage Ta tumors (97). A replication-defective adenovirus delivering a modified form of CD154 with increased membrane stability was injected into lymph nodes of patients with chronic lymphocytic leukemia (CLL), and in a dose-escalation study it reduced lymphocytosis, lymphadenopathy or splenomegaly in most patients (98).

A unique GM-CSF cytokine was identified as promising for cancer immunotherapy in preclinical work. Now, it has emerged as the leading cytokine in the virotherapy field (99). The most notable preclinical study of GM-CSF was an in vivo screen by Dranoff and colleagues on tumor cell lines carrying various immune-stimulatory agents. Investigators immunized mice, and vaccination with the GM-CSF–expressing cells provided the greatest protection against later tumor engraftment when mice were challenged with the parental tumor cell lines (99). Cell-mediated antitumor responses were seen in humans when a replication-competent tumor-selective adenovirus was armed with GM-CSF and injected intratumorally to patients with various metastatic cancers and generated MHC I–dependent T-cell activity against the tumor-associated antigen "survivin" while inducing clinical responses (tumor regression or stabilization) in 7 of 15 patients (100). Several clinical trials on ONCOS-102 (Ad5/3-D24-GMCSF) with triple orphan status for mesothelioma, soft tissue sarcoma and ovarian cancer showed evidence of immune priming on biopsies in phase I clinical trials (101). ONCOS-102 and Ad5 D24 show similar results. However, some differences are (1) the Ad 5 fiber knob domain has been replaced with an Ad 3 fiber knob that binds to cells via a CAR-independent pathway, which is often downregulated in advanced tumors and (2) it is armed with an immunostimulatory GM-CSF transgene in the E3 region.

8.11 POTENTIAL OF VIRUS THERAPY FOR IMMUNOTHERAPY: IMMUNOGENIC EFFECTS

Oncolytic virus therapy has showed limited efficacy in directly treated tumors, as intravenously administered viruses fail to reach distant metastatic disease due to off-target tissue trapping in the liver or spleen, and oncolytic viruses are rapidly cleared by neutralizing antibodies (see Figure 8.4) (102). Furthermore, the immune response is rapidly mobilized to clear the viral infection to minimize systemic spread and proliferative toxicity. On the other hand, it inhibits the therapeutic efficacy. As an alternative, there are many strategies to suppress the immune response and rapid viral clearance. These include PEGylation (103), cell or nanoparticle carriers (104), modification of the tumor vasculature (105) and/or transient immunosuppression (106).

Fortunately, evidence indicates that oncolytic virus therapy shows global antibody release effects in the body (107). This therapy primes an immune response against distant lesions due to cell death, production of cytokines and release of tumor antigens. OVs are presumed both as "direct tumor killers or simply immune adjuvants" based on T-cell and dendritic cell (DC) activation and stimulation of innate and adaptive antitumor immunity reported with adenovirus (108–109) and other oncolytic therapies (27, 36).

In the light of all this, oncolytic adenoviral therapy seems suitable for combination with other potential immunostimulatory/immunomodulatory treatments, including cytokines, transcription regulating (Treg)-depleting chemotherapies like cyclophosphamide, DC-based vaccines like sipuleucel-T (Provenge) and, of course, the checkpoint inhibitors such as cytotoxic T-lymphocyte antigen 4 (CTLA-4) and programmed death 1 receptor (PD-1), which "release the brakes" on the adaptive antitumor immune response (110). This was demonstrated in one small trial where metronomic cyclophosphamide, which selectively depletes Tregs, augmented the activity of an oncolytic adenovirus carrying GM-CSF (111), and trials combining talimogene laherparepvec with checkpoint inhibitors are planned. Furthermore, insertion of immunostimulatory transgenes (e.g., ligand traps, cytokines, costimulatory molecules) from oncolytic viruses and incorporation of GM-CSF into viruses are an emerging source of potential antitumor activity into viruses.

8.12 COMBINATION THERAPIES OF ONCOLYTIC VIRUSES

Oncolytic adenoviruses have meaningful single-agent antitumor activity. Existing complementary mechanisms of action and nonoverlapping toxicity OV profiles also make them ideal and better options to combine with radiation, chemotherapy, kinase inhibitors and/or immunotherapy partner than a stand-alone treatment. For example, the combination of metronomic cyclophosphamide and the oncolytic adenovirus, ONCOS-102, in a phase I solid tumor trial resulted in a significant reduction of T_{regs} in the presence of a Th1-like response. Alone, T_{reg} infiltration not only correlates with a poor prognosis but also compromises the efficacy of immunotherapies (72, 112). The OVs stimulate an antitumor immune response. These OVs in combination with checkpoint inhibitors will improve therapeutic efficacy. Several research groups are evaluating the combination of OVs with traditional chemotherapy agents, multikinase inhibitors and CTLA-4 and PD1 inhibitors.

Autophagy-inducing agents like temozolomide have also been reported to potentiate the activity of oncolytic viruses (113). In addition to temozolomide, another intriguing potential combination is with the experimental pan-epigenetic inhibitor, radiosensitizer (114) and autophagy inducer, RRx-001, which has demonstrated promising activity without systemic toxicity in phase I and phase II metastatic colorectal cancer and brain metastasis (+ whole brain radiation) studies (115). The tumor microenvironment is characterized by aberrant expression of cytokines promoting tumor progression like TGF-β (116), and viruses may be a tool particularly well suited to manipulate the tumor microenvironment itself as represented in Figure 8.5. They offer the possibility to produce therapeutic agents directly within treated tumors, turning the problem of delivering agents to a dense tumor with high interstitial pressure completely around and leading to greater intratumoral activity and fewer systemic side effects. The wild-type adenoviruses are a common cause of respiratory, diarrheal and conjunctival disease and can infect about a billion people worldwide every year (117).

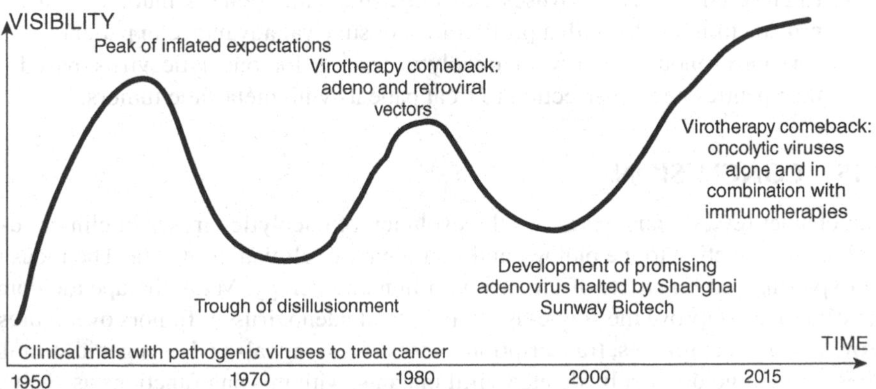

FIGURE 8.5 A graphic presentation of incomplete attempts to develop anticancer virus therapy agents in last century towards a combination therapy to treat cancer. (Modified from Ref. (32)).

8.13 FUTURE DIRECTIONS

Oncolytic viruses now appear to be good anticancer tool. Their inherent tumor-tropic and anticancer properties were recognized at the end of the 20th century. Through the seemingly impossible magic of genetic engineering, viruses have been engineered into tumor destruction vehicles. Viruses particularly target cancer cells because the viruses dismantle the immunosuppression that shields tumors from the innate and adaptive immune system. Viruses also increase their susceptibility to pathogenic attack to "save" the normal cell neighborhoods from high levels of cancer-induced destruction that are far away largely off-limits to the immune-protected surroundings of the tumor. Several infectious viral species have been developed as virus therapy agents. Fortunately, adenoviruses, herpes viruses and others have emerged as most promising because they are intrinsically oncolytic for tumor cells without doing normal tissue loss or being minimally toxic to normal non-transformed cells.

Despite the potential of oncolytic adenoviruses, especially in combination with checkpoint inhibitors or other immunotherapies, several ups and downs have occurred in the quest to label OVs as "magic anticancer agents" (118–119, 120). Unrealistic, unattainable expectations further complicate the issue and burst of the bubble for virus therapy success. Continued incomplete efforts also undermine its potential and lead to a withdrawal of interest or support.

8.14 MAJOR POINTS

1. Clinical trials indicate that oncolytic viruses are safe and effective anticancer agents.
2. The translation of oncolytic viruses from preclinical tumor models to clinical studies on cancer therapy needs multidisciplinary approaches.
3. Novel anticancer strategies facilitate viral evasion of the immune system, the prevention of viral uptake by the liver and an increased specificity for tumor cells, either at the cell surface or through intracellular restriction.
4. Engineered oncolytic viruses can target the same genetic mutations that provide tumor cells with a proliferative or survival advantage in patients.
5. The intravenous delivery of oncolytic viruses for oncolytic virus–based therapeutics needs perfection to treat patients with metastatic tumors.

8.15 CONCLUSION

The chapter reviews and examines the evolution of oncolytic viruses in clinical use with an introduction to the biology and a summary of clinical trial data. The focus is on exploring combinations of viruses with immunotherapy. Many therapeutic combinations may improve the single-agent activity of adenoviruses. Tumors overexpress growth factors, cytokines, transcription factors, stress signals and oncogenic stimuli. These stimuli go defunct by deleted viral mutants, with missing functions as "helper functions" in point deletions of a few base pairs, rather than whole genes. These stimuli are required to impair replication in normal tissue, while permitting near-wild-type levels of replication and expression in cancer cells. Viruses have a small genome with overlapping reading frames and proteins carrying out multiple functions. E1B-19k mediates both p53 neutralization and RNA export. Oncolytic adenoviral engineering is fascinating, with many oncolytic viruses carrying GM-CSF as a therapeutic gene used to fight cancer. The checkpoint inhibitor can be delivered with an oncolytic virus within the tumor. These engineered oncolytic viruses can be readily modified by genetic manipulation as novel therapeutics to exploit various oncogenic mutations. Combined with multimodality therapeutics and modulating the host antitumor response, CRAds have promise for the scientific community and have inspired a multidisciplinary effort to turn laboratory concepts into fully functional and effective therapeutics. In the next several years, several oncolytic genetically engineered adenoviruses will have potential use in cancer therapies and other diseases.

REFERENCES

1. Dock G. The influence of complicating diseases upon leukaemia. *Am J Med Sci.* 1904; 127:561–592.
2. Pack G. Note of the experimental use of rabies vaccine for melanomatosis. *Arch Dermatol Syphilol.* 1950; 62:694–695.
3. Taqi AM, Abdurrahman MB, Yakubu AM and Fleming AF. Regression of Hodgkin's disease after measles. *Lancet.* 1981; 1:11–12.
4. Bluming AZ and Ziegler JL. Regression of Burkitt's lymphoma in association with measles infection. *Lancet.* 1971; 2:105–106.
5. Kelly E and Russell SJ. History of oncolytic viruses: Genesis to genetic engineering. *Mol Ther.* 2007; 15:651–659.
6. Ring CJ. Cytolytic viruses as potential anti-cancer agents. *J Gen Virol.* 2002; 83:491–502.
7. Newman W and Southam CM. Virus treatment in advanced cancer; A pathological study of fifty-seven cases. *Cancer.* 1954; 7:106–118.
8. Southam CM and Moore AE. Induced virus infections in man by the Egypt isolates of West Nile virus. *Am J Trop Med Hyg.* 1954; 3:19–50.
9. Singh PK, Doley J, Kumar GR, Sahoo AP and Tiwari AK. Oncolytic viruses & their specific targeting to tumour cells. *Indian J Med Res.* 2012; 136:571–584.
10. Huebner RJ, Bell JA, Rowe WP, Ward TG, Suskind RG, Hartley JW and Paffenbarger RS, Jr. Studies of adenoidal-pharyngeal-conjunctival vaccines in volunteers. *J Am Med Assoc.* 1955; 159:986–989.
11. Zielinski T and Jordan E. (Remote results of clinical observation of the oncolytic action of adenoviruses on cervix cancer). *Nowotwory.* 1969; 19:217–221.
12. Rowe WP, Huebner RJ, Gilmore LK, Parrott RH and Ward TG. Isolation of a cytopathogenic agent from human adenoids undergoing spontaneous degeneration in tissue culture. *Proc Soc Exp Biol Med.* 1953; 84:570–573.
13. Georgiades J, Zielinski T, Cicholska A and Jordan E. Research on the oncolytic effect of APC viruses in cancer of the cervix uteri; preliminary report. *Biul Inst Med Morsk Gdansk.* 1959; 10:49–57.
14. Huebner RJ, Rowe WP, Schatten WE, Smith RR and Thomas LB. Studies on the use of viruses in the treatment of carcinoma of the cervix. *Cancer.* 1956; 9:1211–1218.
15. Oronsky B, Carter CA, Mackie V, Scicinski J, Oronsky A, Oronsky N, Caroen S, Parker C, Lybeck M and Reid T. The war on cancer: A military perspective. *Front Oncol.* 2014; 4:387.

16. Hemminki A and Alvarez RD. Adenoviruses in oncology: A viable option? *BioDrugs.* 2002; 16:77–87.
17. Orkin SH and Motulsky AG. Report and recommendations of the panel to assess the NIH investment in research on gene therapy. In: Panel to Assess the NIH Investment in Research on Gene Therapy. (Bethesda, MD: National Institutes of Health, 1995). Library Catalog; MMS ID 9910958973406676; NLM ID 101095897.
18. Jia H and Kling J. China offers alternative gateway for experimental drugs. *Nat Biotechnol.* 2006; 24:117–118.
19. Liu TC and Kirn D. Gene therapy progress and prospects cancer: Oncolytic viruses. *Gene Ther.* 2008; 15:877–884.
20. McCormick F. Success and failure on the Ras pathway. *Cancer Biol Ther.* 2007; 6:1654–1659.
21. Garber K. China approves world's first oncolytic virus therapy for cancer treatment. *J Natl Cancer Inst.* 2006; 98:298–300.
22. Theodore F. Oncolytic Virus Therapy. In: Theodore F, ed. *Methods in Enzymology.* (Academic Press, 2012), pp. i–xxi.
23. Friedman GK, Cassady KA, Beierle EA, Markert JM and Gillespie GY. Targeting pediatric cancer stem cells with oncolytic virotherapy. *Pediatr Res.* 2012; 71:500–510.
24. Wollmann G, Ozduman K and van den Pol AN. Oncolytic virus therapy for glioblastoma multiforme: Concepts and candidates. *Cancer J.* 2012; 18:69–81.
25. Van Etten JL, Lane LC and Dunigan DD. DNA viruses: The really big ones (giruses). *Annu Rev Microbiol.* 2010; 64:83–99.
26. Liu BL, Robinson M, Han ZQ, Branston RH, English C, Reay P, McGrath Y, Thomas SK, Thornton M, Bullock P, Love CA and Coffin RS. ICP34.5 deleted herpes simplex virus with enhanced oncolytic, immune stimulating, and anti-tumour properties. *Gene Ther.* 2003; 10:292–303.
27. Kaufman HL, Kim DW, DeRaffele G, Mitcham J, Coffin RS and Kim-Schulze S. Local and distant immunity induced by intralesional vaccination with an oncolytic herpes virus encoding GM-CSF in patients with stage IIIc and IV melanoma. *Ann Surg Oncol.* 2010; 17:718–730.
28. Hu JC, Coffin RS, Davis CJ, Graham NJ, Groves N, Guest PJ, Harrington KJ, James ND, Love CA, McNeish I, Medley LC, Michael A, Nutting CM, Pandha HS, Shorrock CA, Simpson J, et al. A phase I study of OncoVEXGM-CSF, a second-generation oncolytic herpes simplex virus expressing granulocyte macrophage colony-stimulating factor. *Clin Cancer Res.* 2006; 12:6737–6747.
29. Senzer NN, Kaufman HL, Amatruda T, Nemunaitis M, Reid T, Daniels G, Gonzalez R, Glaspy J, Whitman E, Harrington K, Goldsweig H, Marshall T, Love C, Coffin R and Nemunaitis JJ. Phase II clinical trial of a granulocyte-macrophage colony-stimulating factor-encoding, second-generation oncolytic herpesvirus in patients with unresectable metastatic melanoma. *J Clin Oncol.* 2009; 27:5763–5771.
30. Harrington KJ, Hingorani M, Tanay MA, Hickey J, Bhide SA, Clarke PM, Renouf LC, Thway K, Sibtain A, McNeish IA, Newbold KL, Goldsweig H, Coffin R and Nutting CM. Phase I/II study of oncolytic HSV GM-CSF in combination with radiotherapy and cisplatin in untreated stage III/IV squamous cell cancer of the head and neck. *Clin Cancer Res.* 2010; 16:4005–4015.
31. Andtbacka RH, Kaufman HL, Collichio F, Amatruda T, Senzer N, Chesney J, Delman KA, Spitler LE, Puzanov I, Agarwala SS, Milhem M, Cranmer L, Curti B, Lewis K, Ross M, Guthrie T, et al. Talimogene laherparepvec improves durable response rate in patients with advanced melanoma. *J Clin Oncol.* 2015; 33(25): 2780–2788.
32. Parato KA, Senger D, Forsyth PAJ and Bell JC. Recent progress in the battle betweenoncolytic viruses and tumours. *Nature Rev. Cancer.* 2005;5:965–976.

33. Hwang TH, Moon A, Burke J, Ribas A, Stephenson J, Breitbach CJ, Daneshmand M, De Silva N, Parato K, Diallo JS, Lee YS, Liu TC, Bell JC and Kirn DH. A mechanistic proof-of-concept clinical trial with JX-594, a targeted multi-mechanistic oncolytic poxvirus, in patients with metastatic melanoma. *Mol Ther.* 2011; 19:1913–1922.
34. Park BH, Hwang T, Liu TC, Sze DY, Kim JS, Kwon HC, Oh SY, Han SY, Yoon JH, Hong SH, Moon A, Speth K, Park C, Ahn YJ, Daneshmand M, Rhee BG, et al. Use of a targeted oncolytic poxvirus, JX-594, in patients with refractory primary or metastatic liver cancer: A phase I trial. *Lancet Oncol.* 2008; 9:533–542.
35. Breitbach CJ, Burke J, Jonker D, Stephenson J, Haas AR, Chow LQ, Nieva J, Hwang TH, Moon A, Patt R, Pelusio A, Le Boeuf F, Burns J, Evgin L, De Silva N, Cvancic S, et al. Intravenous delivery of a multi-mechanistic cancer-targeted oncolytic poxvirus in humans. *Nature.* 2011; 477:99–102.
36. Heo J, Reid T, Ruo L, Breitbach CJ, Rose S, Bloomston M, Cho M, Lim HY, Chung HC, Kim CW, Burke J, Lencioni R, Hickman T, Moon A, Lee YS, Kim MK, et al. Randomized dose-finding clinical trial of oncolytic immunotherapeutic vaccinia JX-594 in liver cancer. *Nat Med.* 2013; 19:329–336.
37. Strong JE, Coffey MC, Tang D, Sabinin P and Lee PW. The molecular basis of viral oncolysis: Usurpation of the Ras signaling pathway by reovirus. *EMBO J.* 1998; 17(12):3351–3362.
38. Kelly KR, Espitia CM, Mahalingam D, Oyajobi BO, Coffey M, Giles FJ, Carew JS and Nawrocki ST. Reovirus therapy stimulates endoplasmic reticular stress, NOXA induction, and augments bortezomib-mediated apoptosis in multiple myeloma. *Oncogene.* 2012; 31:3023–3038.
39. Vidal L, Pandha HS, Yap TA, White CL, Twigger K, Vile RG, Melcher A, Coffey M, Harrington KJ and DeBono JS. A phase I study of intravenous oncolytic reovirus type 3 Dearing in patients with advanced cancer. *Clin Cancer Res.* 2008; 14:7127–7137.
40. Gollamudi R, Ghalib MH, Desai KK, Chaudhary I, Wong B, Einstein M, Coffey M, Gill GM, Mettinger K, Mariadason JM, Mani S and Goel S. Intravenous administration of Reolysin, a live replication competent RNA virus is safe in patients with advanced solid tumors. *Invest New Drugs.* 2010; 28:641–649.
41. Galanis E, Markovic SN, Suman VJ, Nuovo GJ, Vile RG, Kottke TJ, Nevala WK, Thompson MA, Lewis JE, Rumilla KM, Roulstone V, Harrington K, Linette GP, Maples WJ, Coffey M, Zwiebel J, et al. Phase II trial of intravenous administration of Reolysin((R)) (Reovirus Serotype-3-dearing Strain) in patients with metastatic melanoma. *Mol Ther.* 2012; 20:1998–2003.
42. Morris DG, Feng X, DiFrancesco LM, Fonseca K, Forsyth PA, Paterson AH, Coffey MC and Thompson B. REO-001: A phase I trial of percutaneous intralesional administration of reovirus type 3 Dearing (Reolysin(R)) in patients with advanced solid tumors. *Invest New Drugs.* 2013; 31:696–706.
43. Forsyth P, Roldan G, George D, Wallace C, Palmer CA, Morris D, Cairncross G, Matthews MV, Markert J, Gillespie Y, Coffey M, Thompson B and Hamilton M. A phase I trial of intratumorally administration of reovirus in patients with histologically confirmed recurrent malignant gliomas. *Mol Ther.* 2008; 16:627–632.
44. Lolkema MP, Arkenau HT, Harrington K, Roxburgh P, Morrison R, Roulstone V, Twigger K, Coffey M, Mettinger K, Gill G, Evans TR and de Bono JS. A phase I study of the combination of intravenous reovirus type 3 Dearing and gemcitabine in patients with advanced cancer. *Clin Cancer Res.* 2011; 17:581–588.
45. Comins C, Spicer J, Protheroe A, Roulstone V, Twigger K, White CM, Vile R, Melcher A, Coffey MC, Mettinger KL, Nuovo G, Cohn DE, Phelps M, Harrington KJ and Pandha HS. REO-10: A phase I study of intravenous reovirus and docetaxel in patients with advanced cancer. *Clin Cancer Res.* 2010; 16:5564–5572.

46. Karapanagiotou EM, Roulstone V, Twigger K, Ball M, Tanay M, Nutting C, Newbold K, Gore ME, Larkin J, Syrigos KN, Coffey M, Thompson B, Mettinger K, Vile RG, Pandha HS, Hall GD, et al. Phase I/II trial of carboplatin and paclitaxel chemotherapy in combination with intravenous oncolytic reovirus in patients with advanced malignancies. *Clin Cancer Res.* 2012; 18:2080–2089.
47. Benko M, Harrach B and Russell W. Virus taxonomy; Seventh report of the international committee on taxonomy of viruses. In: Van Regenmortel M, Fauquet C and Bishop D, eds. *Virus Taxonomy; Seventh Report of the International Committee on Taxonomy of Viruses* (New York: Academic Press, 2000).
48. Shenk T. Adenoviridae: The viruses and their replication. In: Fields B, Knipe D and Howley P, eds. *Virology* (Philadelphia: Lippencott-Raven, 1996), pp. 2111–2148.
49. Purkayastha A, Ditty SE, Su J, McGraw J, Hadfield TL, Tibbetts C and Seto D. Genomic and bioinformatics analysis of HAdV-4, a human adenovirus causing acute respiratory disease: Implications for gene therapy and vaccine vector development. *J Virol.* 2005; 79:2559–2572.
50. Cook JL and Lewis AM, Jr. Differential NK cell and macrophage killing of hamster cells infected with nononcogenic or oncogenic adenovirus. *Science.* 1984; 224:612–615.
51. Williams PD, Ranjzad P, Kakar SJ and Kingston PA. Development of viral vectors for use in cardiovascular gene therapy. *Viruses.* 2010; 2:334–371.
52. Schoggins JW and Falck-Pedersen E. Fiber and penton base capsid modifications yield diminished adenovirus type 5 transduction and proinflammatory gene expression with retention of antigen-specific humoral immunity. *J Virol.* 2006; 80:10634–10644.
53. Trotman LC, Mosberger N, Fornerod M, Stidwill RP and Greber UF. Import of adenovirus DNA involves the nuclear pore complex receptor CAN/Nup214 and histone H1. *Nat Cell Biol.* 2001; 3:1092–1100.
54. Chakraborty AA and Tansey WP. Adenoviral E1A function through Myc. *Cancer Res.* 2009; 69:6–9.
55. Frisch SM and Mymryk JS. Adenovirus-5 E1A: Paradox and paradigm. *Nat Rev Mol Cell Biol.* 2002; 3:441–452.
56. Nemajerova A, Talos F, Moll UM and Petrenko O. Rb function is required for E1A-induced S-phase checkpoint activation. *Cell Death Differ.* 2008; 15:1440–1449.
57. Dynlacht BD. E2F and p53 make a nice couple: Converging pathways in apoptosis. *Cell Death Differ.* 2005; 12:313–314.
58. Berk AJ. Recent lessons in gene expression, cell cycle control, and cell biology from adenovirus. *Oncogene.* 2005; 24:7673–7685.
59. Rao L, Debbas M, Sabbatini P, Hockenbery D, Korsmeyer S and White E. The adenovirus E1A proteins induce apoptosis, which is inhibited by the E1B 19-kDa and Bcl-2 proteins. *Proc Natl Acad Sci U S A.* 1992; 89:7742–7746.
60. Harada JN and Berk AJ. p53-Independent and -dependent requirements for E1B-55K in adenovirus type 5 replication. *J Virol.* 1999; 73:5333–5344.
61. McCormick F. ONYX-015 selectivity and the p14ARF pathway. *Oncogene.* 2000; 19:6670–6672.
62. Goodrum FD and Ornelles DA. p53 status does not determine outcome of E1B 55-kilodalton mutant adenovirus lytic infection. *J Virol.* 1998; 72:9479–9490.
63. Au T, Thorne S, Korn WM, Sze D, Kirn D and Reid TR. Minimal hepatic toxicity of Onyx-015: Spatial restriction of coxsackie-adenoviral receptor in normal liver. *Cancer Gene Ther.* 2007; 14:139–150.
64. Sébastien A. Felt et al. Recent advances in vesicular stomatitis virus-based oncolytic virotherapy: A 5-year update. *J Gen Virol.* 2017; 98(12): 2895–2911.
65. Burgert HG and Kvist S. The E3/19K protein of adenovirus type 2 binds to the domains of histocompatibility antigens required for CTL recognition. *EMBO J.* 1987; 6:2019–2026.

66. Deryckere F and Burgert HG. Tumor necrosis factor alpha induces the adenovirus early 3 promoter by activation of NF-kappaB. *J Biol Chem.* 1996; 271:30249–30255.
67. Halbert DN, Cutt JR and Shenk T. Adenovirus early region 4 encodes functions required for efficient DNA replication, late gene expression, and host cell shutoff. *J Virol.* 1985; 56:250–257.
68. Harada JN, Shevchenko A, Shevchenko A, Pallas DC and Berk AJ. Analysis of the adenovirus E1B-55K-anchored proteome reveals its link to ubiquitination machinery. *J Virol.* 2002; 76:9194–9206.
69. Gonzalez RA and Flint SJ. Effects of mutations in the adenoviral E1B 55-kilodalton protein coding sequence on viral late mRNA metabolism. *J Virol.* 2002; 76:4507–4519.
70. Farley DC, Brown JL and Leppard KN. Activation of the early-late switch in adenovirus type 5 major late transcription unit expression by L4 gene products. *J Virol.* 2004; 78:1782–1791.
71. Yiosmaki E, Hakkarainen T, Hemmings A, Visakorpi T, Adding R and Saksela K. Generation of conditionally replicating adenovirus based on targeted destruction of E1A mRNA by a cell type specific microRNA. *J Virol.* 2008; 82(22):11009–11015.
72. Renteln, M. Conditional replication of oncolytic viruses based on detection of oncogenic mRNA. *Gene Therapy* 2018; 25:1–3.
73. Abou El Hassan MA, van der Meulen-Muileman I, Abbas S and Kruyt FA. Conditionally replicating adenoviruses kill tumor cells via a basic apoptotic machinery-independent mechanism that resembles necrosis-like programmed cell death. *J Virol.* 2004; 78:12243–12251.
74. Small EJ, Carducci MA, Burke JM, Rodriguez R, Fong L, van Ummersen L, Yu DC, Aimi J, Ando D, Working P, Kirn D and Wilding G. A phase I trial of intravenous CG7870, a replication-selective, prostate-specific antigen-targeted oncolytic adenovirus, for the treatment of hormone-refractory, metastatic prostate cancer. *Mol Ther.* 2006; 14:107–117.
75. Coughlan L, Vallath S, Gros A, Gimenez-Alejandre M, Van Rooijen N, Thomas GJ, Baker AH, Cascallo M, Alemany R and Hart IR. Combined fiber modifications both to target alpha(v)beta(6) and detarget the coxsackievirus-adenovirus receptor improve virus toxicity profiles *in vivo* but fail to improve antitumoral efficacy relative to adenovirus serotype 5. *Hum Gene Ther.* 2012; 23:960–979.
76. Kim KH, Dmitriev IP, Saddekni S, Kashentseva EA, Harris RD, Aurigemma R, Bae S, Singh KP, Siegal GP, Curiel DT and Alvarez RD. A phase I clinical trial of Ad5/3-Delta24, a novel serotype-chimeric, infectivity-enhanced, conditionally-replicative adenovirus (CRAd), in patients with recurrent ovarian cancer. *Gynecol Oncol.* 2013; 130:518–524.
77. O'Shea CC, Johnson L, Bagus B, Choi S, Nicholas C, Shen A, Boyle L, Pandey K, Soria C, Kunich J, Shen Y, Habets G, Ginzinger D and McCormick F. Late viral RNA export, rather than p53 inactivation, determines ONYX-015 tumor selectivity. *Cancer Cell.* 2004; 6:611–623.
78. Peng, KW et al. Oncolytic measles viruses displaying a single-chain antibody against CD38, a myeloma cell marker. *Blood.* 2003; 101:2557–2562.
79. Raper SE, Chirmule N, Lee FS, Wivel NA, Bagg A, Gao GP, Wilson JM and Batshaw ML. Fatal systemic inflammatory response syndrome in a ornithine transcarbamylase deficient patient following adenoviral gene transfer. *Mol Genet Metab.* 2003; 80:148–158.
80. Au GG, Lindberg AM, Barry RD and Shafren DR. Oncolysis of vascular malignant human melanoma tumors by Coxsackievirus A21. *Int. J. Oncol.* 2005:1471–1476.
81. Reid T, Warren R and Kirn D. Intravascular adenoviral agents in cancer patients: Lessons from clinical trials. *Cancer Gene Ther.* 2002; 9:979–986.
82. Ganly I, Kirn D, Eckhardt G, Rodriguez GI, Soutar DS, Otto R, Robertson AG, Park O, Gulley ML, Heise C, Von Hoff DD and Kaye SB. A phase I study of Onyx-015, an E1B attenuated adenovirus, administered intratumorally to patients with recurrent head and neck cancer. *Clin Cancer Res.* 2000; 6:798–806.

83. Griesenbach U. Progress and prospects: Gene therapy clinical trials (Part 2). *Gene Ther.* 2007; 14:1555–1563.
84. Wolchok JD, Hoos A, O'Day S, Weber JS, Hamid O, Lebbe C, Maio M, Binder M, Bohnsack O, Nichol G, Humphrey R and Hodi FS. Guidelines for the evaluation of immune therapy activity in solid tumors: Immune-related response criteria. *Clin Cancer Res.* 2009; 15:7412–7420.
85. Parvez K, Parvez A and Zadeh G. The diagnosis and treatment of pseudoprogression, radiation necrosis and brain tumor recurrence. *Int J Mol Sci.* 2014; 15:11832–11846.
86. Werewka-Maczuga A, Osinski T, Chrzan R, Buczek M and Urbanik A. Characteristics of computed tomography imaging of gastrointestinal stromal tumor (GIST) and related diagnostic problems. *Pol J Radiol.* 2011; 76:38–48.
87. Reid T, Infante J, Burris III H, Scribner C, Knox S, Oronsky B, Stephens J and Scicinski J. Activity observed in a phase I dose escalation trial of the hypoxia-activated, NO prodrug, RRx-001. *J Clin Oncol.* 2013; 31(suppl 4; abstr 241).
88. Reid TR, Freeman S, Post L, McCormick F and Sze DY. Effects of Onyx-015 among metastatic colorectal cancer patients that have failed prior treatment with 5-FU/leucovorin. *Cancer Gene Ther.* 2005; 12:673–681.
89. Hemminki A. Oncolytic immunotherapy: Where are we clinically? *Scientifica (Cairo).* 2014; 2014: Article ID 862925.
90. Heise C, Hermiston T, Johnson L, Brooks G, Sampson-Johannes A, Williams A, Hawkins L and Kirn D. An adenovirus E1A mutant that demonstrates potent and selective systemic anti-tumoral efficacy. *Nat Med.* 2000; 6:1134–1139.
91. Shayakhmetov DM, Di Paolo NC and Mossman KL. Recognition of virus infection and innate host responses to viral gene therapy vectors. *Mol Ther.* 2010; 18:1422–1429.
92. Smith JS, Xu Z, Tian J, Palmer DJ, Ng P and Byrnes AP. The role of endosomal escape and mitogen-activated protein kinases in adenoviral activation of the innate immune response. *PLoS One.* 2011; 6:e26755.
93. Dummer R, Rochlitz C, Velu T, Acres B, Limacher JM, Bleuzen P, Lacoste G, Slos P, Romero P and Urosevic M. Intralesional adenovirus-mediated interleukin-2 gene transfer for advanced solid cancers and melanoma. *Mol Ther.* 2008; 16:985–994.
94. Rasmussen H, Rasmussen C, Lempicki M, Durham R, Brough D, King CR and Weichselbaum R. TNFerade Biologic: Preclinical toxicology of a novel adenovector with a radiation-inducible promoter, carrying the human tumor necrosis factor alpha gene. *Cancer Gene Ther.* 2002; 9:951–957.
95. MacGill RS, Davis TA, Macko J, Mauceri HJ, Weichselbaum RR and King CR. Local gene delivery of tumor necrosis factor alpha can impact primary tumor growth and metastases through a host-mediated response. *Clin Exp Metastasis.* 2007; 24:521–531.
96. Herman JM, Wild AT, Wang H, Tran PT, Chang KJ, Taylor GE, Donehower RC, Pawlik TM, Ziegler MA, Cai H, Savage DT, Canto MI, Klapman J, Reid T, Shah RJ, Hoffe SE, et al. Randomized phase III multi-institutional study of TNFerade biologic with fluorouracil and radiotherapy for locally advanced pancreatic cancer: Final results. *J Clin Oncol.* 2013; 31:886–894.
97. Malmstrom PU, Loskog AS, Lindqvist CA, Mangsbo SM, Fransson M, Wanders A, Gardmark T and Totterman TH. AdCD40L immunogene therapy for bladder carcinoma—the first phase I/IIa trial. *Clin Cancer Res.* 2010; 16:3279–3287.
98. Castro JE, Melo-Cardenas J, Urquiza M, Barajas-Gamboa JS, Pakbaz RS and Kipps TJ. Gene immunotherapy of chronic lymphocytic leukemia: A phase I study of intranodally injected adenovirus expressing a chimeric CD154 molecule. *Cancer Res.* 2012; 72:2937–2948.
99. Delawer Z, Zhang K, Rennie PS, Zia W. Oncolytic virotherapy for urological cancers. *Nat Rev Urology.* 2016; 13:334–352.

100. Cerullo V, Pesonen S, Diaconu I, Escutenaire S, Arstila PT, Ugolini M, Nokisalmi P, Raki M, Laasonen L, Sarkioja M, Rajecki M, Kangasniemi L, Guse K, Helminen A, Ahtiainen L, Ristimaki A, et al. Oncolytic adenovirus coding for granulocyte macrophage colony-stimulating factor induces antitumoral immunity in cancer patients. *Cancer Res.* 2010; 70:4297–4309.
101. Majumder M, Kumar A, Heckman C, Kankainen M, Pesonen S, Jäger E, Karbach J, Joensuu T, Kairemo K, Partanen K, Alanko T, Hemminki A, Backman C, Dienel K, von Euler M, Hakonen T, et al. Gene expression analysis of tumors demonstrates an induction of Th1 type immune response following intratumorally administration of ONCOS-102 in refractory solid tumor patients. *Journal for Immunotherapy of Cancer.* 2014; 2:P230–P230.
102. Ferguson MS, Lemoine NR and Wang Y. Systemic delivery of oncolytic viruses: Hopes and hurdles. *Adv Virol.* 2012; 2012(6): Article ID 805629. doi.org/10.1155/2012/805629
103. Simpson GR, Horvath A, Annels NE, Pencavel T, Metcalf S, Seth R, et al. Combination of a fusogenic glycoprotein, pro-drug activation and oncolytic HSV as an intravesical therapy for superficial bladder cancer. *Br J Cancer.* 2012; 106:496–507.
104. Bolhassani A, Javanzad S, Saleh T, Hashemi M, Aghasadeghi MR and Sadat SM. Polymeric nanoparticles: Potent vectors for vaccine delivery targeting cancer and infectious diseases. *Hum Vaccin Immunother.* 2014; 10:321–332.
105. Wojton J and Kaur B. Impact of tumor microenvironment on oncolytic viral therapy. *Cytokine Growth Factor Rev.* 2010; 21:127–134.
106. Dhar D, Toth K and Wold WS. Cycles of transient high-dose cyclophosphamide administration and intratumorally oncolytic adenovirus vector injection for long-term tumor suppression in Syrian hamsters. *Cancer Gene Ther.* 2014; 21:171–178.
107. Siva S, MacManus MP, Martin RF and Martin OA. Abscopal effects of radiation therapy: A clinical review for the radiobiologist. *Cancer Lett.* 2015; 356:82–90.
108. Bell J. Oncolytic viruses: Immune or cytolytic therapy? *Mol Ther.* 2014; 22:1231–1232.
109. Koski A, Kangasniemi L, Escutenaire S, Pesonen S, Cerullo V, Diaconu I, Nokisalmi P, Raki M, Rajecki M, Guse K, Ranki T, Oksanen M, Holm SL, Haavisto E, Karioja-Kallio A, Laasonen L, et al. Treatment of cancer patients with a serotype 5/3 chimeric oncolytic adenovirus expressing GMCSF. *Mol Ther.* 2010; 18:1874–1884.
110. Errington F, Steele L, Prestwich R, Harrington KJ, Pandha HS, Vidal L, de Bono J, Selby P, Coffey M, Vile R and Melcher A. Reovirus activates human dendritic cells to promote innate antitumor immunity. *J Immunol.* 2008; 180:6018–6026.
111. Cerullo V, Diaconu I, Kangasniemi L, Rajecki M, Escutenaire S, Koski A, Romano V, Rouvinen N, Tuuminen T, Laasonen L, Partanen K, Kauppinen S, Joensuu T, Oksanen M, Holm SL, Haavisto E, et al. Immunological effects of low-dose cyclophosphamide in cancer patients treated with oncolytic adenovirus. *Mol Ther.* 2011; 19:1737–1746.
112. Adenovirus clinical trial: http://www.sunwaybio.com.cn/newweb01/english.htm; Reovirus clinical trial: http://www.oncolyticsbiotech.com/; Biovex herpes simplex virus clinical trial: http://www.biovex.com; Crusade laboratories herpes simplex virus clinical trial: http://www.crusadelabs.co.uk; Medigene herpes simplex virus clinical trials: http://www.medigene.com; Newcastle-disease virus clinical trial: http://www.wellstat.com/biologics/bioindex.html/; Vaccinia virus information: http://jennerex.com/; Coxsackievirus information: http://www.psiron.com.
113. Liikanen I, Ahtiainen L, Hirvinen ML, Bramante S, Cerullo V, Nokisalmi P, Hemminki O, Diaconu I, Pesonen S, Koski A, Kangasniemi L, Pesonen SK, Oksanen M, Laasonen L, Partanen K, Joensuu T, et al. Oncolytic adenovirus with temozolomide induces autophagy and antitumor immune responses in cancer patients. *Mol Ther.* 2013; 21:1212–1223.
114. Ning S, Bednarski M, Oronsky B, Scicinski J, Saul G and Knox SJ. Dinitroazetidines are a novel class of anticancer agents and hypoxia-activated radiation sensitizers developed from highly energetic materials. *Cancer Res.* 2012; 72:2600–2608.

115. Reid T, Dad S, Korn R, Oronsky B, Knox S and Scicinski J. Two case reports of resensitization to previous chemotherapy with the novel hypoxia-activated hypomethylating anticancer agent RRx-001 in metastatic colorectal cancer patients. *Case Rep Oncol.* 2014; 7:79–85.
116. Mathias Felix Leber et al. Sequencing of serially passaged measles virus affirms its genomic stability and reveals a nonrandom distribution of consensus mutations. *J Gen Virol.* 2020; 101(4):399–409.
117. Shin DH, Nguyen T, Ozpolat B, Lary F, Almao, M, Mandatory CG, Fuel J. Current strategies to circumvent the antiviral immunity to optimize cancer virotherapy. *J Immuno Therapy Cancer.* 2021; 9(4):e002086.
118. Wojciech K. Panek et al. Hitting the nail on the head: Combining oncolytic adenovirus-mediated virotherapy and immunomodulation for the treatment of glioma. *Oncotarget.* 2017; 8(51): 89391–89405.
119. Geon-Tae Park et al. Advanced new strategies for metastatic cancer treatment by therapeutic stem cells and oncolytic virotherapy. *Oncotarget.* 2016; 7:58684–58695.
120. Shafren DR, Sylvester D, Johansson ES, Campbell IG and Barry RD. Oncolysis of human ovarian cancers by echovirus type 1. *Int. J. Cancer.* 2005; 115:320–328.

9 Unilateral Ex Vivo Gene Therapy by GDNF in Neurodegenerative Diseases

Sonia Barua and Yashwant V. Pathak

CONTENTS

9.1 INTRODUCTION

Neurodegenerative diseases commonly occur in the elderly. This heterogeneous group of diseases are mainly characterized by progressive degeneration of the structure and functions of the central nervous system (CNS) and peripheral nerve tissue. Alzheimer's disease (AD) and Parkinson's disease (PD) are common examples of neurodegenerative diseases [1–2]. Since the brain is a complex organ in the body, it is critical to understand the causes of neurodegenerative diseases and develop new strategies for their treatment and prevention. Studies have proven that the risks of neurodegenerative diseases are due to a combination of a person's genes and environmental factors [2–5]. Moreover, the rate of disease progression depends on lifetime exposures to the environment.

Nerve growth factor (NGF) is a neurotrophic factor and comes under the transforming growth factor-β superfamily [4]. NGF mainly controls cell growth and maintains the cell proliferation and survival rate [3–4]. Studies have reported that NGF has been shown to act as a potential therapeutic agent for AD. Delivery of NGF in nerve cells of Alzheimer's patients exhibited a positive effect on the basal forebrain cholinergic neurons, which decline in AD patients [5–9]. Glial cell line–derived

DOI: 10.1201/9781003186069-9

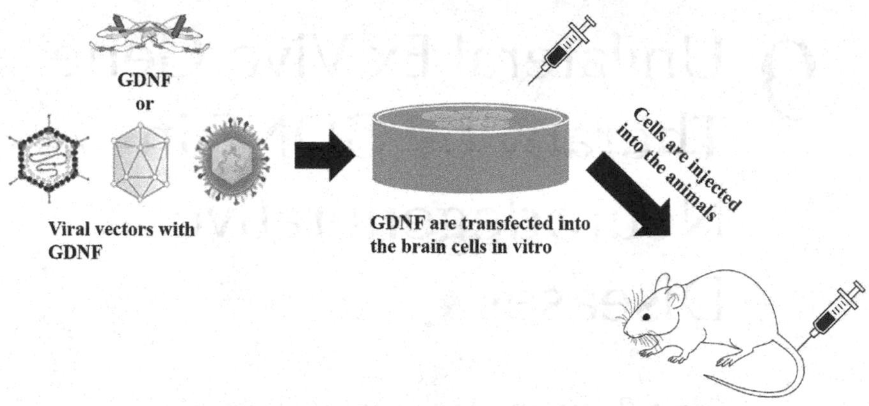

FIGURE 9.1 Ex vivo GDNF cell transfection into brain cell culture.

neurotrophic factor (GDNF) is a neurotrophic factor whose functions is to protect the neurons from degeneration. GDNF was initially recognized as a survival factor for dopaminergic neurons. It is widely distributed in the rat and human CNS, but is expressed highly in the principal pyramidal neurons and the dentate gyrus (DG) granule cells. GDNF has been shown to increase the dopaminergic function in patients with PD [7–8]. These findings have drawn much attention in clinical trials of GDNF therapy for the restoration of PD patients. Gene therapy is a potential agent to deliver the GDNF to the targeted neurons. In transplantation, ex vivo cell-based gene delivery of GDNF shows an advantage in that it removes cells if untoward effects occur [7–9] (Figure 9.1). In addition, the development of cell lines is considered a novel strategy for transplantation into the damaged CNS (cell therapy), which favors the expression and delivery of molecules with therapeutic potential (ex vivo gene therapy) by limiting the challenges associated with the in vivo technique.

Data show that intraventricular infusion or adenoviral vector–mediated overexpression of GDNF in the hippocampus reduces kainic acid (KA), which induces tonic-clonic seizures. Moreover, overexpression of GDNF suppresses acute seizure activity in vivo in animal models [5]. In embryonic midbrain cultures, GDNF enhances the survival and differentiation of dopaminergic neurons as well as dopamine uptake. Although GDNF may not increase the levels of total neurons or astrocytes, it enhances the affinity of y-aminobutyric-containing and serotonergic neurons for neurotransmitter uptake [3]. Pozas and Ilbanez demonstrated that GDNF stimulates the differentiation and migration of cortical GABAergic neurons signaling via GFRα1 receptors. GABAergic cells govern the cell-to-cell communication and induce transmitter activity in the CNS, peripheral nervous system (PNS) and hippocampus. In addition, GDNF effectively stimulates the growth of dopaminergic neurons in the midbrain, thus restoring the patient with PD [10]. Unilateral ex vivo delivery of GDNF using ECB devices effectively suppresses recurrent seizures in rats [5]. Taking all the findings together, unilateral delivery of neurotrophic factors, such as GDNF, using ex vivo gene therapy could be a promising strategy to treat various neurodegenerative diseases. On other hand, unilateral striatal administration of GDNF exerts a bilateral effect on protein, which regulates the functions of DA and GABA neuronal function. GDNF also enhances the release of DA and alters the physiological properties of neurons examined on the rat nigrostriatal system [11].

9.2 EX VIVO VS. IN VIVO GENE THERAPY

In the ex vivo technique, cells are harvested outside of the patient's body and used in the viral transduction in the ex vivo laboratory setting. The transduced cells are then injected back into the patient to deliver the therapeutic genes. On the other hand, with the in vivo method, virus loading with therapeutic genes is directly injected into the patient. Commonly used viral vectors are adenovirus, adeno-associated virus (AAV), lentivirus and retrovirus for both ex vivo and in vivo gene therapy. AAV is considered an ideal vector in gene therapy due to its unique properties. More importantly, it reduces the risk of immune response by containing no viral genes. In addition, AAV provides long-term gene expression. This vector is mostly employed in in vivo gene delivery due to its long-term gene expression, which limits the number of treatment administrations. However, the drawback of AAV is its low carrying capacity—approximately 4.5 kb per particle as compared to other vectors. The major drawbacks of in vivo techniques include low survival rates of grafted cells; it can cause migration and proliferation, in particular for stem-cell lines; immunosuppression may be needed; and the preparation of cells is a time-consuming and complex process. Thus, ex vivo has been considered as a potential gene therapy that overcomes the challenges of in vivo methods.

9.3 APPROACHES TO GDNF DELIVERY

9.3.1 Astrocyte-Derived GDNF

The symptoms of PD are associated with progressive loss of dopaminergic neurons and their functions in the midbrain substantia nigra. Currently, a suitable treatment is not available to treat PD progression. GDNFs are a class of potentially neuroprotective components that have a profound effect in recovering dopaminergic neurons. Endogenous secretion of neurotrophic factors would be promising in the treatment of PD [3–4, 11].

Microglia is the main source of the degeneration of dopaminergic neurons in PD patients. It also has been shown that astrocytes could be suppressed through overexpression of microglia. In addition, astrocyte culture cells silenced GDNF, which was unable to prevent microglial activation in contrast to media with GDNF. Data have shown that GDNF can restore the normal dopaminergic function in PD and inhibits neuroinflammation [12–14]. Cytotoxicity of neuronal cells induce by the lipopolysaccharide can be prevented by GDNF, which suppresses the microglia activation and nitric oxide production shown in the pretreatment of triple cortex–striatum–midbrain organotypic cultures with GDNF. GDNF also inhibits the phosphoinositide 3-kinase (PI3K) in dopaminergic neurons reversibly, thus enhancing its neuroprotective effects [15]. Furthermore, GDNF blocks the accumulation of oxygen radicals in mesencephalic neurons and prevents caspase-dependent apoptosis in the 1-methyl-4-phenylpyridinium (MPP+) model in the PI3K/Akt pathway. Moreover, the activity of the PI3K pathway has been observed in Alzheimer patients [15]. Established data proved that delivery or enhanced expression of GDNF in neurons plays a pivotal role in increasing the survival rate of dopaminergic neurons in PD and blocks the progression of AD. GDNF also has antidyskinetic effects which increase DA levels in the globus pallidus in monkeys. Increased expression of DA is mandatory to reduce dyskinesias. Treatment with antidepressant drugs such as amitriptyline has enhanced the expression of GDNF. In rat astrocytes, amitriptyline raised the expression of GDNF messenger RNA (mRNA), which promotes neuronal survival and protects neurons from the damaging effects of stress. This mechanism could be regulated by the MEK/MAPK signaling pathway [16]. Many drugs can target the functions and secretion of neurotrophic factor GDNF. For example, riluzole, an anti-excitotoxic agent, induces a neuroprotective effect by stimulating GDNF, NGF and BDNF in cultured mouse astrocytes [17]. It also has been reported that expression of GDNF in genetically modified ex vivo astrocytes provides marked neuroprotection of nigral dopaminergic neurons.

9.4 PERICYTE-DERIVED GDNF DELIVERY

Most of the neurological disorders are characterized by the malfunction of the blood–brain barrier (BBB) and blood–nerve barrier (BNB). Such diseases include cerebral ischemia, AD, multiple sclerosis and diabetic neuropathy. Studies have indicated that GDNF secreted from the brain and peripheral nerve pericytes modulate the expression of claudin-5 and transendothelial electrical resistance (TEER) in BBB and BNB. This experiment was carried out in a human brain microvascular endothelial cell (BMEC) line or peripheral nerve microvascular endothelial cell (PnMEC) line. The obtained data revealed that GDNF secreted from pericytes governs the function of the BBB or BNB and induces the regeneration of brain or peripheral nerve cells [5, 18]

9.5 VECTORS FOR GDNF DELIVERY

9.5.1 Viral Vectors

Viral vectors are extensively used in gene therapy because they are naturally efficient to introduce genes into target cells. Delivery of GDNF via a viral vector is promising because it induces long-term expression of these factors in brain cells and has a low immune response and high transduction efficiency in the cells [19]. Studies have reported that delivery of herpes simplex virus (HSV)–mediated GDNF to the striatum produces significant neuroprotection with GDNF in the dopaminergic neurons located at the substantia nigra examined in an intrastriatal 6-hydroxydopamine lesion model [20]. The viral vectors that apply in gene therapy include adenovirus (AdV), AAV and lentivirus (LV). Each of these is highly capable of delivering their genome into nondividing cells such as neurons, aiding their therapeutic application in neuronal gene therapy [19–21].

9.6 ADENO-ASSOCIATED VIRAL VECTORS

These are highly utilized in gene delivery owing to their broad transduction range in tissues such as liver, muscle, retina and the CNS and ability to express genes for a longer period. However, the limitation of these vectors include poor encapsulation capacity, cost-effectiveness in large-scale production and poor stability in biological systems; thus it is restricted to use as a vehicle for therapeutic agents. Other drawbacks include preexisting immunity in humans to AAV and the random integration into the host genome [20–21].

Amyotrophic lateral sclerosis (ALS) is a relentlessly progressive lethal disease that involves selective annihilation of motoneurons. Studies have showed AAV-mediated delivery of GDNF protects motoneurons from degeneration, preserves their axons innervating the muscle, and helps recover from muscle atrophy [22]. Subsequently, four-limb injection of AAV-GDNF reduces disease onset, delays the progression of motor dysfunction and prolongs the survival rate of treated ALS mice [22].

9.7 LENTIVIRUS VECTORS

LVs are an attractive tool in gene therapy because they transfer genes slowly in the brain. Additional benefits include less interaction with retroviruses, the lack of expression of viral gene and its large cloning capacity. Various ex vivo and in vivo studies have been carried out using LVs, including neurons, astrocytes, adult neuronal stem cells, oligodendrocytes and glioma cells. Studies have reported that LV-mediated GDNF induces neuroprotection in mice midbrains examined by using a 6-hydroxydopamine model of PD [23]. Other than this, genetically modified astrocytes expressing GDNF provide neuroprotection in a rat model of PD following transplantation to the substantia nigra (SN). However, studies have also demonstrated that LV-mediated GDNF into the striatum fails to produce behavioral and neuropathological changes in R6/2 Huntington mice [24]. Transplantation of GDNF-expressing astrocytes to the SN provided a significant protection of nigral TH-positive cells, demonstrating that lentivirally transduced rat astrocytes have good potential for neuroprotection in a rat model of PD [25]. However, some research studies have reported that direct injection of a lentiviral vector can cause unwanted side effects such as anterograde transport.

Ex vivo GDNF gene transfer is a promising approach for treating various neurodegenerative disorders that are difficult to treat with traditional therapy. In various clinical trials, it has showed well-tolerated and long-lasting effects to cure neurodegenerative diseases, including PD, AD and Huntington disease (HD). Moreover, advancement of GDNF-based gene therapy promotes its application in the human use, although many investigations are still taking place in terms of its safety and efficacy to treat diseases. Viral vectors are an attractive approach to deliver the GDNF; however, some unwanted side effects could be a major concern. Several initiatives has been undertaken to advance GDNF delivery to the brain with neurodegenerative diseases and its acceptability in clinical trials. The continued development of GDNF-based gene transfection leads to promising therapeutic application of gene therapy in neurodegenerative disorders. Safety profile such as overcomes the insertional mutagenesis and genotoxicity are taken for dosing adjustment in animal models and various phases of clinical investigations. Therefore, it is mandatory to carefully scrutinize all the strategies of GDNF-based gene therapy for its potential therapeutic effects in various neurological disorders.

REFERENCES

1. Nikitidou Ledri, Christiansen SH et al. Translational approach for gene therapy in epilepsy: Model system and unilateral overexpression of neuropeptide Y and Y2 receptors. *Neurobiol. Dis.* 2016;86: 52–61.
2. McGrath J, Linz E, Hoffer BJ et al. Adeno-associated viral delivery of GDNF promotes recovery of dopaminergic phenotype following a unilateral 6-hydroxydopamine lesion. *Cell Transplant.* 2002;11:215–227.
3. Lin LFH, Doherty DH, Lile JD et al. GDNF: A glial cell line—Derived neurotrophic factor for midbrain dopaminergic neurons. *Science.* 1993;260 (80):1130–1132.
4. Nanobashvili A, Melin E, Emerich D et al. Unilateral ex vivo gene therapy by GDNF in epileptic rats. *Gene Ther.* 2019;26:65–74.
5. Jakobsson J and Lundberg C. Lentiviral vectors for use in the central nervous system. *Mol. Ther.* 2006;13:484–493.
6. Bensadoun JC, Deglon N, Tseng JL et al. Lentiviral vectors as a gene delivery system in the mouse midbrain: Cellular and behavioral improvements in a 6-OHDA model of Parkinson's disease using GDNF. *Exp. Neurol.* 2000;164:15–24.
7. Jezierski A, Rennei K, Zurakowski B et al. Neuroprotective Effects of GDNF-expressing human amniotic fluid cells. *Stem Cell Rev. Reports.* 2014;10:251–268.
8. Ebert AD, Barber AE, Heins BM et al. Ex vivo delivery of GDNF maintains motor function and prevents neuronal loss in a transgenic mouse model of Huntington's disease. *Exp. Neurol.* 2010;224:155–162.
9. Fjord-Larsen L, Kusk P, Emerich DF et al. Increased encapsulated cell biodelivery of nerve growth factor in the brain by transposon-mediated gene transfer. *Gene Ther.* 2012;19:1010–1017.
10. Pozas E and Ibáñez CF. GDNF and GFRα1 promote differentiation and tangential migration of cortical GABAergic neurons. *Neuron.* 2005;45:701–713.
11. Salvatore MF, Gerhardt GA, Dayton RD et al. Bilateral effects of unilateral GDNF administration on dopamine- and GABA-regulating proteins in the rat nigrostriatal system. *Exp. Neurol.* 2009;219:197–207.
12. Zhao Y, Haney MJ, Gupta R et al. GDNF-transfected macrophages produce potent neuroprotective effects in parkinson's disease mouse model. *PLoS One.* 2014;9:1–11.
13. Fjord-Larsen L, Julius B, Tornoe J et al. Long-term delivery of nerve growth factor by encapsulated cell biodelivery in the göttingen minipig basal forebrain. *Mol. Ther.* 2010;18:2164–2172.
14. Ericson C, Georgievska B and Lundberg C. Ex vivo gene delivery of GDNF using primary astrocytes transduced with a lentiviral vector provides neuroprotection in a rat model of Parkinson's disease. *Eur. J. Neurosci.* 2005;22:2755–2764.
15. Xing B, Xin T, Zhao L et al. Glial cell line-derived neurotrophic factor protects midbrain dopaminergic neurons against lipopolysaccharide neurotoxicity. *J. Neuroimmunol.* 2010;225:43–51.
16. Hisaoka K, Nishida A, Koda T et al. Antidepressant drug treatments induce glial cell line-derived neurotrophic factor (GDNF) synthesis and release in rat C6 glioblastoma cells. *J. Neurochem.* 2001;79:25–34.
17. Mizuta I, Ohta M, Ohta K et al. Riluzole stimulates nerve growth factor, brain-derived neurotrophic factor and glial cell line-derived neurotrophic factor synthesis in cultured mouse astrocytes. *Neurosci. Lett.* 2001;310:117–120.

18. Shimizu F, Sanu Y, Saito K et al. Pericyte-derived glial cell line-derived neurotrophic factor increase the expression of claudin-5 in the blood-brain barrier and the blood-nerve barrier. *Neurochem. Res.* 2012;37:401–409.
19. Lundstrom K and Boulikas T. Viral and non-viral vectors in gene therapy: Technology development and clinical trials. *Technol. Cancer Res. Treat.* 2003;2:471–485.
20. Monville C, Torress E, Thoams E et al. HSV vector-delivery of GDNF in a rat model of PD: Partial efficacy obscured by vector toxicity. *Brain Res.* 2004;1024:1–15.
21. Kelly MJ, O'Keeffe GW and Sullivan AM. Viral vector delivery of neurotrophic factors for Parkinson's disease therapy. *Expert Rev. Mol. Med.* 2015;17:1–14.
22. Wang L, Lu MY, Ikeguchi K et al. Delayed delivery of AAV-GDNF prevents nigral neurodegeneration and promotes functional recovery in a rat model of Parkinson's disease. *Gene Ther.* 2002;9:381–389.
23. Bensadoun JC, Deglon N, Tseng JL et al. Lentiviral vectors as a gene delivery system in the mouse midbrain: Cellular and behavioral improvements in a 6-OHDA model of Parkinson's disease using GDNF. *Exp. Neurol.* 2000;164:15–24.
24. Ebert AD, Barber AE, Heins BM et al. Ex vivo delivery of GDNF maintains motor function and prevents neuronal loss in a transgenic mouse model of Huntington's disease. *Exp. Neurol.* 2010;224:155–162.
25. Chen W, Hu Y, Ju D. Gene therapy for neurodegenerative disorders: Advances, insights and prospects. *Acta Pharm. Sin. B.* 2020;10:1347–1359.
26. Peel AL and Klein RL. Adeno-associated virus vectors: Activity and applications in the CNS. *J. Neurosci. Methods.* 2000;98:95–104.

10 Gene Therapy for Cancer Treatment

Recent Trends and Clinical Evidence

Manish P. Patel, Mansi S. Shah, Mansi N. Athalye and Jayvadan K. Patel

CONTENTS

10.1 INTRODUCTION

Cancer is the second leading cause of death worldwide [Hassanpour and Dehghani 2017]. The rate of new cases of cancer is 442.4 per 100,000 men and women per year (based on 2013–2017 cases); the cancer death rate is 158.3 per 100,000 men and women per year (based on 2013–2017 deaths) [www.cancer.gov]. It is an irregular cell development with the possibility to attack or spread to different parts of the body [Bansode 2019]. The cells multiply over and over as cancer grows. The initiation

DOI: 10.1201/9781003186069-10

of cancer occurs when gene changes make one cell or a few cells start to grow and multiply too much and rapidly, forming a tumor. Primarily small tumor formation is where a cancer starts. Sometimes cancer can spread to other parts of the body also, which is called a secondary tumor or metastasis [Bansode et al. 2019]. An idea of how rapidly cancer may grow and which treatments may work best, in addition to staging and grading, are necessary. The stage of a cancer means how big it is and whether it has spread. Grading means how abnormal the cancer cells are. The basic reason for sporadic (non-familial) cancers is DNA damage and genomic instability. A minority of cancers are caused by inherited genetic mutations. Many of the cancers are related to environmental, lifestyle or behavioral exposures [Doll and Peto 1981]. The indication sof cancer are self-sufficiency in growth signals, ability for tissue invasion and metastasis, insensitivity to antigrowth signals, sustained angiogenesis, limitless replicative potential and evasion of apoptosis [Fouad and Aanei 2017]. Conventional therapy aims to destroy tumor while leaving as much of the normal host tissue as possible undamaged. The limitation of surgery and radiotherapy is tumor invasion and its spread outside the tumor area, whereas some limitations with chemotherapy is its low therapeutic ratio [Gutierrez et al. 1992].

The new human genome era is creating an increase in possibilites for genomics-based medicine, which is known as "personalized medicine." In medicine, gene therapy is defined as a therapeutic strategy that transfers DNA to a patient's cells to correct a defective/imperfect gene or a gene product in order to treat diseases which are not curable with conventional drugs [Shahryari et al. 2019]. Gene therapies can work by several mechanisms, like replacing a disease-causing gene with a healthy copy of the gene, inactivating a disease-causing gene that is not functioning properly or introducing a new or modified gene into the body to help in treatment of a disease. Studies have shown that gene therapy techniques have broad potential applications in cancer, and almost over 65% of all ongoing clinical gene trials are related to cancerous diseases [DAS et al. 2015].

See Figure 10.1 for currently approved gene therapy protocols from US and European databases [Cooper and Lemoine 2020].

Gene therapy aims at delivering genetic material to target tissue/cells and express it with the intention to gain a better therapeutic effect. It has the benefit over other conventional therapies because it can be administered locally and thereby deliver a high therapeutic dose without risking systemic adverse effects.

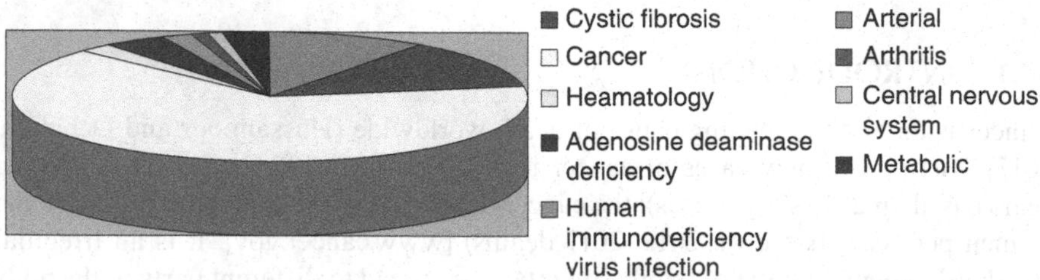

FIGURE 10.1 Currently approved gene therapy protocols from US and European databases (From Cooper and Lemoine 2020).

Additionally, gene therapy can be cost-effective in the long run, since many of the gene therapies are one-time applications. The success of gene therapy highly depends on an efficient means of delivering genes into target cells with minimum toxicity [Hunt et al. 2007].

In 1989 the US Food and Drug Administration (USFDA) approved the protocol for the first gene therapy, in which tumor-infiltrating lymphocytes from metastatic melanoma patients were collected and transduced with a marker gene ex vivo (i.e., not a therapeutic gene), expanded in vitro and reinfused to the patients. The first clinical trial on cancer with a therapeutic intent took place, wherein patients with metastatic melanoma were treated with tumor-infiltrating lymphocytes that are genetically modified ex vivo to manifest tumor necrosis factor [Rosenberg et al. 1990]. In the study conducted by Cline and colleagues, they extracted bone marrow cells from thalassemia patients and transfected ex vivo with plasmids containing the human globulin gene, which was an important milestone in the history of gene therapy. Cells were administered back to the patients after being transfected. The purpose behind this study presents a milestone in the history not because of the failure of the study itself, but because the study was completed without the consent to perform it from the University of California, Los Angeles (UCLA) institutional review board (IRB). This case shows that knowledge was limited and that human gene therapy would be ethically, as well as technically, much more complex than expected [Wirth and Ylä-Herttuala 2014].

10.2 GENE THERAPY PROCESS: RELEASE OF THE GENE

An abnormal gene is responsible for causing a certain disease; that abnormal or muted gene is then replaced by a healthy copy of the gene [Gonçalves et al. 2017]. Various challenges are involved in the gene therapy processes—the difficulty in releasing the gene into the stem cell is the most significant one. Hence, a vector is used to release the gene as a molecular carrier, which must be specific, display efficiency in the release of one or more genes of the sizes required for clinical applications, should not be recognized by the immune system and purified in huge quantities and high concentrations so it can be available on a large scale. After inserting the vector into the patient, it should not induce inflammatory reactions or allergic reactions; it should correct deficiencies, improve the normal functions and inhibit deleterious activities. It should be safe not only for patients but for the environment and the professionals who manipulate it. In general, for the patient's entire life, the vector should be capable of expressing the gene [Gonçalves et al. 2017; Misra 2013].

10.3 METHODS OF GENE TRANSFER

There are two main methods of gene transfer: non-viral and viral mediated.

10.3.1 Non-Viral Vectors

Non-viral vectors are favorable alternatives because of their ease of preparation and reduced immunogenicity and toxicity to patients. There are various approaches like direct injection, electroporation, gene gun, ultrasonic technique, liposomes, etc.

The simplest approach to non-viral vectors is direct injection of naked DNA. Naked DNA is not associated with proteins, lipids or any other molecules to help to protect it. Naked DNA is produced by the release of genetic information into the surrounding environment, such as from bursting cells [David P. Clark and Nanette J. Pazdernik 2013]. The promise of direct injection of naked DNA was first shown in Wolff's study on the expression of a reporter gene following direct intramuscular (IM) injection of DNA. The study disclosed that the reporter gene delivered with the naked DNA could lead to long-term expression of the gene in the muscle [Hunt et al. 2007].

The electroporation technique involves applying electrical pulses to the skin, thereby creating transient pores in the skin promoting the entry of DNA into the cell by increasing the cell permeability. On removal of the electrical energy, the skin regains its structure and holds the entrapped immunogenic agent because the pores have closed [Saroja et al. 2011]. Enhancement of gene transfer using electroporation is generally about 100- to 1000-fold greater than the delivery of naked DNA alone [Hunt et al. 2007].

The gene gun is a biolistic device that enables DNA to directly enter into the cell following bombardment of target DNA in the gene gun chamber kept against the target site [Saroja et al. 2011]. The gene gun delivers DNA-coated gold beads at high pressure, and this allows the transgene access to subcutaneous tissues, such as muscle or tumor, and consequently one can achieve long-term gene expression [Hunt et al. 2007]. Generally, gold, tungsten or silver microparticles are used as the gene carrier. Recently, biodegradable polymer-based delivery has been developed to increase the efficiency of gene transfer of naked DNA. The polymers, such as hyaluronan matrix, polyvinylpyrrolidone (PVP) and poly [α-(4-aminobutyl)-L-glycolic acid] (PAGA), act as release carriers of DNA and provide protection of DNA from damage or enzyme degradation. It has been reported that the lifespan of DNA is prolonged using these polymers in vitro and in vivo [Saroja et al. 2011]. Also, a significant improvement in tissue penetration has been achieved using a new design of the gene gun by Dileo and colleagues [Hunt et al. 2007].

The ultrasonic energy technique is used to disrupt the cell membrane temporarily. The transfection efficiency of this system is based on the frequency, time of ultrasound treatment, plasmid DNA mount used, etc. In a phase II study, repeated intranodal injections of adenovirus- CD 154 (Ad-ISF35) were given by ultrasound to subjects with chronic lymphocytic leukemia/small lymphocytic lymphoma. Ultrasound and laser are emerging techniques for the delivery of DNA vaccines [Saroja et al. 2011].

Liposomes have come a long way as a vehicle for gene delivery. There are three kinds of liposomes: anionic, neutral and cationic. Since DNA is a negatively charged molecule, it has the ability to form complexes with positively charged liposomes. DNA can also be trapped inside the aqueous interior cavity of the liposomes [Seth 2005]. The addition of cationic liposome to DNA decreases its negative charge and reduces the repulsion between cell surfaces and DNA. Thus, cationic lipid is important to facilitate DNA binding to cell membranes for internalization [Wirth and Ylä-Herttuala 2014]. Molecular conjugates, which consist of protein or synthetic ligands to which a nucleic acid– or DNA-binding agent has been attached for the specific targeting of nucleic acids (i.e., plasmid DNA) to cells, have also been studied. Once the DNA is combined with the molecular conjugate, it results in a protein–DNA complex [Roth and Cristiano 1997].

10.3.2 Viral Vectors

Viruses have a natural ability to deliver genetic material within its own genome to specific cell types like cancer cells. This ability makes them popular and attractive as gene delivery vehicles [Akbulut et al. 2015].

10.3.2.1 Adeno-Associated Viruses

AAVs are a type of genome that is linear and have single-stranded DNA of 4680 base pairs. AAV needs a helper virus such as herpes virus or adenovirus, although wild-type AAV have the ability to integrate into the host cell genome in the absence of a helper virus. This property also makes it an attractive and useful vector for gene therapy [Bulcha et al. 2021]. Although not all 13 AAV serotypes isolated use the same receptor repertoire on the host cell surface for infection, every serotype has the capacity to infect cells, transport it to the nucleus, uncoat and introduce its genome into the host's chromosome or leave it in the episomal form. This makes AAV a very beneficial system for a specific cell or tissue type transduction [Goswami et al. 2019]. Glybera (alipogene tiparvovec) was the world's first AAV-based gene therapy to gain regulatory approval for commercialization from the European Medicines Agency (EMA) in 2012. It is an AAV1-based gene therapy that delivers lipoprotein lipase (LPL) to patients deficient in it [Seth et al. 2005].

10.3.2.2 Adenoviruses

Adenoviruses are linear and non-enveloped double-stranded DNA viruses [Cai et al. 2017]. Around 57 serotypes of human Ad exist (Ad1 to Ad57), with seven species (A to G). The human Ad genome contains five early transcription units (E1A, E1B, E2, E3 and E4), four intermediate and one late transcription unit [Mozhei et al. 2020]. Type 5 (Ad5) and type 2 (Ad2) are the most commonly used serotypes of adenoviruses for the development of vectors in humans for cancer gene therapy studies [Akbulut et al. 2015]. They have the capacity of approximately 8 to 10 kb and up to 36 kbp of therapeutic genes with first-generation vectors and third-generation adenoviral vectors, respectively. Based on expression of AV genes during infection and multiplication, its genome is organized into early genes like E1, E2a, E2b, E3 and E4; intermediate genes like IVA2 and IX; and late genes like L1, L2, L3, L4 and L5. Also, its genome has non-coding inverted terminal repeat (ITR) sequences, ψ packaging sequences and many viral RNAs. Several variations have been used to develop safe and economical vectors of genome adenoviruses for gene therapy applications. The first-generation vectors with a partial deletion of E1 or E3 gene sequences don't replicate or show oncogenicity; however, they can deliver less than an 8-kb gene and show leaky expression of viral proteins, immune response and contamination with a replication-competent virus. After the first-generation adenovirus vectors, second-generation vectors were developed by deleting E2A, E2B and E4. The third-generation vectors, also known as "helper dependent or gutless AV vectors," lack all viral genes except the ψ and ITR sequences. Because of their larger capacity to carry therapeutic genes up to 37 kb, they have received much attention, and they were able to show long-term transgene expression and lesser contamination with replicating virus particles. They are also less immunogenic as compared to first- and second-generation vectors [Mozhei et al. 2020; Goswami et al. 2019]. Adenoviruses enter the cells by a mechanism called receptor-mediated endocytosis. When the virus genome is released inside the nucleus, the viral genes are transcribed, which cause replication of DNA, late transcription, synthesis of viral structural proteins and virus assembly [Seth et al. 2005]. However, the transgene expression is limited up to 7 to 10 days post infection. Hence, further repeated vector administrations are required to achieve sustainable responses in cancer treatment [Ortiz et al. 2012]. In addition, transgene transduction has been prevented with the help of adenovirus vectors to undergo sequestration in the liver during systemic administration, displayed severe hepatotoxicity and even caused the death of a clinical trial participant. This was because of the binding of blood coagulation factor FV and FX to the hypervariable region (HPV) of the adenovirus hexon subunit. Therefore, by mutation of the HPV region site, it neither activates the complementary pathway nor interacts with FX, so it could be an ideal way to solve the liver sequestration issue. By treating with chemicals and developing chimeric and hybrid vectors, changes are carried out to increase the safety of adenovirus vectors and to decrease inflammation and immunogenicity [Goswami et al. 2019]. Adenoviruses do not commonly causes serious illness and death in healthy persons, but immunocompromised patients may develop a wide range of illnesses, including diarrhea, conjunctivitis, fever, common cold, sore throat, bronchitis, pneumonia and neurologic disease [Goswami et al. 2019].

10.3.2.3 Herpes Simplex Virus

Herpes simplex virus (HSV) is an enveloped, double-stranded, large DNA virus, with approximately 152 kb of a double-stranded DNA (dsDNA) genome. Herpes viruses are classified into different subfamilies, and HSV-1 is used for gene therapy applications. It cannot integrate into the host genome and has a natural response to nerve tissues. The HSV vectors can be designed in three different types as amplicons, replication-defective and replication-competent vectors. Generally, this type of vectors is used as oncolytic agents in cancer gene therapy studies [Rothand Cristiano 1997].

10.3.2.4 Retroviral Vectors

Retroviral vectors are primarily used by approved gene transfer protocols [Rothand Cristiano 1997]. Retroviruses have a linear single-stranded RNA of around 7 to 10 kb and have a lipid envelope. It consists of a double0stranded RNA genome, on which there are two long terminal repeats (LTRs), namely 5' and 3'. Adjacent to the 5' LTR is the region at which the transfer RNA (tRNA) primer binds and then gives signals for the reverse transcription process [Seth 2005]. Unlike other RNA viruses, these viruses are able to reverse-transcribe their genetic blueprint of positive, single-stranded RNA into dsDNA and insert it into the host cell genome. A major benefit of retroviral vectors for cancer gene therapy is their ability for transgene expression

TABLE 10.1
Advantages and Limitations of the Vectors Used in Different Anti-Cancer Gene Therapies [Ortiz et al. 2012; Bulcha et al. 2021; Seth 2005]

Vectors	Advantages	Limitations
Adeno-associated virus	- No viral gene expression - Can infect non-dividing cells - Low immunogenicity - Long-term gene expression - Non-pathogenic	- Low capacity for insertion of foreign DNA fragments (5 kb) - Tedious to prepare large quantities - Decreased efficacy of repeat administration
Lentivirus	- Reduced insertional mutagenesis - Can infect non-dividing cells - Low immunogenicity - High capacity for insertion of foreign DNA fragments (8 kb)	- Low capacity for insertion of foreign DNA fragments - Insertional mutagenesis - Random integration into host genome
Retrovirus	- Easy to prepare - Well characterized - Currently in clinical trials - Stable expression - High capacity for insertion of foreign DNA fragments (8 kb)	- Can only infect dividing cells - Low capacity for insertion of foreign DNA fragments - Risk of replication - Random integration into host genome
Adenovirus	- High transduction efficiency - Epichromosomal persistence in the host cell - Broad tropism for different tissue targets - Availability of scalable production systems	- High immunogenicity - Cellular toxicity - Limited duration of in vivo gene expression - Risk of replication - Limited repeat administration
Herpes virus	- High capacity for insertion of foreign DNA fragments (25 kb) - Wide host range	- High immunogenicity - Limited duration of in vivo gene expression

in only dividing cells to prevent undesired expression in non-dividing cells of surrounding tissues. The most notable disadvantages are less ability for cell specificity and the chances of insertional mutagenesis. However, this type of vector has been the most commonly used vehicle for gene transfer in the clinic. The risk of insertional oncogenesis has been seen in a clinical trial of X-linked severe combined immunodeficiency (X-SCID) infants in 2003, which has limited the use of retroviral gene transfer systems in human subjects [Akbulut et al. 2015]. A new technique called non-integrating retrovirus-based CRISPR/Cas9 vectors has been developed for targeted gene knockout. Creating vectors that target specific genes would help in developing therapeutic strategies by avoiding insertional mutagenesis issues [Goswami et al. 2019].

10.3.2.5 Baculoviruses

Baculoviruses are enveloped viral particles with a large dsDNA of about 80 to 180 kb. They naturally infect insect cells. There have been no diseases related to baculoviruses in humans. Accompanying their high safety profile in humans, they appear to be very useful vehicles in gene therapy with their high capacity of approximately 40 kb with possible multiple inserts, easy manipulation and production [Airenne et al. 2013]. *Autographa californica* multiple nucleopolyhedron virus (*Ac*MNPV) is the most commonly used type of baculovirus in gene therapy studies. It has a circular dsDNA genome of around 135 kb. They can readily transduce mammalian cells, including various types of cancerous cells, and cause high transgene expression in the host cell. Earlier they were approved for the production of human vaccine components such as Cervarix (GlaxoSmithKline) used in cervical cancer and Provenge (Dendreon) used in prostatic cancer [Akbulut et al. 2015].

10.3.2.6 Poxviruses

In gene therapy, poxviruses were the first viruses used as vectors. By fusing with the plasma membrane, viruses enters the cell. After entry of viruses into the cytosol, DNA replicates and virions are assembled and ultimately released from the cells [Seth 2005]. They have been used in the in vitro production of proteins and live vaccines; also the attenuated forms of poxviruses have been developed, and they were used in the development of genetic cancer vaccine trials [Moss 1996]. Poxviruses are more suitable agents to induce immunity against tumors due to their immune stimulatory properties [Akbulut et al. 2015].

Refer to Figure 10.2 for different methods of gene therapy treatment.

10.4 GENE TARGETING APPROACHES IN CANCER GENE THERAPY

In order to increase the therapeutic index of cancer gene therapy, the expression of therapeutic genes could be restricted to the target tissues only. Hence, the targeting of gene therapy vectors is the major key for the success of those treatments [Akbulut et al. 2015]. The tumor deposits in the body cavities such as pleura, peritoneum and meninges and in subcutaneous (SC) tissues are the potential areas for physical targeting of the gene therapy vectors in the clinic [Li et al. 2006]. There are various approaches to targeting, which are discussed in the following sections.

10.4.1 Physical Targeting

This means uses such physical methods as local injections, catheters, gene guns and electroporation [Akbulut et al. 2015]. But this strategy is generally used for local delivery of gene therapy vectors and is hence not suitable for most of the cancer patients, who may have cancer spread throughout the body. The supercoiled DNA molecules and oligonucleotides are also successfully delivered to the cells of the skin through intradermal injection to the tumor deposits accessible by local injections, although intratumoral injection might have only the transducing capacity of the cells near the needle [Li et al. 2006].

10.4.2 Biological Targeting

In the second strategy, the viral or non-viral carriers of the genes are modified so that they can only bind to tumor cells and not to the normal cells. The specific transgene

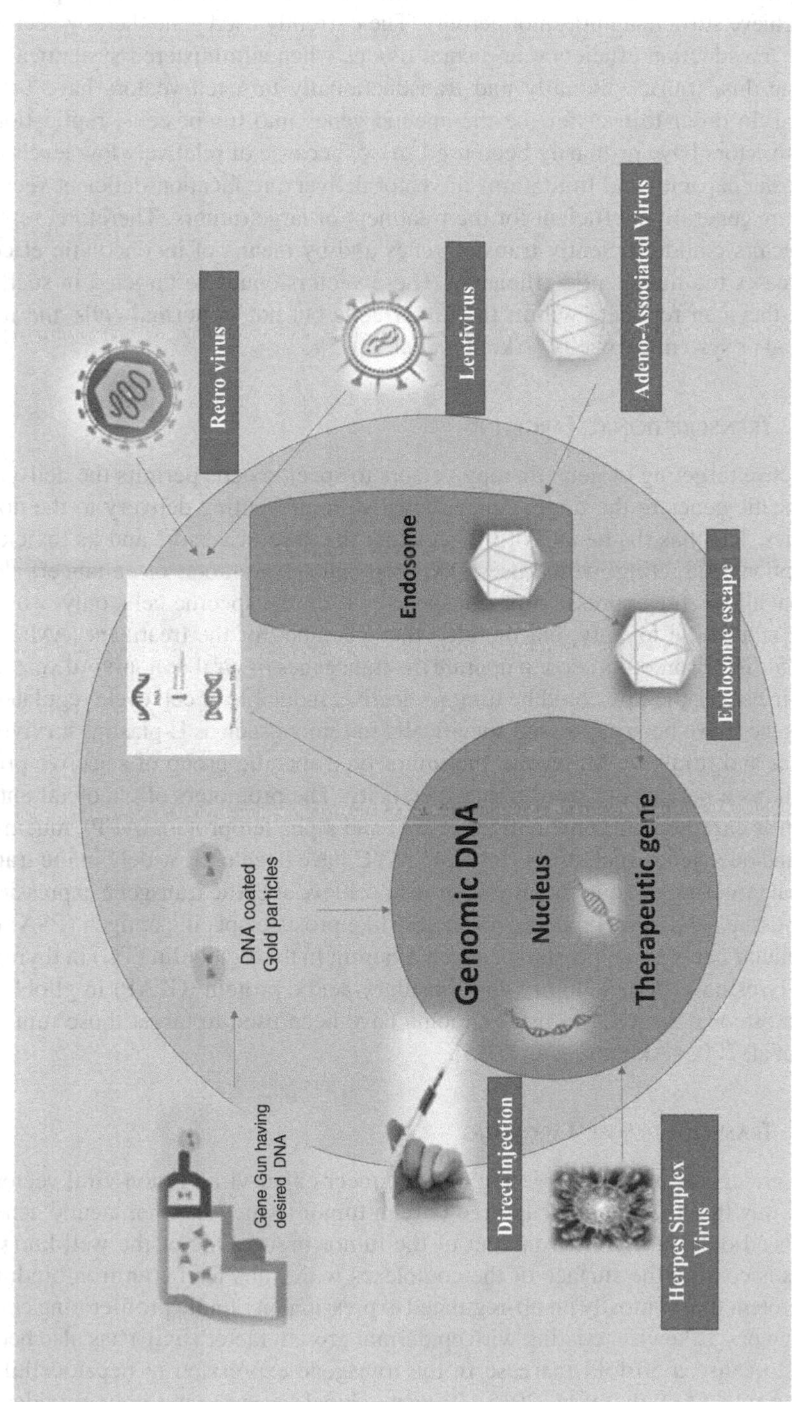

FIGURE 10.2 Different methods for gene therapy treatment.

expression or viral replication into targeted cells or tissues could provide an opportunity to achieve sufficient antitumor activity. The currently used gene therapy vectors have low transduction efficiency in distant tissues when administered systemically. To change this, transcriptionally and transductionally targeted vectors have been developed. In order to transfer the therapeutic genes into tumor cells, replication-defective vectors have primarily been used. Also, because of relatively low levels of gene transfer capacity and limitations of vector delivery, replication-deficient vector systems are generally inefficient for the treatment of large tumors. Therefore, replicating vectors could efficiently transfer genes and by means of its oncolytic effect also increases the therapeutic efficiency. These vectors could be targeted in such a way that they can replicate within the tumor cells but not in normal cells and not cause local or systemic toxicity [Akbulut et al. 2015].

10.4.3 Transcriptional Targeting

The selective targeting of gene therapy vectors to specific cells permits the delivery of therapeutic genes to the target cancer cells while preventing delivery to the normal tissues. This has the benefit of the reducing the dose of vectors and its toxicity. Transcriptional targeting, which uses DNA regulatory (promoter or enhancer) elements that allows the expression of transgenes within the specific cells only, would probably reduce the toxicity and increase the specificity of the treatment [Akbulut et al. 2015]. The promoters used to operate the transgenes in viral or non-viral vectors targeted in cancer therapy could be tumor selective, inducible or cell cycle regulated. Certain genes have been expressed specifically in tumors such as L-plastin, survivin, telomerase and midkine. Moreover, the tumor type specific group of selective promoters shows a pattern of tumor tissue specificity. The promoters of oncofetal antigens such as carcinoembryonic antigen (CEA) and alpha fetoprotein (AFP), mucin-1 (mucl), and oncogenes such as c-erbB2 and MYC have been used widely in the transcriptional targeting of gene therapy vectors to achieve specific transgene expression in tumor tissue. The tissue-specific promoters like prostate specific antigen (PSA) in hepatocellular carcinoma, prostatic cancer, albumin in thyroglobulin (TG) in thyroid cancers, tyrosinase in melanoma, glial fibrillary acidic protein (GFAP) in glioblastoma and osteocalcin (OC) in osteosarcoma have been used to target those tumors [Barker et al. 2003; Akbulut et al. 2015].

10.4.4 Transductional Targeting

Another strategy of biologic targeting is to engineer either viral or non-viral vectors in such a way that they can be captured only in tumor tissues and therapeutic genes are produced only in the environment of the tumor tissue. One of the well-known strategies is coating the surface of the complexes with trans ferrin, an iron-binding plasma protein that is mostly an up-regulated expression on rapidly proliferating cells such as tumors. Likewise, coating with epidermal growth factor (EGF) has also been reported to cause a 50-fold increase in the transgene expression in hepatocellular carcinoma cells [Akbulut et al. 2015]. Transductional targeting not only provides a higher degree of infection specificity but also a higher degree of infection efficiency. The most common promoters used to direct expression in the context of Ad gene delivery have been the cytomegalovirus (CMV) immediate early and Rous sarcoma virus promoters [Barker et al. 2003].

10.4.5 Anti-Angiogenic Gene Therapy

This therapy targets the development of new vessels in tumor tissue, thus inhibiting tumor growth [Ortiz et al. 2012]. Anti-angiogenic factors include fragments of proteins like angiostatin and endostatin, thrombospondin, tissue inhibitors of metalloproteinases (TIMPs) and interferon (IFN)-α and -β, among other factors. Hence, the activation of oncogenes and the loss of tumor suppressor genes are essential to the angiogenic phenotype that supports tumorigenicity [Ortiz et al. 2012]. Jo and colleagues (2011) patented the use of a cell-permeable recombinant endostatin protein with a macromolecule transduction domain (MTD) for use against tumor cells by gene therapy. As per this invention, the cell-permeable endostatin recombinant protein has the ability to block the formation of micro vessels and inhibit the migration, proliferation, penetration and subsequent tube formation of vascular endothelial cells present in tumor tissue with high efficiency [Liu et al. 2006].

10.4.6 Genetic Immunopotentiation

Active immunotherapy (vaccine therapies) aims to stimulate the patient's immune response through cytokines and gene vaccines. In contrast, to augment immunological recognition of neo-plastic cells, genetic immunopotentiation efforts are involved in the modifications. In addition, to enhance the therapeutic index or sensitivity of cells to chemotherapy, investigators have utilized a variety of strategies. The patent titled "Methods of stimulating an immune response against prostate specific antigen" describes the immunization of T cells with the prostate specific antigen oligoepitope peptide (PSA-OP) [Mansoor et al. 2005]. This application of the PSA-specific cytotoxic T-cell lines enhances anticancer immune responses. This approach is useful for the prevention or treatment of prostate cancer and the inhibition of the establishment of prostatic cancer [Mansoor et al. 2005].

10.4.7 Genetic Modulation of Resistance/Sensitivity

Tumor cells can develop resistance mechanisms after an unpredictable period, which results in a failure of chemotherapy. This phenomenon is termed multidrug resistance (MDR), and it is a major obstacle in successful cancer treatment. Classic MDR has been associated with *MDR1*, the most commonly analyzed resistance gene and one of the most used in cancer gene therapy [Callaghan et al. 2006]. The P-glycoprotein (P-gp), a 170-kDa protein product of the *MDR1* gene, is an energy-dependent transport protein that has a physiological function in cellular detoxification and has a connection with major histocompatibility complex (MHC) molecule expression. One of the last trials undertaken by the Clinical Center of the National Institutes of Health (USA) demonstrated the prevention of chemotherapy's toxic effects using *MDR1* gene therapy in patients with metastatic breast cancer (NCT00001493) [Ortiz et al. 2012].

10.4.8 Molecular Chemotherapy

Also known as suicide or pro-drug gene therapy, this is the selective delivery or expression of genes encoding a pro-drug–activating enzyme for tumor cell eradication. Approaches tested in the clinic include herpes simplex virus thymidine kinase (HSVTK) and *Escherichia coli* cytosine deaminase (*E. coli* CD), which convert non-toxic prodrugs (e.g., ganciclovir for HSVTK or 5-fluorocytosine for *E. coli* CD) into potent cell poisons, which helps alleviate the daunting task of transduction of each tumor cell. Some advances in gene-directed enzyme pro-drug therapy have been patented such as a new plasmid construct in which the *HSV-tk* toxic gene is translationally repressed in normal cells by placing a complex 5' untranslated region (UTR) in front of its reading frame. This is discussed in the patent "Cancer gene therapy based on translational control of a suicide gene" [Ortiz et al. 2012] (Figure 10.3).

An advantage of the genetic pro-drug activation therapy is that its effect is not only on transfected cells but also on neighboring non-transfected cells. This phenomenon is called the bystander effect. The "bystander effect is the lateral diffusion of the activated drug into untransduced neighbouring cells [causing] additional cell killing."

Another approach uses the suicidal capacities of plants (e.g., saporins) or bacterial toxins for gene therapy. The use of *Clostridium perfringens* enterotoxin (CPE) is a recent example that acts as a pore-forming toxin that selectively kills claudin-3 and claudin-4 overexpressing epithelial tumor cells. Walther and colleagues demonstrated that CPE gene transfer exerts targeted and efficient tumor killing in vitro and in vivo associated with massive necrosis in xeno-transplant models. Such studies lead to the emerging potential of toxin gene therapy for tumor eradication [Walther and Schlag 2013] (Figure 10.4).

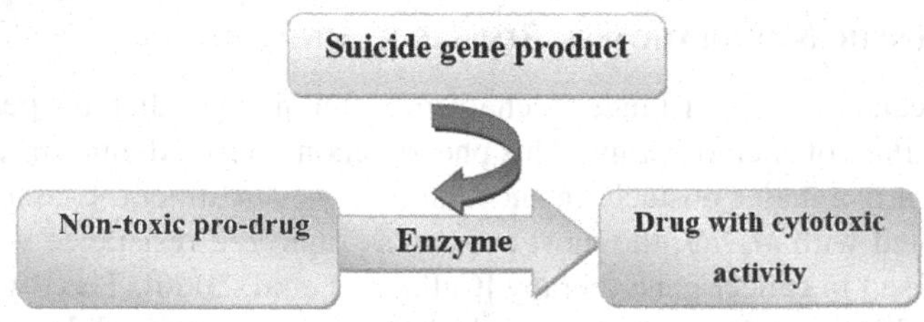

FIGURE 10.3 Mechanism of suicide/pro-drug gene therapy.

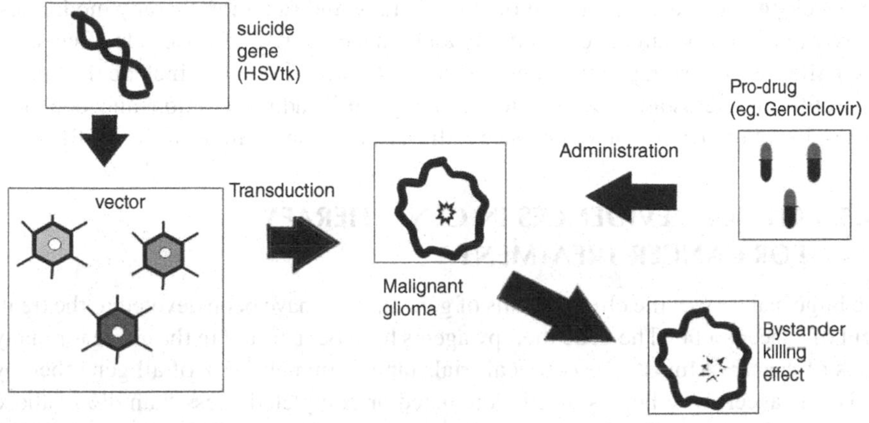

FIGURE 10.4 Molecular gene therapy: a unique approach.

10.4.9 Combination of Gene Therapy With Radiation

Conventional radiotherapy in cancer is generally limited by a narrow therapeutic index [Hunt et al. 2007]. However, a growing body of evidence suggests that manipulation of the genes involved in tumor progression and radiation resistance represents a promising approach for therapeutic intervention in combination with radiation therapy [Kaliberovand Buchsbaum 2012].

Gene therapy approaches offer the potential for specific targeting at several levels, including transcriptional targeting. Transcriptional control of therapeutic gene expression using promoters that are responsive to ionizing radiation provides an attractive approach for the combination of radiation therapy and gene therapy. Transcriptional regulatory elements are composed of both cis acting and trans acting elements. The cis acting components include promoters and enhancer regions that also regulate expression of a particular gene, whereas the trans acting elements belong to a growing group of transcription factors that bind to specific sites within promoter and/or enhancer regions [Hallahan et al. 1991]. The promoters from many stress response genes related to cellular fate following DNA damage are potential candidates for cancer gene therapy.

In the last two decades, several radiation-inducible promoters, including tissue plasminogen activator (TPA), *p21/WAF-1* and *GADD45α*, were proposed for gene therapy in combination with radiation therapy strategies. The ability of radiation to activate pathways relies on the levels of DNA damage, generation of reactive oxygen species/reactive nitrogen species (ROS/RNS), activation of a variety of transcriptional factors and alterations in the expression of growth factor receptors and their cognate ligands. A growing body of evidence suggests that the interaction between tumor cells and another surrounding normal cell controls local tumor development and is involved in the development of radiation resistance. Intervention against the interaction between tumor cells and their microenvironment is a promising area for the development of a combination of gene therapy and radiation therapy modalities. These modifications enhance specificity and reduce the risk of toxic side effects.

Challenges regarding current approaches and future directions include the uptake of vectors in metastatic tumor sites after systemic administration and adequate expression of the transgene to produce radiosensitization [Kaliberov et al. 2012].

10.5 CLINICAL EVIDENCES IN GENE THERAPY FOR CANCER TREATMENT

The huge majority of the clinical trials of gene therapy have been devoted to the treatment of cancer so far. The gene therapy agents have been tested in the clinic for many types of cancer. Almost 1200 clinical trials (approximately 65% of all gene therapy trials) in cancer have been started, conducted or completed. Less than 4% of those are phase II or III, and only a few of them are phase IV trials [Akbulut et al. 2015]. The most dominant factor that has limited the success of clinical gene therapy trials in human subjects is the delivery of the vector genetic elements or their products to the target cancer cells and their vasculature. A second problem has been toxicity.

The first commercialized gene therapy, Gendicine, is a recombinant adenovirus engineered to express wild-type p53 under a Rous sarcoma virus promoter, which was effective in treatment of head and neck squamous cell carcinoma [DAS et al. 2015]. Oncorine is the second gene therapy product which was developed by Chinese Shanghai Sunway Biotech and also received market approval by the Chinese State Food and Drug Administration (SFDA). Oncorine is a conditionally replicative adenovirus developed by E1B 55K deletion. Through deletion of this gene, it prevents the virus from binding and inactivating wild-type p53 protein, which is a crucial self defense mechanism of the host against virus infection [DAS et al. 2015].

Glybera, an adeno-associated vector (AAV)–based therapy for familial lipoprotein lipase deficiency, received conditional marketing approval from the EMA in 2012. Imlygic, a genetically modified HSV-1 for local treatment of unresectable lesions in patients with melanoma, was approved by the USFDA in 2015. Strimvelis, a γ-retrovirus–based therapy for the treatment of severe combined immune deficiency due to adenosine deaminase deficiency (ADA-SCID), gained EMA approval in 2016.

Some pharmaceutical companies have developed several medications; such as Novartis-LBH589, cIAP1 and cIAP2, which inhibit the Bcl-2 protein, thus promoting apoptosis and tumor regression, prevent or delay tumor resistance and prolong remission following gene therapy [Amer 2014]. Notably, clinical trials for the treatment of cervical dysplasia (high-grade squamous intraepithelial lesions) caused by human papilloma virus with the DNA vaccine VGX-3100 are in advanced stages (phase III, NCT03185013) [Ginn et al. 2017]. Most commonly, HSV thymidine-kinase has been used to convert the non-toxic pro-drug ganciclovir into the cytotoxic triphosphate ganciclovir [Ginn et al. 2017]. Therapies that are targeting CD19, an antigen present in most B-cell malignancies but absent in normal tissues other than the B-cell lineage, are at the forefront of CAR-based technology. A turning point occurred when the positive outcomes from three CAR therapy trials were published in 2010 and 2011. These studies showed unprecedented antitumor activity in patients with B-cell lymphoma, chronic lymphocytic leukemia (NCT01029366, NCT00466531) or B-cell acute lymphoblastic leukemia. This success concluded with the recent USFDA and EMA approval of two CAR T-cell therapies targeting CD19-expressing B cells.

Further, both Kymriah and Yescarta are indicated for the treatment of adult patients with relapsed or refractory large B-cell lymphoma, and Kymriah is also indicated for the treatment of relapsed and refractory B-cell acute lymphoblastic leukemia in pediatric and young adult patients [Anguela and High 2019]. It is clear from this discussion that huge potential remains for more improvement in clinical cancer gene therapy. In this field, future directions should include more efforts on improved understanding of the biological activities of the gene therapy agents in vivo in patients, enhancing efficacy and reducing side effects.

10.6 CHALLENGES IN GENE THERAPY

Gene therapy has some potential risks—a gene can't be easily inserted into the cells. The major barrier for successful cancer gene therapy is optimal transgene expression for suppressing a cancer-associated gene or delivery of a cancer therapeutic gene to diseased tissue at efficacious doses. Recognition of an appropriate therapeutic genes that have capability of inhibiting disease progression will also influence success. The most common side effects following gene therapy include transient fever and flulike symptoms [Amer 2014]. Retroviral (i.e., lentiviruses) mediated gene therapy directs viral integration into the host genome; hence, it may cause mutagenic incidence with possible second malignancies. This was reported in earlier investigations on the murine leukemia retrovirus vector in the treatment of severe combined immunodeficient patients and in which 5 out of 30 cases developed leukemia [Gaspar et al. 2011]. Another crucial problem associated with gene therapy for cancer is the resistance to treatment with subsequent tumor recurrences and shorter survival. A potential mechanism is intrinsic and possibly acquired tumor cell resistance to therapy-induced cell death, also called apoptosis, by dysregulation and release of anti-apoptotic inhibitor of apoptosis protein or Bcl-2 proteins [Amer 2014].

10.7 RECENT TRENDS IN CANCER GENE THERAPY

Recently, new advancements in improving the delivery and specificity of vectors in gene therapy have suggested these trials may be more successful in the upcoming years. This is especially true of the attempts to use vectors for activation of the immune response against the tumor tissue. Continued testing of these approaches in the context of clinical trials may result in new opportunities for individuals engaged in a personal struggle with cancer to control their disease condition. Actually, the nature of the distant spread of disease, which causes the failure of conventional treatment modalities, is also one of the major drawbacks of gene therapy for cancer. It is anticipated that gene therapy will play a major role in future cancer therapy as part of a multimodality treatment, in combination with cancer therapy such as surgery, radiation and chemotherapy [Amer 2014].

TABLE 10.2
Future Directions for Genetic Therapy Improvement [Hunt et al. 2007]

Directions	Solutions
Disclosing the in vivo activities of gene therapy agents	Improving the design of new vectors to allow in vivo monitoring
	Proper patient selection/trial design
Enhancing efficacy	Transgene-armed, replication- selective oncolytic viruses
	Targeting tumor stroma/connective tissues to improve transfection efficiency
	Proper patient selection
	Combination treatment with existing modalities
Reducing side effects	More thorough understanding of vectorology
	Decrease vector binding by antibodies and/or uptake into reticuloendothelial (RE) cells
	More sophisticated toxicology studies

Current progress in developing safe and effective vectors for gene transfer, like the use of synthetic viral and non-viral mediated methods, along with the success of using autologous and allogenic chimeric antigen receptor–integrated T cells from healthy individuals are considered universal effector cells in mediating adoptive immunotherapy and will enhance the effectiveness and safety profile of gene therapy. Through improvements in biological research, much cheaper gene vectors will become commercially available, and that will make gene therapy more economical and easily available to cancer patients. This in turn will lead to a major change in the future of cancer therapy from conventional cancer treatments, based on their tumor size, nature and site, to a more preferable personalized cancer therapy, based on a patient's specific genomic structures, immune status and genetic profile of the underlying malignancy. Therapy should be fast and more effective, with less toxicity, and cost-effective, with higher cure rates, and may even prevent cancer altogether.

REFERENCES

Airenne, Kari J., Yu-Chen Hu, Thomas A. Kost, Richard H. Smith, Robert M. Kotin, Chikako Ono, Yoshiharu Matsuura, Shu Wang, and Seppo Ylä-Herttuala. "Baculovirus: An insect-derived vector for diverse gene transfer applications." *Molecular Therapy* 21, no. 4 (2013): 739–749.

Akbulut, Hakan, Muge Ocal, and Gizem Sonugur. "Cancer gene therapy." In *Gene Therapy-Principles and Challenges*. IntechOpen, 2015.

Amer, Magid H. "Gene therapy for cancer: Present status and future perspective." *Molecular and Cellular Therapies* 2, no. 1 (2014): 1–19.

Anguela, Xavier M., and Katherine A. High. "Entering the modern era of gene therapy." *Annual Review of Medicine* 70 (2019): 273–288.

Bansode, Sudha. "Cancer biology-causes & biomarkers of cancer." (2019).

Barker, Shannon D., I. P. Dmitriev, Dirk M. Nettelbeck, Bin Liu, Angel A. Rivera, Ronald D. Alvarez, David T. Curiel, and Akseli Hemminki. "Combined transcriptional and transductional targeting improves the specificity and efficacy of adenoviral gene delivery to ovarian carcinoma." *Gene Therapy* 10, no. 14 (2003): 1198–1204.

Bulcha, Jote T., Yi Wang, Hong Ma, Phillip WL Tai, and Guangping Gao. "Viral vector platforms within the gene therapy landscape." *Signal Transduction and Targeted Therapy* 6, no. 1 (2021): 1–24.

Cai, Zhonglin, Haidi Lv, Wenjuan Cao, Chuan Zhou, Qiangzhao Liu, Hui Li, and Fenghai Zhou. "Targeting strategies of adenovirus-mediated gene therapy and virotherapy for prostate cancer." *Molecular Medicine Reports* 16, no. 5 (2017): 6443–6458.

Callaghan, Richard, Robert C. Ford, and Ian D. Kerr. "The translocation mechanism of P-glycoprotein." *FEBS Letters* 580, no. 4 (2006): 1056–1063.

Clark, David P., and Nanette J. Pazdernik. *Chapter 25 - Bacterial Genetics, Molecular Biology* (Second Edition). Page no. 641–646, 2013.

Cooper, David, and Nick Lemoine, eds. *Gene Therapy*. Garland Science, page no. 2, 2020.

Das, Swadesh K., Mitchell E. Menezes, Shilpa Bhatia, Xiang-Yang Wang, Luni Emdad, Devanand Sarkar, and Paul B. Fisher. "Gene therapies for cancer: Strategies, challenges and successes." *Journal of Cellular Physiology* 230, no. 2 (2015): 259–271.

Doll, Richard, and Richard Peto. "The causes of cancer: Quantitative estimates of avoidable risks of cancer in the United States today." *JNCI: Journal of the National Cancer Institute* 66, no. 6 (1981): 1192–1308.

Fouad, Yousef Ahmed, and Carmen Aanei. "Revisiting the hallmarks of cancer." *American Journal of Cancer Research* 7, no. 5 (2017): 1016.

Gaspar, H. Bobby, Samantha Cooray, Kimberly C. Gilmour, Kathryn L. Parsley, Stuart Adams, Steven J. Howe, Abdulaziz Al Ghonaium et al. "Long-term persistence of a polyclonal T cell repertoire after gene therapy for X-linked severe combined immunodeficiency." *Science Translational Medicine* 3, no. 97 (2011): 97ra79.

Ginn, Samantha L., Anais K. Amaya, Ian E. Alexander, Michael Edelstein, and Mohammad R. Abedi. "Gene therapy clinical trials worldwide to 2017: An update." *The Journal of Gene Medicine* 20, no. 5 (2018): e3015.

Gonçalves, Giulliana Augusta Rangel, and Raquel de Melo Alves Paiva. "Gene therapy: Advances, challenges and perspectives." *Einstein (Sao Paulo)* 15, no. 3 (2017): 369–375.

Goswami, Reena, Gayatri Subramanian, Liliya Silayeva, Isabelle Newkirk, Deborah Doctor, Karan Chawla, Saurabh Chattopadhyay, Dhyan Chandra, Nageswararao Chilukuri, and Venkaiah Betapudi. "Gene therapy leaves a vicious cycle." *Frontiers in Oncology* 9 (2019): 297.

Gutierrez, Andres A., Nick R. Lemoine, and Karol Sikora. "Gene therapy for cancer." *The Lancet* 339, no. 8795 (1992): 715–721.

Hallahan, Dennis E., Subbulakshmi Virudachalam, Michael Beckett, Matthew L. Sherman, Donald Kufe, and Ralph R. Weichselbaumi. "Mechanisms of X-ray-mediated protooncogene c-iun expression in radiation-induced human sarcoma cell lines." *International Journal of Radiation Oncology* Biology* Physics* 21, no. 6 (1991): 1677–1681.

Hassanpour, Seyed Hossein, and Mohammadamin Dehghani. "Review of cancer from perspective of molecular." *Journal of Cancer Research and Practice* 4, no. 4 (2017): 127–129.

Hunt, Kelly K., Stephan A. Vorburger, and Stephen G. Swisher, eds. *Gene Therapy for Cancer*. Springer Science & Business Media, page no. 4, 2007.

Hunt, Kelly K., Stephan A. Vorburger, and Stephen G. Swisher, eds. *Gene Therapy for Cancer*. Springer Science & Business Media, page no. 158, 2007.

Hunt, Kelly K., Stephan A. Vorburger, and Stephen G. Swisher, eds. *Gene Therapy for Cancer*. Springer Science & Business Media, page no. 159–160, 2007.

Hunt, Kelly K., Stephan A. Vorburger, and Stephen G. Swisher, eds. *Gene Therapy for Cancer*. Springer Science & Business Media, page no. 243, 2007.

Hunt, Kelly K., Stephan A. Vorburger, and Stephen G. Swisher, eds. *Gene Therapy for Cancer*. Springer Science & Business Media, page no. 376, 2007.

Kaliberov, Sergey A., and Donald J. Buchsbaum. "Cancer treatment with gene therapy and radiation therapy." *Advances in Cancer Research* 115 (2012): 221–263.

Li, Li, Ran-Yi Liu, Jia-Ling Huang, Qi-Cai Liu, Yan Li, Pei-Hong Wu, Yi-Xin Zeng, and Wenlin Huang. "Adenovirus-mediated intra-tumoural delivery of the human endostatin gene inhibits tumour growth in nasopharyngeal carcinoma." *International Journal of Cancer* 118, no. 8 (2006): 2064–2071.

Liu, Ching-Chiu, Zan Shen, Hsiang-Fu Kung, and Marie CM Lin. "Cancer gene therapy targeting angiogenesis: An updated review." *World Journal of Gastroenterology: WJG* 12, no. 43 (2006): 6941.

Mansoor, Was, David E. Gilham, Fiona C. Thistlethwaite, and Robert E. Hawkins. "Engineering T cells for cancer therapy." *British Journal of Cancer* 93, no. 10 (2005): 1085–1091.

Misra, Sanjukta. "Human gene therapy: A brief overview of the genetic revolution." *Journal of the Association of Physicians of India* 61, no. 2 (2013): 127–133.

Moss, Bernard. "Genetically engineered poxviruses for recombinant gene expression, vaccination, and safety." *Proceedings of the National Academy of Sciences* 93, no. 21 (1996): 11341–11348.

Mozhei, Oleg, Anja G Teschemacher, and Sergey Kasparov. "Viral vectors as gene therapy agents for treatment of glioblastoma." *Cancers* 12, no. 12 (2020): 3724.

NATIONAL CANCER INSTITUTE https://www.cancer.gov/about-cancer/understanding/statistics U.S. Department of Health and Human Services (Access on 1st July 2021).

Ortiz, Raul, Consolación Melguizo, José Prados, Pablo J Alvarez, Octavio Caba, Fernando Rodríguez-Serrano, Fidel Hita, and Antonia Aránega. "New gene therapy strategies for cancer treatment: A review of recent patents." *Recent Patents on Anti-Cancer Drug Discovery* 7, no. 3 (2012): 297–312.

Rosenberg, Steven A., Paul Aebersold, Kenneth Cornetta, Attan Kasid, Richard A. Morgan, Robert Moen, Evelyn M. Karson et al. "Gene transfer into humans—immunotherapy of patients with advanced melanoma, using tumour-infiltrating lymphocytes modified by retroviral gene transduction." *New England Journal of Medicine* 323, no. 9 (1990): 570–578.

Roth, Jack A., and Richard J. Cristiano. "Gene therapy for cancer: What have we done and where are we going?" *Journal of the National Cancer Institute* 89, no. 1 (1997): 21–39.

Saroja, C. H., P. K. Lakshmi, and Shyamala Bhaskaran. "Recent trends in vaccine delivery systems: A review." *International Journal of Pharmaceutical Investigation* 1, no. 2 (2011): 64.

Seth, Prem. "Vector-mediated cancer gene therapy: An overview." *Cancer Biology & Therapy* 4, no. 5 (2005): 512–517.

Shahryari, Alireza, Marie Saghaeian Jazi, Saeed Mohammadi, Hadi Razavi Nikoo, Zahra Nazari, Elaheh Sadat Hosseini, Ingo Burtscher, Seyed Javad Mowla, and Heiko Lickert. "Development and clinical translation of approved gene therapy products for genetic disorders." *Frontiers in Genetics* 10 (2019): 868.

Walther, Wolfgang, and Peter M. Schlag. "Current status of gene therapy for cancer." *Current Opinion in Oncology* 25, no. 6 (2013): 659–664.

Wirth, Thomas, and Seppo Ylä-Herttuala. "Gene therapy used in cancer treatment." *Biomedicines* 2, no. 2 (2014): 149–162.

11 Gene Therapy for Retina and Eye Diseases

Khushboo Faldu and Jigna Shah

CONTENTS

11.1 INTRODUCTION

Gene therapy manipulates the mutated host cells to compensate for the mutation via the introduction of alien wild-type DNA. Gene therapy can be employed to enhance the immune system response for the recognition of specific tumor markers and infections and to transform the host cells into a "bio-factory" via gene introduction to express a therapeutic protein (1).

Gene therapy prerequisites are:

a) Wild-type gene clone specific for the disorder.
b) A promoter system for gene transcription in the targeted tissue.

DOI: 10.1201/9781003186069-11

c) Viral or a non-viral vector that acts as a carrier of genetic material into the host cells.
d) A recipient host carrying the genetic mutation or condition to be treated (1).

The eyes are ideal organs for gene therapy research and development. It is easy to develop targeted treatments for ocular and retinal diseases, as the eyes are conveniently accessible for surgical interventions and intraocular and intravitreal injections. The eyes are considered immune-favored and can hold the viral vector antigenicity. The tight blood–ocular barriers diminish contamination to other organs (1–2).

The first successful preclinical retinal gene therapy was performed on mice for retinitis pigmentosa (RP). Mice with a phosphodiesterase gene defect were treated by a wild-type gene delivered in an adenovirus vector through subretinal injection. Subretinal injection proved an efficient delivery route and become the gold standard for future research (3).

Leber congenital amaurosis (LCA) is a rare ocular disorder. It develops due to the inheritance of autosomal recessive genetic conditions causing severe loss of vision in infants. Vision loss is the result of retinal degeneration causing dysfunction of photoreceptors that precipitate an inability to capture images. Electroretinography (ERG) measures electrical retinal activity in response to impingement by light. The ERG tracings show diminished activity. Additional symptoms include cataracts, strabismus, photophobia, keratoconus, and/or nystagmus (4–5).

The defect is central to the RPE65 (retinal pigment epithelium-specific 65 kDa protein) gene essential for the visual cycle. 11-cis retinal is a derivative of vitamin A, which through light activation, is converted to all-trans-retinal by the photoreceptors. This converts light input into electrical signals. To reinitiate the visual circle, RPE65 transforms all-trans-retinal to 11-cis retinal (2).

In the Briard dog model of LCA, subretinal administration of a wild-type LCA gene improved ambulation in the agility course, recovered electrical retinal activity, and developed a pupillary response (6). The mice model of LCA exhibited comparable positive outcomes. The preclinical results pointed out that the treatment in younger animals was more effective than older animals, thus proving treatment in the early disease stage preserves unimpaired photoreceptors and has favorable outcomes due to stable gene expression for over a decade (1).

A phase I safety and efficacy trial established gene therapy as a safe option in juvenile patients suffering from LCA. The dose-escalation trial enrolled 12 patients wherein the RPE65 gene was administered subretinally via an adenoviral vector and the treated eyes were compared to untreated eyes. The treatment improved vision in the dim light—sensitivity to light increased three times. Pupillary light reflex improved to an extent that an afferent pupillary defect was observed. As compared with baseline, visual field testing was improved, and it covered the subretinal injection anatomic area. The patients could efficiently cross an obstacle trail with subdued lighting using the treated eye as compared with using the untreated eye. A phase III placebo-controlled trial with 16 patients is currently being conducted (7).

Gene therapy in eye care received a boost in 2017 when Luxturna (voretigene neparvovec-rzyl) of Spark Therapeutics acquired marketing authorization from the U.S. Food and Drug Administration (FDA), becoming the first gene therapy to receive an FDA nod (2). Luxturna repairs the defective biallelic RPE652 gene mutation responsible for the genetically derived retinal disease LCA (8).

Ophthalmology gene therapy phase I clinical trials are in the conduction phase for neovascular macular degeneration (AMD), choroideremia, retinitis pigmentosa, Usher's syndrome, and Stargardt's disease (1).

11.2 GENE THERAPY VECTORS

Two types of vectors are utilized in the gene therapy: viral and non-viral vectors.

11.2.1 Viral Vectors

Adenoviruses, adeno-associated viruses (AAVs), lentiviruses, and herpes simplex viruses act as viral vectors and are devoid of their replicative and virulence characteristics (9).

Luxturna is the first gene therapy to procure authorization of marketing from the FDA for LCA, a type of genetically derived retinal disease (IRD) that utilizes a serotype 2 AAV2-based vector (2).

Despite the success, researchers are still conservative towards the usage of viral vectors. Viral vectors like AAV require subretinal administration, and thus bring up an important issue of surgical considerations. Subretinal administration requires trained surgeons to perform pars plana vitrectomy, sometimes under subretinal optical coherence tomography (OCT) (10). Subretinal injection complications include macular holes, unresolved retinal detachment, choroidal effusion, hypotonia, and retinal tears (11–14). Formation of a subretinal bleb limits the benefit to that anatomical area and does not transduce the entire retina (10).

Intravitreal injection (IVT) is less invasive, but AAV vectors are unsuccessful in transducing photoreceptors and retinal pigment epithelium (RPE) cells (15).

AAV vectors have limited capacity, which restricts the packaging of large transgenes (16). To overcome the capacity issue, a dual AAV8 vector was used in patients with Usher syndrome 1B (USHIB) to target the myosin 7A (MYO7A) gene. This gene therapy was designated as an orphan drug by the European Medicines Agency (EMA) (17–18). The efficacy was limited due to lower protein expression as compared to a single AAV vector (19–20).

The long-term expression and efficacy in patients are questionable. Spark therapeutics reported that Luxturna had constant efficacy, but similar AAV2-RPE65 vector studies are indicative of progressive retinal degeneration (21–22). Long-term suppression of therapeutic proteins by transgene expression might aggravate a condition like wet AMD, and choroidal neovascularization (CNV) requires suppression of vascular endothelial growth factor (VEGF), which may aggravate choroidal vascular atrophy (15).

The cost of production of AAV gene therapies is exorbitant, which limits access to patients and creates an economic burden on healthcare systems (23).

11.2.2 Non-Viral Vectors

Oligonucleotides, naked plasmid DNA, and RNA are utilized as non-viral vectors in gene therapy and facilitate repeated administration due to lower risks of immunogenicity and insertional mutagenesis. They have a larger cargo capacity and are easily produced on large scales (15). However, transduction of naked DNA into the host cells is not effective unless it is used in combination with other chemical methods, such as DNA nanoformulations (24), polymers (25), lipid-based delivery systems (26), functionalized cell-penetrating peptides (27), or physical particles (28), and physical methods, such as iontophoresis (29), bioballistic (30), electrotransfection (31), magnetofection (32), sonoporation (33), and optoporation (34), to facilitate cellular and nuclear entry.

An in-depth understanding of the non-viral vectors mechanism of action still requires research. Recent research suggested that electroporation utilizes endocytosis instead of transient pore creation theory (35). Thus, methods to improve endocytosis could improve electrotransfection, and a delay in endosomal escape may protect naked plasmid DNA from endonuclease degradation (35).

Non-viral gene delivery will require continuous improvement with the use of plasmid engineering for the addition of a scaffold/matrix attachment region (S/MAR) that maintains replication while preventing epigenetic silencing (36). Minimizing CpG motifs and nonessential sequences from plasmid (minicircle DNA, Nanoplasmid) showed a reduction in gene silencing (15). Plasmid DNA with a combination of multiple transgenes in one vector can give an added advantage of multigene targeting in a disease like macular edema (15).

Antisense oligonucleotides (AONs), small interfering RNAs (siRNAs), and microRNA (miRNA) are also promising candidates for ophthalmic treatment. Fomivirsen (Vitravene) is the first AON to receive FDA approval as a cytomegalovirus retinitis treatment (37).

Clinical trials are underway for QR-110 (Sepofarsen), an AON for the treatment of patients with LCA10 with ciliopathy gene encoding centrosomal protein 290 (CEP290) point mutation and siRNAs for AMD, nonarteritic anterior ischemic optic neuropathy (NAION), and glaucoma treatment through targeting of the RT801 gene or caspase-2 (QPI-1007) (38).

Non-viral gene delivery requires delivery of gene therapy product into the system and a medical device (a pulse generator and/or electrodes or liposomes) for target facilitation and thus makes research and development and regulatory approval tricky (39).

TABLE 11.1
Gene Therapy Delivery Systems (15, 40)

Vector	Features	Advantages	Limitations
Viral Vectors			
Adenoviral vectors (Ad)	• Contains double-stranded DNA genome • Vector DNA does not integrate into the target cells • More than 50 human serotypes have been identified • Ad5 is widely used.	• It has the largest transgene capacity of up to 37 kb • It has high transduction efficiency in dividing and non-dividing cells	• Long-term expression limited to postmitotic/non-dividing cells • It can elicit a strong antiviral inflammatory and immune response

Vector	Features	Advantages	Limitations
Adeno-associated viral vectors (AAV)	• Contains single-stranded DNA genome • It is derived from replication-defective non-pathogenic parvovirus • Vector DNA does not integrate into the target cells • 12 naturally occurring serotypes and more than 100 variants have been identified in primates • AAV2, AAV5, and AAV8 have been widely researched in ocular gene therapy	• It has long-term transgene expression in non-dividing cells • AAV1, AAV2, AAV4, AAV5, AAV6, AAV7, AAV8, and AAV9 all display tropism for retinal tissue, including retinal pigment epithelium and photoreceptors	• Small capacity of ~3 kb of transgene DNA limits usefulness in many inherited retinal degenerations (e.g., Stargardt) • Long-term expression is confined to postmitotic/non-dividing cells • High incidence of preexisting immunity to AAV in humans may limit transduction capabilities, especially via an intravitreal route
Second-generation AAV	• Backbone of naturally occurring AAVs with altered capsid proteins • Designed (via rational design) or isolated (via directed evolution) to have greater transduction efficiency, altered tropism, and/or less immunogenicity compared to naturally occurring AAVs	• Vectors generated via directed evolution can easily cross biological barriers to target specific cell types (e.g., AAV2.7m8 crosses the internal limiting membrane following intravitreal injection) • Site-directed mutagenesis via rational design of AAV2, AAV8, and AAV9 capsids tyrosine residues can result in augment nuclear transport and transgene expression	• Capacity constraints and potential immune/inflammatory response remain, as with naturally occurring AAVs
Lentiviral vectors (LV)	• Single-stranded RNA genome • Vector DNA fits into target cell genome	• Low immunogenicity • Genomic integration permits prolonged expression of transgene even in dividing cells • Cargo space up to 10 kb	• Chances of insertional mutagenesis is increased due to random genomic integration • Transgene production yields are low
Non-Viral Vectors			
Non-viral gene delivery (chemical methods and physical methods)	• Liposome- and polymer-based nanoparticle carriers • Physical methods (e.g., electroporation, iontophoresis)	• Lower risk for immunogenicity compared to viral vectors • No risk of insertional mutagenesis	• Less transfection efficiency than viral vectors • Limited duration of effect due to lack of persistent gene expression

11.3 MOLECULAR APPROACHES FOR GENE THERAPY

The gene therapy utilizes the molecular approaches for gene targeting discussed in the following sections.

11.3.1 Gene Augmentation

This is also referred to as gene replacement or addition and is widely researched for targeting monogenic recessive disorders/X-linked inherited diseases by introducing functional genes to replace the dysfunctional host gene. It provides long-lasting single-dose therapy due to continuous transgene expression. Clinical trials of choroideremia, achromatopsia, Leber hereditary optic neuropathy (LHON), and RP have employed the gene augmentation approach and deployed a recombinant AAV vector (21).

11.3.2 Specific Gene Targeting

DNA or RNA segments are employed for the incorporation of new genes or obstruction of gene expression (33).

11.3.3 Genetic Modification

This utilizes clustered regularly interspaced short palindromic repeats (CRISPR) to restore mutated genes so that they attain normal functionality and sequence. It enables in situ gene editing, which increases the efficacy by providing long-lasting single-dose therapy. CRISPR is utilized in the modeling of diseases like RP (via deletion of the Rho gene) and CNV (suppression of VEGFA or HIF1A by AAV CRISPR-mediated modulation and CRISPR nucleases) (33).

11.4 ROUTES OF VECTOR DELIVERY

The target tissue in ophthalmic gene therapy is the photoreceptor layer and RPE. The anatomically internal limiting membrane (ILM), choroid, and sclera protect the photoreceptor layer, and RPE acts as a rate-limiting factor for conventional drug delivery systems, and thus, surgical interventions are utilized in gene therapy for the targeted delivery of gene therapeutic material (41–42).

11.5 OPHTHALMIC INDICATIONS ADDRESSED BY GENE THERAPY

Gene therapy has been researched for the conditions discussed in the following sections.

11.5.1 Hereditary Diseases

11.5.1.1 Retinitis Pigmentosa

RP is a rare, hereditary disorder with biphasic rod–cone progressive pathology causing loss of rods and eventually cones, impairing night and peripheral vision and ultimately causing day vision loss (41).

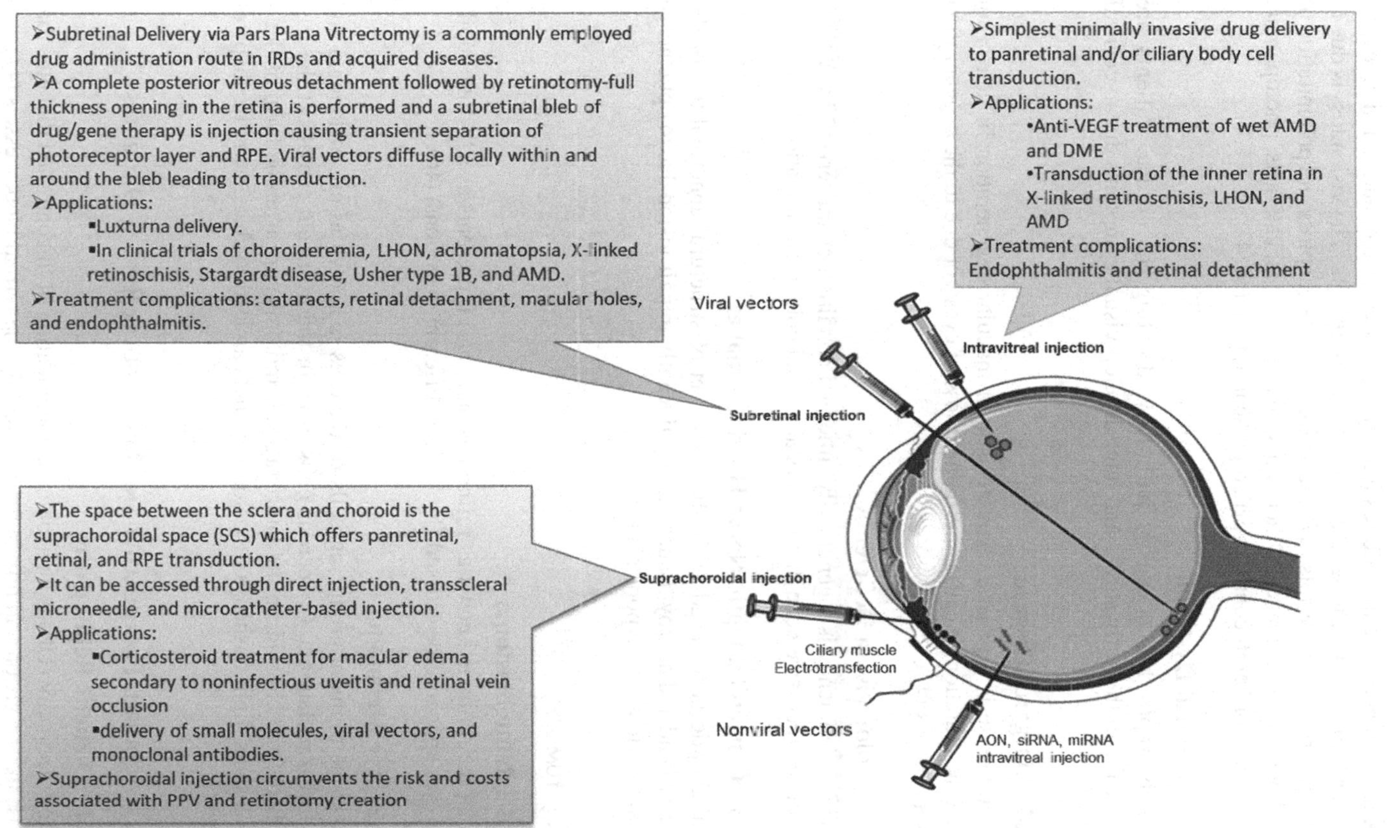

➢Subretinal Delivery via Pars Plana Vitrectomy is a commonly employed drug administration route in IRDs and acquired diseases.
➢A complete posterior vitreous detachment followed by retinotomy-full thickness opening in the retina is performed and a subretinal bleb of drug/gene therapy is injection causing transient separation of photoreceptor layer and RPE. Viral vectors diffuse locally within and around the bleb leading to transduction.
➢Applications:
▪Luxturna delivery.
▪In clinical trials of choroideremia, LHON, achromatopsia, X-linked retinoschisis, Stargardt disease, Usher type 1B, and AMD.
➢Treatment complications: cataracts, retinal detachment, macular holes, and endophthalmitis.
➢Simplest minimally invasive drug delivery to panretinal and/or ciliary body cell transduction.
➢Applications:
•Anti-VEGF treatment of wet AMD and DME
•Transduction of the inner retina in X-linked retinoschisis, LHON, and AMD
➢Treatment complications: Endophthalmitis and retinal detachment
Viral vectors
Intravitreal injection
Subretinal injection
➢The space between the sclera and choroid is the suprachoroidal space (SCS) which offers panretinal, retinal, and RPE transduction.
➢It can be accessed through direct injection, transscleral microneedle, and microcatheter-based injection.
➢Applications:
▪Corticosteroid treatment for macular edema secondary to noninfectious uveitis and retinal vein occlusion
▪delivery of small molecules, viral vectors, and monoclonal antibodies.
➢Suprachoroidal injection circumvents the risk and costs associated with PPV and retinotomy creation
Suprachoroidal injection
Ciliary muscle
Electrotransfection
Nonviral vectors
AON, siRNA, miRNA
intravitreal injection

FIGURE 11.1 Routes of vector delivery.

11.5.1.2 Leber Congenital Amaurosis

LCA is a rare genetic eye disorder caused by the inheritance of autosomal recessive genetic conditions leading to severe loss of vision in infants. The vision loss is due to retinal degeneration that results in dysfunction of photoreceptors and precipitation of an inability to capture images. Other signs, like strabismus, cataracts, photophobia, nystagmus, and/or keratoconus, are also present in patients (43).

11.5.1.3 Corneal Dystrophy

Corneal dystrophy has a genetic pathology affecting the cornea. Patients are asymptomatic in the early stages and later develop visual symptoms due to corneal erosion (9).

11.5.1.4 Stargardt Disease

Stargardt disease is a genetic characteristic of macular degeneration in lieu of an *ABCA4* gene mutation. It causes permanent loss of eyesight due to the degeneration of rods and cones (43).

11.5.1.5 Color Vision Deficiency

Color vision deficiency is a genetically inherited condition characterized by a common X-linked recessive gene that confers abnormal color discrimination (44).

11.5.1.6 Congenital Optic Nerve Head Anomalies

Congenital optic nerve head anomalies are a set of structural abnormalities of the optic nerve head and nearby tissues that significantly impair vision due to optic nerve pitting and optic nerve hypoplasia (45).

11.5.2 Tumors

11.5.2.1 Retinoblastoma

Cancer of the retina is known as retinoblastoma, and it presents as a "white pupil" and the eyes appear to be crossed (looking in different directions) (46).

11.5.2.2 Eye Melanoma

Cancer in the pigment-producing cells of the eyes is known as eye melanoma and also as uveal melanoma. Cancerous cells grow in the uvea and can affect the iris, ciliary body, and choroid. In the later stages, symptoms appear in the form of floating black spots, light flashes, and vision loss and can lead to changes in the shape of the pupil (1).

11.5.3 Acquired Proliferative and Neovascular Retinal Disorders

11.5.3.1 Diabetic Retinopathy

Diabetic retinopathy (DR) is an avoidable complication of uncontrolled diabetes that can cause loss of vision and blindness by affecting the retinal blood vessels (47).

11.5.3.2 Diabetic Macular Edema

DR leads to a complication known as diabetic macular edema (DME) that causes retinal thickening, accumulation of intraretinal fluid, and hyperpermeability of the retinal vasculature leading to vision loss in patients (48).

11.5.4. Keratoconus

Keratoconus gives rise to visual impairment due to gradual corneal thinning and steepening. The cornea becomes cone-shaped, which leads to refractive abnormalities, blurry vision, diplopia, impaired night vision, and visual acuity and can lead to myopia (49).

11.5.5 Glaucoma

Glaucoma leads to the development of permanent blindness. Initially, the retinal nerve and optic nerve are damaged, causing optic neuropathy. Intraocular pressure management may provide therapeutic relief. The drainage angle formed by the cornea and iris divide glaucoma into open-angle and angle-closure forms. Congenital glaucoma is a birth defect (50).

11.5.6 Cataract

A cataract primarily causes visual impairment due to development of a cloudy or opaque area in the eye lens. The disease presents itself as blurry vision, increased sensitivity to lights, decreased sensitivity to colors, and difficulty seeing at night. It can be corrected by cataract surgery (51).

11.5.7 Age-Related Macular Degeneration

AMD leads to permanent loss of central vision. Dry AMD leads to the accumulation of waste products of rods and cones in the RPE, which leads to the development of yellow spots, also known as drusen. Advanced stages of dry AMD also develop chorioretinal atrophy (52).

Wet AMD occurs due to CNV in which new abnormal blood vessels develop under the retina and cause localized macular edema or hemorrhage affecting a macular area or causing RPE detachment. If left untreated, it can lead to the development of a disciform scar under the macula (52).

11.5.8 Non-Arteritic Anterior Ischemic Optic Neuropathy

Small vessel infarction of the anterior optic nerve leads to the development of optic neuropathy, also identified as non-arteritic anterior ischemic optic neuropathy. Risk factors include old age, diabetes mellitus, obstructive sleep apnea, and hypertension. It causes loss of vision (53).

11.5.9 Noninfectious Uveitis

Noninfectious uveitis (NIU) is the major source of preventable blindness. Intraocular inflammation of the uvea (choroid, iris, and ciliary body) leads to inflammation owing to a T-cell–mediated autoimmune reaction. Symptoms include redness, eye pain, floaters, and light sensitivity (54).

TABLE 11.2
Ongoing Ocular Gene Therapy Clinical Trials (55)

Conditions	Targeted Gene	Vector	Route of Administration	Phases	NCT Number
Viral Vectors					
Advanced retinitis pigmentosa	Channelrhopodsin-2 (ChR2)	AAV2	Intravitreal	Phase I | Phase II	NCT02556736
X-Linked retinitis pigmentosa	Retinitis pigmentosa GTPase regulator (RPGR)	rAAV	Intravitreal	Phase I | Phase II	NCT04517149
Retinitis pigmentosa due to mutations in PDE6B gene	Rod cGMP phosphodiesterase 6 β subunit (or PDE6β)	AAV 2/5	Subretinal	Phase I | Phase II	NCT03328130
X-linked retinitis pigmentosa	Retinitis pigmentosa GTPase regulator (RPGR)	AAV 2/5	Subretinal	Phase I | Phase II	NCT03252847
RLBP1 retinitis pigmentosa	Retinaldehyde binding protein 1 (RLBP1)	AAV8	Subretinal	Phase I | Phase II	NCT03374657
Retinitis pigmentosa	Phosphodiesterase 6A (PDE6A)	rAAV	Subretinal	Phase I | Phase II	NCT04611503
X-linked retinitis pigmentosa	Retinitis pigmentosa GTPase regulator (RPGR)	rAAV2	Subretinal	Phase I | Phase II	NCT03316560
Non-syndromic retinitis pigmentosa	Channelrhopodsin-2 (ChR2)	rAAV2.7m8	Intravitreal	Phase I | Phase II	NCT03326336
X-linked retinitis pigmentosa	Retinitis pigmentosa GTPase regulator (RPGR)	AAV5	Subretinal	Phase III	NCT04671433
X-linked retinitis pigmentosa	Retinitis pigmentosa GTPase regulator (RPGR)	AAV5	Subretinal	Phase III	NCT04794101
Refractory retinoblastoma	-	Oncolytic AAV5	Intravitreal	Not applicable	NCT03284268
X-linked retinoschisis	Retinoschisin 1 (RS1)	AAV	Intravitreal	Phase I | Phase II	NCT02317887

Conditions	Targeted Gene	Vector	Route of Administration	Phases	NCT Number
X-linked retinoschisis	Retinoschisin 1 (RS1)	rAAV2	Intravitreal	Phase I | Phase II	NCT02416622
Non-Viral Vectors					
Autosomal dominant retinitis pigmentosa	P23H mutation in the RHO gene	Antisense oligonucleotide, no vectors needed for delivery	Intravitreal	Phase I | Phase II	NCT04123626
Retinitis pigmentosa	Exon 13 of the USH2A (Usherin) gene	Naked molecules, no vectors needed for delivery	Intravitreal	Phase I | Phase II	NCT03780257

11.6 CONCLUSIONS

The present review focuses on gene therapy, which will prove to be the "magic bullet" in the therapeutic arsenal with continued research and development in genetic engineering. Despite several scientific and clinical evidences, the success of gene therapy lies in exploration of quite a few other research areas. It will be a breakthrough success to develop a therapy that can eradicate blindness and other eye-related disorders completely.

REFERENCES

1. Samiy N. Gene therapy for retinal diseases. *J Ophthalmic Vis Res.* 2014;9(4):506–509.
2. Gene Therapy: The Future is Now. 2020 Apr:2020. Steve Silberberg, OD, Optometry Times Journal, April digital edition 2020, Volume 12, Issue 4.
3. Bennett J, Tanabe T, Sun D, Zeng Y, Kjeldbye H, Gouras P. et al. Photoreceptor cell rescue in retinal degeneration (rd) mice by in vivo gene therapy. *Nat Med* [Internet]. 1996 [cited 2021 Mar 28];2(6):649–654. Available from: https://pubmed.ncbi.nlm.nih.gov/8640555/.
4. Leber Congenital Amaurosis (LCA)—The American Society of Retina Specialists [Internet]. [cited 2021 Mar 27]. Available from: https://www.asrs.org/patients/retinal-diseases/37/leber-congenital-amaurosis-lca.
5. Leber Congenital Amaurosis—NORD (National Organization for Rare Disorders) [Internet]. [cited 2021 Mar 27]. Available from: https://rarediseases.org/rare-diseases/leber-congenital-amaurosis/.
6. Acland GM, Aguirre GD, Ray J, Zhang Q, Aleman TS, Cideciyan AV. et al. Gene therapy restores vision in a canine model of childhood blindness. *Nat Genet* [Internet]. 2001 [cited 2021 Mar 28];28(1):92–95. Available from: https://pubmed.ncbi.nlm.nih.gov/11326284/.
7. Maguire AM, High KA, Auricchio A, Wright JF, Pierce EA, Testa F. et al. Age-dependent effects of RPE65 gene therapy for Leber's congenital amaurosis: A phase 1 dose-escalation trial. *Lancet* [Internet]. 2009 [cited 2021 Mar 28];374(9701):1597–1605. Available from: https://pubmed.ncbi.nlm.nih.gov/19854499/.

8. FDA Approves Novel Gene Therapy to Treat Patients with a Rare Form of Inherited Vision Loss | FDA [Internet]. [cited 2021 Mar 28]. Available from: https://www.fda.gov/news-events/press-announcements/fda-approves-novel-gene-therapy-treat-patients-rare-form-inherited-vision-loss.
9. Gavrilova NA, Tishchenko OI, Zinov'eva AV. Results and possible prospects of genetic technology in ophthalmology (literature review). Part I. *Oftalmol Zh.* 2021;90(1):70–75.
10. Ramachandran PS, Lee V, Wei Z, Song JY, Casal G, Cronin T, et al. *Evaluation of dose and safety of AAV7m8 and AAV8BP2 in the non-human primate retina* [Internet]. Vol. 28, Human Gene Therapy. Mary Ann Liebert Inc.; 2017 [cited 2021 Mar 28]. pp. 154–167. Available from: https://pubmed.ncbi.nlm.nih.gov/27750461/.
11. Maguire AM, Simonelli F, Pierce EA, Pugh EN, Mingozzi F, Bennicelli J, et al. Safety and efficacy of gene transfer for leber's congenital amaurosis. *N Engl J Med* [Internet]. 2008 May 22 [cited 2021 Mar 28];358(21):2240–2248. Available from: https://pubmed.ncbi.nlm.nih.gov/18441370/.
12. Hauswirth WW, Aleman TS, Kaushal S, Cideciyan AV., Schwartz SB, Wang L, et al. Treatment of leber congenital amaurosis due to RPE65 mutations by ocular subretinal injection of adeno-associated virus gene vector: Short-term results of a phase I trial. *Hum Gene Ther* [Internet]. 2008 Oct 1 [cited 2021 Mar 28];19(10):979–990. Available from: https://pubmed.ncbi.nlm.nih.gov/18774912/.
13. Jacobson SG, Cideciyan A V., Ratnakaram R, Heon E, Schwartz SB, Roman AJ, et al. Gene therapy for leber congenital amaurosis caused by RPE65 mutations: Safety and efficacy in 15 children and adults followed up to 3 years. *Arch Ophthalmol* [Internet]. 2012 Jan [cited 2021 Mar 28];130(1):9–24. Available from: https://pubmed.ncbi.nlm.nih.gov/21911650/.
14. Simonelli F, Maguire AM, Testa F, Pierce EA, Mingozzi F, Bennicelli JL, et al. Gene therapy for leber's congenital amaurosis is safe and effective through 1.5 years after vector administration. *Mol Ther* [Internet]. 2010 Mar [cited 2021 Mar 28];18(3): 643–650. Available from: /pmc/articles/PMC2839440/.
15. Bordet T, Behar-Cohen F. Ocular gene therapies in clinical practice: Viral vectors and nonviral alternatives. *Drug Discov Today* [Internet]. 2019;24(8):1685–1693. Available from: https://doi.org/10.1016/j.drudis.2019.05.038.
16. Grieger JC, Samulski RJ. Packaging capacity of adeno-associated virus serotypes: Impact of larger genomes on infectivity and postentry steps. *J Virol* [Internet]. 2005 Aug 1 [cited 2021 Mar 29];79(15):9933–9944. Available from: https://pubmed.ncbi.nlm.nih.gov/16014954/.
17. Maddalena A, Tornabene P, Tiberi P, Minopoli R, Manfredi A, Mutarelli M. et al. Triple vectors expand AAV transfer capacity in the retina. *Mol Ther* [Internet]. 2018 Feb 7 [cited 2021 Mar 29];26(2):524–541. Available from: https://pubmed.ncbi.nlm.nih.gov/29292161/.
18. Medicines Agency E. Public summary of opinion on orphan designation [Internet]. 2015 [cited 2021 Mar 29]. Available from: www.ema.europa.eu/contact.
19. Lopes VS, Boye SE, Louie CM, Boye S, Dyka F, Chiodo V. et al. Retinal gene therapy with a large MYO7A cDNA using adeno-associated virus. *Gene Ther* [Internet]. 2013 Aug [cited 2021 Mar 29];20(8):824–833. Available from: https://pubmed.ncbi.nlm.nih.gov/23344065/.
20. Trapani I, Colella P, Sommella A, Iodice C, Cesi G, de Simone S, et al. Effective delivery of large genes to the retina by dual AAV vectors. *EMBO Mol Med* [Internet]. 2014 Feb [cited 2021 Mar 29];6(2):194–211. Available from: https://pubmed.ncbi.nlm.nih.gov/24150896/.
21. Cideciyan AV., Jacobson SG, Beltran WA, Sumaroka A, Swider M, Iwabe S, et al. Human retinal gene therapy for Leber congenital amaurosis shows advancing retinal degeneration despite enduring visual improvement. *Proc Natl Acad Sci U S A* [Internet]. 2013 Feb 5 [cited 2021 Mar 29];110(6). Available from: https://pubmed.ncbi.nlm.nih.gov/23341635/.

22. Jacobson SG, Cideciyan AV, Roman AJ, Sumaroka A, Schwartz SB, Heon E, et al. Improvement and decline in vision with gene therapy in childhood blindness. *N Engl J Med* [Internet]. 2015 May 14 [cited 2021 Mar 29];372(20):1920–1926. Available from: http://www.nejm.org/doi/10.1056/NEJMoa1412965.
23. Kaemmerer WF. How will the field of gene therapy survive its success? *Bioeng Transl Med* [Internet]. 2018 May [cited 2021 Mar 29];3(2):166–177. Available from: /pmc/articles/PMC6063870/.
24. Wang R, Gao Y, Liu A and Zhai G. A review of nanocarrier-mediated drug delivery systems for posterior segment eye disease: Challenges analysis and recent advances [Internet]. *Journal of Drug Targeting. Taylor and Francis Ltd.* 2021 [cited 2021 Mar 29]. Available from: https://www.tandfonline.com/doi/abs/10.1080/1061186X.2021.1878366.
25. Tsai CH, Wang PY, Lin IC, Huang H, Liu GS, Tseng CL. Ocular drug delivery: Role of degradable polymeric nanocarriers for ophthalmic application [Internet]. *International Journal of Molecular Sciences. MDPI AG.* 2018 [cited 2021 Mar 29];19:2830. Available from: /pmc/articles/PMC6164366/.
26. Battaglia L, Serpe L, Foglietta F, Muntoni E, Gallarate M, Del Pozo Rodriguez A, et al. *Application of lipid nanoparticles to ocular drug delivery* [Internet]. Vol. 13. Expert Opinion on Drug Delivery. Taylor and Francis Ltd; 2016 [cited 2021 Mar 29]. pp. 1743–1757. Available from: https://pubmed.ncbi.nlm.nih.gov/27291069/.
27. Reissmann S, Filatova MP. New generation of cell-penetrating peptides: Functionality and potential clinical application. *J Pept Sci* [Internet]. 2021 Feb 21 [cited 2021 Mar 29];e3300. Available from: https://onlinelibrary.wiley.com/doi/10.1002/psc.3300.
28. Masse F, Ouellette M, Lamoureux G, Boisselier E. *Gold nanoparticles in ophthalmology* [Internet]. Vol. 39, Medicinal Research Reviews. John Wiley and Sons Inc.; 2019 [cited 2021 Mar 29]. pp. 302–327. Available from: https://pubmed.ncbi.nlm.nih.gov/29766541/.
29. Souied EH, Reid SNM, Piri NI, Lerner LE, Nusinowitz S, Farber DB. Non-invasive gene transfer by iontophoresis for therapy of an inherited retinal degeneration. *Exp Eye Res* [Internet]. 2008 Sep [cited 2021 Mar 29];87(3):168–175. Available from: https://pubmed.ncbi.nlm.nih.gov/18653181/.
30. Sharma A, Tandon A, Tovey JCK, Gupta R, Robertson JD, Fortune JA, et al. Polyethylenimine-conjugated gold nanoparticles: Gene transfer potential and low toxicity in the cornea. *Nanomedicine Nanotechnology, Biol Med* [Internet]. 2011 Aug [cited 2021 Mar 29];7(4):505–513. Available from: /pmc/articles/PMC3094737/.
31. Cervia LD, Yuan F. *Current progress in electrotransfection as a nonviral method for gene delivery* [Internet]. Vol. 15, Molecular Pharmaceutics. American Chemical Society; 2018 [cited 2021 Mar 29]. pp. 3617–3624. Available from: /pmc/articles/PMC6123289/.
32. Czugala M, Mykhaylyk O, Böhler P, Onderka J, Stork B, Wesselborg S, et al. Efficient and safe gene delivery to human corneal endothelium using magnetic nanoparticles. *Nanomedicine* [Internet]. 2016 Jul 1 [cited 2021 Mar 29];11(14):1787–1800. Available from: https://pubmed.ncbi.nlm.nih.gov/27388974/.
33. Wan C, Li F, Li H. *Gene therapy for ocular diseases meditated by ultrasound and microbubbles (review)* [Internet]. Vol. 12, Molecular Medicine Reports. Spandidos Publications; 2015 [cited 2021 Mar 29]. pp. 4803–4814. Available from: /pmc/articles/PMC4581786/.
34. Batabyal S, Kim Y-T, Mohanty S. Ultrafast laser-assisted spatially targeted optoporation into cortical axons and retinal cells in the eye. *J Biomed Opt* [Internet]. 2017 Jun 29 [cited 2021 Mar 29];22(6):060504. Available from: https://pubmed.ncbi.nlm.nih.gov/28662241/.

35. Cervia LD, Chang C-C, Wang L, Yuan F. Distinct effects of endosomal escape and inhibition of endosomal trafficking on gene delivery via electrotransfection. Ceña V, editor. *PLoS One* [Internet]. 2017 Feb 9 [cited 2021 Mar 29];12(2):e0171699. Available from: https://dx.plos.org/10.1371/journal.pone.0171699.
36. Koirala A, Conley SM, Naash MI. Episomal maintenance of S/MAR-containing non-viral vectors for RPE-based diseases. *Adv Exp Med Biol* [Internet]. 2014 [cited 2021 Mar 29];801:703–709. Available from: https://pubmed.ncbi.nlm.nih.gov/24664761/.
37. Cideciyan AV., Jacobson SG, Drack AV., Ho AC, Charng J, Garafalo AV, et al. Effect of an intravitreal antisense oligonucleotide on vision in Leber congenital amaurosis due to a photoreceptor cilium defect. *Nat Med* [Internet]. 2019 Feb 1 [cited 2021 Mar 29];25(2):225–228. Available from: https://pubmed.ncbi.nlm.nih.gov/30559420/.
38. Nguyen QD, Schachar RA, Nduaka CI, Sperling M, Basile AS, Klamerus KJ, et al. Phase 1 dose-escalation study of a siRNA targeting the RTP801 gene in age-related macular degeneration patients. *Eye* [Internet]. 2012 May 25 [cited 2021 Mar 29];26(8): 1099–1105. Available from: www.clinicaltrials.gov.
39. Tsourounis M, Stuart J, Smith MA, Toscani M, Barone J. Challenges in the development of drug/device and biologic/device combination products in the United States and European Union: A summary from the 2013 DIA meeting on combination products. *Ther Innov Regul Sci* [Internet]. 2015 Mar 15 [cited 2021 Mar 29];49(2):239–248. Available from: https://link.springer.com/article/10.1177/2168479014553033.
40. Retinal Physician—Vector Considerations for Ocular Gene Therapy [Internet]. [cited 2021 Mar 28]. Available from: https://www.retinalphysician.com/issues/2020/special-edition-2020/vector-considerations-for-ocular-gene-therapy.
41. Xu D, Khan MA, Ho AC. Creating an ocular biofactory. *Asia-Pacific J Ophthalmol.* 2021;Publish Ah:5–11.
42. Rodrigues GA, Shalaev E, Karami TK, Cunningham J, Slater NKH, Rivers HM. *Pharmaceutical development of AAV-based gene therapy products for the eye* [Internet]. Vol. 36, Pharmaceutical Research. Springer New York LLC; 2019 [cited 2021 Mar 30]. Available from: https://pubmed.ncbi.nlm.nih.gov/30591984/.
43. Ku CA, Pennesi ME. The new landscape of retinal gene therapy. *Am J Med Genet Part C Semin Med Genet.* 2020;184(3):846–59.
44. El Moussawi Z, Boueiri M, Al-Haddad C. *Gene therapy in color vision deficiency: A review* [Internet]. International Ophthalmology. Springer Science and Business Media B.V.; 2021 [cited 2021 Mar 30]. pp. 1–11. Available from: https://link.springer.com/article/10.1007/s10792-021-01717-0.
45. Amador-Patarroyo MJ, Pérez-Rueda MA, Tellez CH. *Congenital anomalies of the optic nerve* [Internet]. Vol. 29, Saudi Journal of Ophthalmology. Elsevier; 2015 [cited 2021 Mar 30]. pp. 32–38. Available from: /pmc/articles/PMC4314572/.
46. National Cancer Institute. *Retinoblastoma treatment (PDQ®): Patient version* [Internet]. PDQ Cancer Information Summaries. National Cancer Institute (US); 2002 [cited 2021 Mar 30]. Available from: http://www.ncbi.nlm.nih.gov/pubmed/26389197.
47. Kumar A, Agarwal D, Kumar A. *Diabetic retinopathy screening and management in India: Challenges and possible solutions* [Internet]. Vol. 69, Indian Journal of Ophthalmology. Wolters Kluwer Medknow Publications; 2021 [cited 2021 Mar 30]. p. 479–81. Available from: /pmc/articles/PMC7942083/.
48. Browning D, Stewart M, Lee C. Diabetic macular edema: Evidence-based management. *Indian J Ophthalmol* [Internet]. 2018 Dec 1 [cited 2021 Mar 30];66(12):1736. Available from: http://www.ijo.in/text.asp?2018/66/12/1736/245608.
49. Crahay F-X, Debellemanière G, Tobalem S, Ghazal W, Moran S, Gatinel D. Quantitative comparison of corneal surface areas in keratoconus and normal eyes. *Sci Rep* [Internet]. 2021 Dec 25 [cited 2021 Mar 31];11(1):6840. Available from: http://www.nature.com/articles/s41598-021-86185-3.

50. Stein JD, Khawaja AP, Weizer JS. *Glaucoma in adults—screening, diagnosis, and management: A review* [Internet]. Vol. 325, JAMA—Journal of the American Medical Association. American Medical Association; 2021 [cited 2021 Mar 31]. pp. 164–174. Available from: https://jamanetwork.com/journals/jama/fullarticle/2774838.
51. Chen PW, Liu PPS, Lin SM, Wang JH, Huang HK, Loh CH. Cataract and the increased risk of depression in general population: A 16-year nationwide population-based longitudinal study. *Sci Rep* [Internet]. 2020 Dec 1 [cited 2021 Mar 31];10(1):1–8. Available from: https://doi.org/10.1038/s41598-020-70285-7.
52. Han X, Gharahkhani P, Mitchell P, Liew G, Hewitt AW, MacGregor S. Genome-wide meta-analysis identifies novel loci associated with age-related macular degeneration. *J Hum Genet* [Internet]. 2020 Aug 1 [cited 2021 Mar 31];65(8):657–665. Available from: https://www.nature.com/articles/s10038-020-0750-x.
53. Berry S, Lin W V., Sadaka A, Lee AG. *Nonarteritic anterior ischemic optic neuropathy: Cause, effect, and management* [Internet]. Vol. 9, Eye and Brain. Dove Medical Press Ltd.; 2017 [cited 2021 Mar 31]. pp. 23–28. Available from: /pmc/articles/PMC5628702/.
54. Yeh S, Khurana RN, Shah M, Henry CR, Wang RC, Kissner JM, et al. Efficacy and safety of suprachoroidal CLS-TA for macular edema secondary to noninfectious uveitis: Phase 3 randomized trial. In: *Ophthalmology* [Internet]. Elsevier Inc.; 2020 [cited 2021 Mar 30]. pp. 948–955. Available from: https://pubmed.ncbi.nlm.nih.gov/32173113/.
55. Search of: Gene therapy | Ocular—List Results—ClinicalTrials.gov [Internet]. [cited 2021 Mar 31]. Available from: https://clinicaltrials.gov/ct2/results?recrs=&cond=Ocular&term=Gene+therapy&cntry=&state=&city=&dist.

12 COVID-19 Vaccine Development and Applications

Kavita Trimal and Kalpana Joshi

CONTENTS

12.1 INTRODUCTION

In December 2019, a novel coronavirus now known as severe acute respiratory syndrome coronavirus 2 (SARS-CoV-2) emerged in Wuhan, a city in the Hubei Province of China, and rapidly spread globally due to the high transmission rate, which resulted in a global pandemic. On February 11, 2020, the World Health Organization named the disease as coronavirus disease 2019 (COVID-19) and declared a pandemic on March 11, 2020. The dramatic increase in the virus's spread and the mortality rate due to the high transmissibility and pathogenicity of SARS-CoV-2 meant there was an urgent need for safe and efficacious vaccines against COVID-19 to prevent the deadly infection and for the induction of herd immunity to successfully manage the pandemic. Globally, many academic, government, bio-pharma, and non-profit organizations have collaborated to tackle this crisis. Developments of vaccines against SARS-CoV-2 that elicit protective immune responses are essential to prevent and mitigate the morbidity and mortality caused by SARS-CoV-2 infection.

DOI: 10.1201/9781003186069-12

The immune system plays a pivotal role in the pathogenesis of SARS-CoV-2 infection; thus, understanding the immune response and the underlying mechanism is very crucial to develop successful prophylactic vaccines against the virus. The development of an effective vaccine requires a proper antigen and the delivery system to achieve robust cellular and humoral immune responses following vaccination. In case of SARS-CoV-2, previous experiences with severe acute respiratory syndrome coronavirus (SARS-CoV) and Middle East respiratory syndrome coronavirus (MERS-CoV) have enabled rapid development of vaccine candidates. The major antigenic target for SARS-CoV-2 is a spike glycoprotein (S) or its receptor-binding domain (RBD), which mediates viral entry into the host cells. Thus, antibodies against the S protein are capable of neutralizing the virus, suggesting S protein as a promising target for vaccination against SARS-CoV-2.

As of August 2021, several vaccines had become available for use in different parts of the world, more than 20 vaccine candidates have been approved for emergency use, 110 are in human trials, and more than 184 are in preclinical trials (1–2). These COVID-19 vaccine candidates can be mainly classified into two broad categories: protein-based or gene-based vaccines. Protein-based vaccines deliver the immune system–stimulating antigen to the body, whereas gene-based vaccines take different approach—they carry the gene instruction to the host cells to produce a viral antigen and safely trigger an immune response by using the cell's machinery, which more closely mimics a natural infection. For the successful transfer of gene instruction to the host cells, effective gene delivery systems are required. In this current situation of an pandemic outbreak, many companies and research institutions have utilized various viral and non-viral gene delivery systems in designing effective COVID-19 vaccines.

The purpose of this chapter is to highlight the various strategies applied and steps followed for fast-track development of COVID-19 vaccines under different platforms and their applications. In this chapter we also discuss some gene delivery systems and their applications in gene-based COVID-19 vaccine development.

12.2 STRATEGIES FOR COVID-19 VACCINE DEVELOPMENT

The best solution to overcome this pandemic is the development of suitable and effective vaccines. To develop effective SARS-CoV-2 vaccines, a multifaceted strategic approach for vaccine development is being attempted worldwide. Understanding the molecular structure of the virus, disease pathogenesis, host immune response triggered by SARS-CoV-2, and previous research experience of SARS-CoV and MERS-CoV vaccines paved the way for rapid development of COVID-19 vaccines.

SARS-CoV-2 belongs to the Coronavirdae family and Beta-coronavirus genus. SARS-CoV-2 is an enveloped, positive-sense, single-stranded RNA virus with a 30-kb genome, with 14 open-reading frames (ORFs) consisting of four major structural proteins, namely the spike (S) protein, which mediates viral entry into the host cells; the envelope (E) and membrane (M) proteins, which are critical components for the production of coronavirus-like particles; and the nucleocapsid (N) protein, which forms the capsid to pack genomic RNA (3). The RBD of the S1 subunit of the S protein interacts with human angiotensin-converting enzyme 2 (ACE2), followed by membrane fusion mediated by the S2 subunit allowing the delivery of the viral genome into the cellular cytoplasm. Thus, the S protein is a critical component of SARS-CoV-2 for host cellular infection (4). Also, neutralizing antibodies generated in COVID-19 patients were found to be mostly targeting the epitopes within S protein; therefore, S protein is considered a primary target for vaccine design against SARS-CoV-2 (5).

COVID-19 is mainly transmitted through respiratory droplets from coughing and sneezing; however, some other transmission routes have also been described, such as conjunctival mucosa or alimentary transmission (6). Severe and deadly forms of disease pathogenesis have been reported. Underlying health conditions seen in the infected patients were life-threatening, and thus, the COVID-19 pandemic represents an enormous threat to the elderly and immune-compromised patients, particularly those suffering from severe obesity, diabetes, arterial hypertension, asthma, or chronic kidney disease (7–8).

The elucidation of the molecular and cellular mechanisms behind the immune response triggered by SARS-CoV-2 will help to develop vaccines and therapeutic strategies to control the infection or to improve the clinical progression of patients. SARS-CoV-2 infection has an impact on both innate and adaptive immune responses. In some cases, the innate immune cells may contribute to the excessive inflammation and therefore to the disease progression. The inability to control the infection may result in dysregulated inflammatory responses that are potentially lethal. The antibody response particularly leads to the production of neutralizing antibodies to the S protein and to the nucleoprotein. S protein is also the main target of the majority of newly designed vaccines (9).

The first lethal coronavirus, SARS-CoV, emerged in 2002 in Guangdong Province, China (10). The second lethal coronavirus, MERS-CoV, emerged in Saudi Arabia in 2012, in South Korea in 2015, and again in Saudi Arabia in 2018 and is still circulating in the Middle East (11). Compared with SARS-CoV and MERS-CoV, SARS-CoV-2 is more transmissible and contagious (12). Even though COVID-19 is a novel disease, SARS and MERS-CoV research has helped investigators to understand how the host immune system may deal with viral infection and how the virus may evade such host responses (13). The genomic sequence analysis reveals SARS-CoV-2 shares approximately 79.5% sequence similarity with SARS-CoV and 50% with MERS-CoV (14). The genomic analysis also reveals similarities in SARS-CoV and SARS-CoV-2 S proteins, which directly bind to ACE2, while the S protein of MERS-CoV uses dipeptidyl peptidase-4 (DPP4) as its cellular receptor to enter target cells (15).

Based on the knowledge acquired on SARS-CoV and MERS-CoV vaccine development, several research groups were able to start SARS-CoV-2 vaccine development immediately after the outbreak. The target antigen selection and vaccine platform were supported by evidence from previous SARS-CoV and MERS-CoV vaccine development (16–17). The previous vaccine research carried out with SARS-CoV and MERS-CoV also helped to establish suitable animal models for vaccine efficacy testing (18–19). In previous experiments, many vaccines protected animals from a challenge with SARS-CoV or MERS-CoV, although many of them did not induce long-term immunity (20). Several S protein–based vaccines against SARS and MERS-CoV have been shown to elicit potent immune responses and protective effects in preclinical models (21–22). Furthermore, numerous studies have also demonstrated that the anti-S antibody can neutralize SARS and MERS-CoV and provides protective effects in humans as well (23–24). Taken together, these biological and clinical lessons learned from the basic research that was carried out for SARS-CoV and MERS-CoV has facilitated the rapid development of vaccine candidates for COVID-19.

12.3 STEPS AND PROCESSES INVOLVED IN COVID-19 VACCINE DEVELOPMENT

Vaccine development is highly imperative for preventing the spread of SARS-CoV-2 infection and reducing the morbidity and mortality of COVID-19. A successful COVID-19 vaccine should be extremely safe and pure and have high efficacy and potency rates. Typically, any vaccine development begins with exploratory and preclinical stages and progresses sequentially as phase 1, phase 2, and phase 3, followed by its licensure. Phase 4 studies help in continuous monitoring of the safety and immunogenicity of the candidate vaccines.

Generally, the conventional vaccine development pipeline usually takes up to 10 years or more—the increasing mortality rates due to COVID-19 infections resulted in the development of fast-track strategies for accelerated vaccine development. This urgent need led to many different approaches in vaccine development considerations, such as the use of unconventional vaccine platforms like a viral vector and nucleic acid vaccines (DNA and mRNA) due to their ability to be developed using sequence information alone (25). Bioinformatics tools also played critical roles in the acceleration of COVID-19 vaccine development (26). The clinical development process was accelerated by performing trials in parallel rather than following a linear sequence of steps. For example, parallel studies of screening trials at the equivalent of the phase 2 and phase 3 trials were initiated to reduce the time to develop a vaccine. Several vaccine candidates directly entered clinical trials before having preclinical data in animal models, and many vaccine trials used an integrated phase 1/2 or phase 2/3 approach to save time (27).

12.4 TYPES OF COVID-19 VACCINES DEVELOPED

To combat the devastating spread of SARS-CoV-2, many pharmaceutical companies and research laboratories have focused on the development of effective and safe vaccines and have come up with a number of candidates. These candidates can be classified into two broad categories: gene-based vaccines and protein-based vaccines. Gene-based vaccines deliver gene sequences that encode protein antigens that are produced by host cells. These include live attenuated virus vaccines, recombinant viral vector vaccines, and nucleic acid vaccines such as DNA and RNA vaccines, whereas protein-based vaccines directly deliver the immune system–stimulating antigen to the body, which include whole inactivated viruses, individual viral proteins or protein subunits, or virus-like particles (VLPs), all of which are manufactured in vitro. Recombinant vaccine vectors and nucleic acid vaccines are best suited for speed because they can be more easily adapted to platform manufacturing technologies in which upstream supply chains and downstream processes are the same for each product. Precision is achieved by knowing the atomic structure of the vaccine antigen and preserving the epitopes targeted by the vaccine.

12.4.1 Protein-Based Vaccines

12.4.1.1 Inactivated Vaccines

Inactivated/whole-cell killed vaccines are produced by growing a virus in cell culture, which is then inactivated by physical (heat) or chemical (formaldehyde) methods (28–29). This type of vaccine is more stable than live attenuated vaccines, but their limit is mainly related to the short duration of immune memory, which requires reminders of the immune system by multiple doses or an inoculation of higher amounts of vaccine. They are often combined with alum or another adjuvant in the vaccine to stimulate a robust immune response (30). Immune responses elicited by a SARS-CoV-2 inactivated vaccine would target not only the spike protein but also other antigens of the virus. Many inactivated COVID-19 vaccines are developed in China, India, and Kazakhstan (see Table 12.1).

12.4.1.2 Recombinant Protein-Based Vaccines

Recombinant protein-based vaccines are viral proteins that have been expressed in vitro in one of various systems, such as mammalian, insect, plant, and yeast cells, by using recombinant DNA technology. They can be administered intramuscularly. The production process of these types of vaccines does not require replication of a live virus. This form of vaccine involves whole proteins, a fragment of a protein, or an outer shell that mimics the coronavirus, such as VLPs. Subunit protein vaccines require multiple dosing regimens with adjuvants to achieve strong immune responses; comparatively, VLPs may induce a strong immune response. However, VLPs are usually difficult to manufacture, especially at a clinical grade on a large scale. Several recombinant protein-based COVID-19 vaccines have been developed, which include recombinant spike protein vaccines, recombinant RBD vaccines, and VLP vaccines (see Table 12.1).

12.4.2 Gene-Based Vaccines

12.4.2.1 Live Attenuated Vaccines

Traditional live-attenuated vaccines are produced by growing the virus in suboptimal conditions or through successive passage in cultures or by generating a genetically weakened version of the virus. These weakened viruses replicate in the recipient to induce an immune response but do not cause disease (31). These vaccines are very effective in stimulating both humoral and cellular immune responses and are efficacious in preventing infection. They can be administered intranasally or orally, which could induce a mucosal immunity based on secretory IgA and IgM. Several COVID-19 vaccines have been developed using this platform (see Table 12.2). However, safety concerns related to live attenuated vaccines include occurrence of

TABLE 12.1
Protein-Based COVID-19 Vaccines Approved for Emergency Use [Ref: (2)]

Sr. No.	Candidate Vaccines	Antigenic Target	Developer Organization	Vaccine Name	Route of Administration	Number of Doses	Developmental Stage
1.	Inactivated	Whole virus	Sinovac Biotech, China	CoronaVac	Intramuscular	2	Approved
			Beijing Institute of Biological Products and Sinopharm, China	BBIBP-CorV	Intramuscular	2	Approved
			Bharat Biotech, India and ICMR, India	Covaxin (BBV152)	Intramuscular	2	Approved
			Wuhan Institute of Biological Products and Sinopharm, China	WIBP-CorV	Intramuscular	2	Approved
			Chumakov Federal Scientific Center for Research and Development, Russia	CoviVac	Intramuscular	2	Approved
			Research Institute for Biological Safety Problems, Kazakhstan	QazVac/ QazCovid-in	Intramuscular	2	Approved
			Minhai Biotechnology Co./Kangtai Biological Products Co. Ltd., China	SARS-CoV-2 Vaccine (Vero Cells), Inactivated	Intramuscular	2	Approved
			Shifa Pharmed Industrial Group, Iran	COVIran Barekat	Intramuscular	2	Approved
			Chinese Academy of Medical Sciences, Institute of Medical Biology, China	-	Intramuscular	2	Approved
2.	Peptide vaccine	S Protein	Federal Budgetary Research Institution State Research Center of Virology and Biotechnology, Russia	EpiVacCorona	Intramuscular	2	Approved
		RBD of S Protein	Center for Genetic Engineering and Biotechnology, Cuba	Abdala (CIGB 66)	Intramuscular	3	Approved
		S Protein	Medigen Vaccine Biologics Corp., Taiwan and Dynavax, USA	MVC-COV1901	Intramuscular	2	Approved
		S Protein	Novavax, USA	NVX-CoV2373	Intramuscular	2	Phase 3
3.	Recombinant protein vaccine	RBD of S Protein	Anhui Zhifei Longcom Biopharmaceutical, Institute of Microbiology of the Chinese Academy of Sciences, China	ZF2001 (ZIFIVAX)	Intramuscular	1	Approved
		S protein	Sanofi Pasteur, France and GlaxoSmithKline, UK	Vidprevtyn	Intramuscular	2	Phase 3
4.	Virus-like particle (VLP)	S protein	Medicago, Canada and GlaxoSmithKline, UK	Co-VLP	Intramuscular	2	Phase 3

TABLE 12.2
Gene-Based COVID-19 Vaccines Under Different Developmental Stages and Approved for Emergency Use [Ref: (2)]

Sr. No.	Candidate Vaccines	Antigenic Target	Developer Organization	Vaccine Name	Route of Administration	Gene Delivery System	Number of Doses	Developmental Stage
1.	Live attenuated	Whole virus	Codagenix, USA and Serum Institute of India	COVI-VAC	Intranasal	-	1	Phase 1
			University of Melbourne and Murdoch Children's Research Institute, Australia	Bacillus Calmette-Guerin (BCG) vaccine	Intradermal	-	1	Phase 2/3
2.	Viral vector-based	S protein	CanSino Biologics, China	Ad5-nCoV/ PakVac / Convidicea	Intramuscular	Ad5	1	Approved
		S protein	Gamaleya National Research Centre, Russia	Sputnik V	Intramuscular	Ad26 and Ad5	2	Approved
		S protein	The Gamaleya Research Institute in Russia and Health Ministry of the Russian Federation, Russia	Sputnik Light	Intramuscular	Ad26	1	Approved
		S protein	Janssen Pharmaceutical and Johnson and Johnson (J&J), USA	Ad26.COV2.S/ JNJ-78436735	Intramuscular	Ad26	1	Approved
		S protein	University of Oxford, UK and AstraZeneca, UK	ChAdOx1 nCoV-19/ AZD1222/Vaxzevria/ Covishield	Intramuscular	Chimpanzee adenovirus ChAdOx1	2	Approved
		S protein	Biotechnology companies ReiThera, Italy and Leukocare, Germany and Univer Cells, Belgium	GRAd-COV2	Intramuscular	Replication-defective gorilla adenoviral vector (GRAd)	1/2	Phase 2/3

(Continued)

TABLE 12.2 (Continued)

Sr. No.	Candidate Vaccines	Antigenic Target	Developer Organization	Vaccine Name	Route of Administration	Gene Delivery System	Number of Doses	Developmental Stage
		S and N protein	ImmunityBio and NantKwest, Inc., USA	hAd5-S-Fusion+N-ETSD	Intranasal+ subcutaneous	Human adenovirus serotype 5 (hAd5)	1/2/3	Phase 2/3
		S protein	Cellid Co, South Korea	AdCLD-CoV19	Intramuscular	Replication-defective human adenovirus type 5/35	1	Phase 1/2a
		S protein	Israel Institute for Biological Research	IIBR-100	Intramuscular	Replicating vesicular stomatitis virus (rVSV)	1/2	Phase 1/2
		RBD protein	Xiamen University, China and University of Hong Kong and Beijing Wantai Biological Pharmacy, China	DelNS1-nCoV-RBD LAIV	Intranasal	Influenza virus	2	Phase 1/2
		S protein	Meissa Vaccines, Inc., USA	MV-014–212	Intranasal	Respiratory syncytial virus (RSV)	1/2	Phase 1
		S protein	Tetherex Pharmaceuticals Corporation, USA	SC-Ad6–1	Intramuscular/ Intranasal	Replicating single-cycle Ad6	1/2	Phase 1
		S protein	LaboratorioAvi-Mex, S.A. de C.V., Mexico and National Council of Science and Technology, Mexico	Recombinant NDV vectored vaccine for SARS-CoV-2	Intramuscular/ Intranasal	Newcastle disease virus (NDV)	2	Phase 1
		S protein	Bharat Biotech, India	BBV154	Intranasal	Non-replicating adenovirus	1/2	Phase 1
		S protein	Gritstone Oncology, USA and NIAID, USA	ChAdV68-S	Intramuscular	Chimpanzee adenovirus serotype 68 (ChAdV68)	2*	Phase 1

		S + T cell epitopes	Gritstone Oncology, USA and NIAID, USA	ChAdV68-S-TCE	Intramuscular	Chimpanzee adenovirus serotype 68 (ChAdV68)	2*	Phase 1
		S protein	University Medical Center Hamburg-Eppendorf, Germany	MVA-SARS-2-S	Intramuscular	Modified Vaccinia Ankara (MVA)	2	Phase 1
		S and N protein	City of Hope Medical Center, USA and National Cancer Institute, USA	COH04S1	Intramuscular	Synthetic modified Vaccinia Ankara (MVA)	2	Phase 1
		S and N protein	Vaxart, Inc., USA	VXA-CoV2–1	Oral	Non-replicating Ad5	2	Phase 1
3.	DNA	S protein	Zydus Cadila, India	ZyCoV-D	Intradermal	Needle-free injectors (Pharmajet)	3	Phase 3
		S protein	Inovio Pharmaceuticals, USA	INO-4800	Intradermal	Electroporation	2	Phase 2/3
		S protein	Takis and Rottapharm Biotech, Italy	COVID-eVax	Intramuscular	Injection and electroporation	2	Phase 1/2
		S protein	Genexine Consortium, South Korea	GX-19	Intradermal	PharmaJet's jet injector	2	Phase 1/2
		S protein	GeneOne Life Science, Inc., South Korea	GLS-5310	Intradermal	-	2	Phase 1/2
		S protein	Entos Pharmaceuticals, Inc. and Canadian Institutes of Health Research (CIHR), Canada and Aegis Life, Inc., USA	Covigenix VAX-001	Intramuscular	Needle injection	2	Phase 1/2
		S protein	AnGes Inc., Japan & Japan Agency for Medical Research and Development	AG0301-COVID-19	Intramuscular	Needle injection	2	Phase 1/2
		S protein	OncoSec, USA and Providence Cancer Institute, USA	CORVax12	Intramuscular/ intradermal	Injection and electroporation	2	Phase 1
		S protein	Symvivo, Canada	bacTRL-Spike	Oral	*Bifidobacterium longum*	1	Phase 1

(*Continued*)

TABLE 12.2 (Continued)

Sr. No.	Candidate Vaccines	Antigenic Target	Developer Organization	Vaccine Name	Route of Administration	Gene Delivery System	Number of Doses	Developmental Stage
4.	RNA	S protein	Pfizer, USA and BioNtech, Germany	BNT162b2	Intramuscular	Lipid nanoparticle	2	Approved
		S protein	Moderna, USA	mRNA-1273	Intramuscular	Lipid nanoparticle	2	Approved
		S protein	CureVac, Germany	CVnCoV vaccine (CV07050101)	Intramuscular	Lipid nanoparticle	2	Phase 2b/3
		RBD of S protein	Walvax Biotechnology Co., Ltd., China	ARCoV	Intramuscular	Lipid nanoparticle	1	Phase 3
		S protein	University of Washington, USA	HDT-301/HGCO19	Intramuscular	Lipid-Inorganic Nanoparticle (LION)	2	Phase 1/2
		S protein	Sanofi, France and Translate Bio, USA	MRT5500	Intramuscular	Lipid nanoparticle	2	Phase 1/2
		RBD of S protein	Fujita Health University, Japan and Elixirgen Therapeutics, Inc., USA	EXG-5003	Intradermal	–	–	Phase 1/2
		S protein	Daiichi Sankyo Co., Ltd., Japan	DS-5670a	Intramuscular	Lipid nanoparticle	2	Phase 1/2
		S protein	Arcturus Therapeutics Inc., USA and Duke-NUS Medical School, Singapore	ARCT-021 / LUNAR-COV19	Intramuscular	Lipid nanoparticle	1	Phase 1/2
		S protein	Gritstone Oncology, USA and NIAID, USA	SAM-LNP-S	Intramuscular	Lipid nanoparticle	1/2	Phase 1
		S + T cell epitopes	Gritstone Oncology, USA and NIAID, USA	SAM-LNP-S-TCE	Intramuscular	Lipid nanoparticle	1/2	Phase 1
		S protein	Providence Therapeutics and Canadian government, Canada	PTX-COVID-19-B	Intramuscular	Lipid nanoparticle	2	Phase 1

* Second dose is with self-amplifying mRNA–lipid nanoparticles–spike (SMA-S) or self-amplifying mRNA–lipid nanoparticles–spike T-cell epitopes (SAM-S-TCE).

mutations or recombination with the wild-type virus, which may lead to virulence reversal, so that this type of vaccine is not recommended for immune-compromised patients.

12.4.2.2 Viral Vector–Based Vaccines

Viral vector–based vaccines are constructed by engineering a viral vector to carry antigenic full-length or truncated viral surface protein-encoding genes and slowly replicate in the host cells. In this scenario, viral vectors serve as gene transfer vehicles generating immune responses by way of heterologous gene transfer (32). Because they are naturally immunogenic and well-characterized, they soon became the preferred vector of choice in vaccine development and translational research on gene therapy (33).

Commonly, these virus-based vaccines are injected intramuscularly; however, several projects are looking at administering the vaccine into the nose by inhalation to induce a mucosal immunity for neutralizing the virus and inhibiting its ability to enter the human body. Potential viral vectors include a broad spectrum of both DNA and RNA viruses. These viral vectors are divided into different categories depending on replication competency in host cells, which we have explained in detail, with its applications in COVID-19 vaccine development discussed later in this chapter (see Section 12.5.1).

12.4.2.3 DNA Vaccines

DNA vaccines consist of bacterial plasmids that encode vaccine antigens driven by eukaryotic promoters (34). Once injected into the muscle or skin, DNA plasmids enter human cells and then plasmid DNA induces the cell to produce the target protein temporarily. The produced antigens are either released by exosomes or apoptotic bodies, which leads to a recognition by antigen-presenting cells and further activates humoral or cytotoxic immune responses. Depending on the route of vaccine administration (intramuscular or intradermal), either myocytes or keratinocytes are addressed, but in antigen-presenting cells near the injection site (35). These vaccines are stable and can easily be produced in large amount in bacteria such as *Escherichia coli*, which is a major production advantage. However, DNA vaccines often have low immunogenicity, probably due to the low amount of administered plasmid DNA. To overcome this problem, DNA vaccines usually need some special delivery and transfection systems (36). Different strategies used for DNA vaccine delivery and its applications in COVID-19 vaccine development are explained in detail later in this chapter (see Section 12.5.2). The main safety concerns regarding use of this type of vaccine are possible integration of transfected DNA into somatic and/or germ cells of the host. In such cases, dysregulation of gene expression might occur and lead to various mutations, and currently there are not any Food and Drug Administration (FDA)–approved DNA vaccines for human use.

12.4.2.4 mRNA Vaccines

The messenger RNA (mRNA) encodes genetic information to produce an antigen, and thus, mRNA vaccines also lead to production of virus proteins in vivo. mRNA must be transported by various in vivo delivery systems to enter the human cell. Once administered, the mRNA is translated into the target protein, which is intended to elicit an immune response (37). The mRNA remains in the cell cytoplasm and does not enter into the nucleus; it also does not integrate into the recipient's genome, so there is no potential risk of infection or insertional mutagenesis (38). These vaccines are produced completely in vitro, which simplifies production. The immunogenicity and half-life of the mRNA in cells can be controlled through genetic modification and delivery methods. Moreover, mRNA vaccines can be administered repeatedly without any concern over antivector immunity. These vaccines can be designed and manufactured within a short time scale. However, mRNA vaccine development does have some limitations, such as the fact that mRNA without a proper formulation is unstable and can be quickly degraded, mRNA is impermeable to cell membranes and cannot be efficiently internalized into cytosol for translation, and mRNA could trigger the innate immune system and potentially induce cytotoxicity and inflammation. mRNA vaccines require a strict cold-chain condition for storage and distribution (39). To overcome these problems, it is crucial to design appropriate mRNA delivery systems that can protect mRNA from degradation; transport mRNA to the target cell cytosol; and increase mRNA vaccine efficacy, safety, and thermal stability. Although mRNA vaccines are a newly emerging technology, many SARS-CoV-2 mRNA vaccines are produced using various formulations and delivery systems that we discuss in detail later in this chapter (see Section 12.5.3).

12.5 APPLICATION OF GENE DELIVERY SYSTEMS IN COVID-19 VACCINE DEVELOPMENT

Gene delivery is the process of introducing foreign genetic material into host cells. The successful design of a gene delivery system requires complete understanding of the interactions between the delivery system and target cell. For effective gene delivery of foreign genetic material, gene delivery systems need to remain stable within the host cell and either integrate into the host genome or replicate independently to induce gene expression (40–41).

Gene delivery systems are broadly categorized into two types: viral-based and non-viral-based. Viral-based gene delivery systems consist of viruses that can be modified as replicating or non-replicating vectors (42). Adenoviruses, lentiviruses, and retroviruses are commonly used as viral gene delivery vectors (43). Non-viral gene delivery systems comprise all the physical and chemical systems except viral systems. One of the most important benefits of these systems is improved transfection. Non-viral systems are mainly categorized as physical or chemical types according to their preparation. Physical methods refer to delivery of the gene through the application of physical force to increase permeability of the cell membrane, and the most common physical methods are electroporation, microinjection, gene gun, ultrasound, and hydrodynamic applications. In contrast, in chemical methods, natural or synthetic carriers are utilized to deliver foreign genes into the host cells, and the most common chemical methods involve the use of liposomes, polymers, cationic lipid systems, and dendrimers as gene delivery systems (44–45).

In this current situation of a pandemic outbreak, many companies and research institutions have used various viral and non-viral gene delivery systems in designing effective COVID-19 vaccines. Here we will discuss the applications of these gene delivery systems in gene-based COVID-19 vaccine development.

12.5.1 Viral Vector–Based Vaccines

Viral vector–based vaccines have emerged as a promising alternative to conventional vaccine platforms. In this type of vaccine, a harmless, unrelated attenuated viral vector is used as a gene delivery system, which delivers genetic instructions (DNA) to host cells to produce a viral antigen and safely trigger an immune response by using host cell machinery (46–48). Depending on the type of vector used, viral vector–based vaccines are divided into three categories: non-replicating, self-replicating, and inactivated viral vector–based vaccines. Non-replicating viral vector are genetically engineered so that they are unable to replicate in infected host cells. The viral vector enters host cells and uses the cell machinery to express the viral protein that is the intended immune target; once this is accomplished, the viral vector is cleared (25, 46). Self-replicating viral vectors are derived from attenuated or vaccine strains of viruses. They are able to replicate in infected host cells and infect additional host cells, which further produce more viral antigen and a more robust immune response than non-replicating viral vectors. Inactivated viral vectors are genetically modified to express the target antigen but have been inactivated. They are safe because they cannot replicate even in the immune-compromised host. Commonly used potential viral vectors for vaccination studies are adenovirus (Ad), adeno-associated virus (AAV), lentiviruses, modified Vaccinia Ankara (MVA), influenza virus, measles virus, human parainfluenza virus, Sendai virus, vesicular stomatitis virus (VSV), and Newcastle disease virus (NDV). These viral vectors can be modified as replicating or non-replicating vectors (42).

Recent advances in viral vector–based vaccine technology offer several benefits over conventional vaccine platforms, including less stringent storage and handling conditions due to greater product stability, and they induce a more robust immune response. One drawback to viral vector vaccines is that preexisting immunity to the vector can diminish the immunogenicity and effectiveness of the vaccine (49). This can be avoided by using viral vectors that are uncommon in humans or vectors derived from animal viruses, such as a chimpanzee adenovirus, or vectors that do not induce self-immunity, such as AAV (50–51). In the challenge of rapid vaccine development for COVID-19, an Ad vector has been utilized, which is a non-replicating viral vector. Compared to other viral vectors, Ad vector–based vaccines are easy to design and produce on a mass scale. Ad vector–based vaccines are highly immunogenic and trigger strong antibody and cell-mediated immune system responses that are anticipated to provide longer-term protection (25, 47–48).

Most COVID-19 non-replicating viral vector–based vaccines are administered intramuscularly and are engineered to express the spike protein (see Table 12.2). In case of COVID-19 non-replicating viral vector–based vaccines, viral vectors such as adenovirus, measles vaccine strain vectors, influenza virus-based vectors, VSV, and NDV have been engineered to express the spike protein (52–53). NDV-based vector vaccines could also be given intranasally to stimulate mucosal immunity at the site of viral entry.

China-based CanSino Biologics have developed a vaccine candidate Ad5-nCoV/Convidicea to administer intramuscularly as a single dose. This vaccine is based on non-replicating adenovirus serotype 5 (Ad5) that expresses the SARS-CoV-2 full-length spike glycoprotein (49). In the interim analysis of an international phase 3 trial, Ad5-nCoV vaccine showed 65.7% efficacy against symptomatic COVID-19 and 90.98% efficacy against severe/critical COVID-19 (54). The data reported by phase 1 and phase 2 trials indicated that the Ad5-nCoV vaccine induces significant immune responses after a single dose in healthy adults age 18 and older (49, 55). Humoral responses against SARS-CoV-2 peaked at day 28 post-vaccination and rapid specific T-cell responses from day 14 post-vaccination (49). Phase 1 trial data of an aerosolized version of Ad5-nCoV reported that two doses of aerosolized Ad5-nCoV induced neutralizing antibody responses, similar to one dose of intramuscular injection. Furthermore, an aerosolized booster dose 28 days after the first intramuscular injection elicited strong IgG and neutralizing antibody responses (56).

The Gamaleya National Research Centre for Epidemiology and Microbiology (Russian Federation) developed a vaccine candidate Gam-COVID-Vac/Sputnik V (rAd26-S + rAd5-S) based on two non-replicating adenovirus vectors adenovirus 26 (Ad26) and adenovirus 5 (Ad5) that express a full-length spike glycoprotein of SARS-CoV-2. The vaccine is designed to be administered intramuscularly as an initial Ad26 vector dose followed by an Ad5 vector boosting dose 21 days to 3 months later (57). According to interim analysis of the phase 3 trial, efficacy of Gam-COVID-Vac is 91.6% against COVID-19 starting at 21 days after first dose and 100% efficacious against severe/critical COVID-19 in individuals 18 years and older (58). This vaccine has a good safety profile and induces a strong humoral and cellular immune response (57). The study of seroconversion and the neutralizing capacity of the Gam-COVID-Vac vaccine 21 days after a single dose showed a 94% seroconversion rate in naive individuals. Notably, a single dose of Gam-COVID-Vac vaccine induced a fast and robust immune response in seropositive participants, with higher neutralizing titers than those found in seronegative participants who received two doses (59).

Janssen Pharmaceutical and Johnson and Johnson (J&J) research teams in collaboration with Beth Israel Deaconess Medical Centre developed a vaccine candidate Ad26.COV2.S (5×10^{10} viral particles) to administer intramuscularly as a single dose. This vaccine is based on a non-replicating adenovirus 26 (Ad26) that expresses a full-length spike glycoprotein of SARS-CoV-2 (60). A single dose at 5×10^{10} viral particles was safe and induced excellent humoral and cellular immune responses in healthy individuals 18 to 85 years. The level of neutralizing and binding antibodies was high but slightly lower than those in convalescent plasma (61–62). A longitudinal evaluation study of Ad26.CoV2.S vaccine suggested that binding and neutralizing antibody responses were largely stable over eight months (63). Ad26.COV2.S vaccine efficacy against moderate to severe COVID-19 was 66.9% with onset at least 14 days after administration and 66.1% with onset 28 days after administration. Higher efficacy against severe/critical COVID-19 was observed: 77% with onset at least 14 days after administration and 85% with onset at least 28 days after administration (64). The onset of efficacy was evident as of 14 days after administration for moderate to severe disease and as of 7 days after administration for severe/critical disease. Efficacy continued to increase through approximately 8 weeks after administration, especially for severe/critical COVID-19. No evidence of declining efficacy was observed (64).

The University of Oxford, UK in collaboration with AstraZeneca, UK developed a vaccine candidate ChAdOx1 nCoV-19/AZD1222 (5×10^{10} viral particles) to administer intramuscularly as two doses 4 to 12 weeks apart. This vaccine is based on a non-replicating chimpanzee adenovirus vector encoding the spike glycoprotein of SARS-CoV-2 (65). The ChAdOx1 nCoV-19 vaccine elicits both humoral and cellular responses against SARS-CoV-2 without serious adverse reactions, but booster immunization was needed to enhance neutralizing antibody titers, and 28 days after the second dose neutralizing antibody titers were comparable to those detected in convalescent plasma (65). ChAdOx1 nCoV-19 has similar immunogenicity across all age groups after a boost dose (66). The interim results from a multinational phase 3 randomized trial showed that this vaccine had 70.4% efficacy against symptomatic COVID-19 at or after 14 days following the second dose (67). In a subsequent analysis of this trial, vaccine efficacy for symptomatic COVID-19 was 76% from 21 days after first dose until the second dose or day 90 after vaccination, with no significant waning of protection during this period (67). Additionally, vaccine efficacy after the second dose was higher in those with a longer prime-boost interval: 81.3% in those with a dosing interval of 12 weeks or more and 55.1% in those with an interval of less than 6 weeks (68). Largely similar outcomes were reported in primary analysis of a placebo-controlled trial conducted in the United States, Chile, and Peru (69). ChAdOx1 nCoV-19 vaccine efficacy against symptomatic COVID-19 was 76% starting 15 days or more after receiving two doses, four weeks apart, and this vaccine showed 100% efficacy against severe/critical disease and hospitalization. In addition, results were comparable across all age groups with 85% efficacy against symptomatic COVID-19 in adults 65 years and older. Further findings of a study on antibody response for a delayed second dose or a third booster dose showed that a longer delay before the second dose leads to an increased antibody titer after the second dose, and a third dose of ChAdOx1 nCoV-19 vaccine induces antibodies to a level that correlate with high efficacy after a second dose and boosts T-cell responses (70).

12.5.2 DNA-Based Vaccines

In response to the COVID-19 pandemic, DNA vaccines have been explored as one of the primary vaccine technologies (71). The DNA vaccine platform is highly suitable for rapid and large-scale manufacturing during infectious disease outbreaks due to its several advantages, including easy design and production, stability at a range of temperatures, and low production cost. However, the major challenge of DNA vaccines is the poor efficiency of DNA delivery into cells for antigen expression and consequently poor efficacy of the vaccines. To overcome this problem and to increase the DNA delivery efficiency, physical methods or chemical methods can be used. The physical methods include electroporation, high-pressure air stream, gold particle-coated DNA delivery by gene gun, microneedle array, and dermal patches. The chemical methods include liposomes, nanoparticles, cell-penetrating peptides, and virosomes (72).

Inovio Pharmaceuticals, USA developed a DNA vaccine candidate INO-4800 to administer intradermally through electroporation. This DNA vaccine is based on a plasmid pGX9501 encoding the SARS-CoV-2 spike protein as the antigen (73). The data reported by preclinical and phase 1 trials indicated that the INO-4800 vaccine elicits neutralizing antibodies as well as humoral and T-cell responses (73–74). Results from the phase 2 portion of the phase 2/3 INNOVATE trial showed INO-4800 to be well-tolerated and immunogenic in all age groups, which involved two doses of INO-4800 (1.0 mg and 2.0 mg) administered by intradermal injections and followed with electroporation in SARS-CoV-2–seronegative adults. Based on comparative immunogenicity outcomes, the 2.0-mg dose was selected for further phase 3 efficacy evaluation (75). Recently, Inovio announced a partnership with Advaccine Company to conduct a phase 3 portion of the INNOVATE trial (76).

Symvivo, Canada has developed a vaccine candidate, bacTRL-Spike, which is a lyophilized gel capsule of genetically modified probiotic bacteria *Bifidobacterium longum* that can colonize in the gut; bind directly to intestinal epithelial cells; and constitutively replicate, secrete, and deliver plasmid DNA molecules encoding the SARS-CoV-2 Spike protein antigen (77). bacTRL-Spike is orally delivered; room temperature stable; and currently being evaluated in a phase 1 trial for its safety, tolerability, and immunogenicity in healthy adult volunteers (78).

Genexine Consortium, South Korea has developed a vaccine candidate GX-19, which is delivered by PharmaJet's jet injector and uses a high-pressure narrow stream of fluid to penetrate the skin instead of a needle (79). An animal study demonstrated that the GX-19 vaccine induces a durable protective immune response (80). Further in a phase 1 trial, Genexine investigated the safety and immunogenicity of two recombinant COVID-19 DNA vaccine candidates, GX-19 and GX-19N, in healthy adults aged 19 to 55 years. GX-19 contains plasmid DNA encoding SARS-CoV-2 spike protein, and GX-19N contains plasmid DNA encoding SARS-CoV-2 RBD fold-on, N protein and spike protein. GX-19 trial participants received two vaccine injections (1.5 mg or 3.0 mg, 1:1 ratio) four weeks apart. GX-19N trial participants received two 3.0-mg vaccine injections four weeks apart. Preliminary results of the study showed that GX-19N is able to induce both humoral and cellular responses, more focused on T-cell responses rather than neutralizing antibody responses; thus, GX-19N was selected as a vaccine candidate for phase 2 immunogenicity trials (81).

AnGes, Inc., in collaboration with the Japan Agency for Medical Research and Development and Osaka University developed a plasmid DNA vaccine candidate AG0301-COVID-19 to administer intramuscularly by a needle injection (82). A phase 1/2 trial of 30 healthy adults of age 20–65 years for evaluating the safety and immunogenicity of two doses of intramuscular AG0301-COVID-19 (1 mg/2 mg) vaccine is underway at Osaka City University Hospital in Japan (83).

ZydusCadila, India also developed a plasmid DNA vaccine candidate, ZyCoV-D, to administer intradermally by needle-free injectors (84). The study in rhesus macaques demonstrated immunogenicity and protective efficacy of the vaccine. Phase 1 of a phase 1/2 trial indicated that the ZyCoV-D vaccine is safe, well-tolerated, and immunogenic (85). Recently, ZydusCadila announced that in an interim analysis the ZyCoV-D vaccine showed 66.6% efficacy (86).

12.5.3 mRNA-Based Vaccines

The mRNA vaccine is a powerful technology to fight against a pandemic outbreak such as COVID-19. mRNA vaccines are a new form of vaccines that trigger immune responses by transfecting synthetic mRNA encoding viral antigens into human cells. These types of vaccines have several advantages such as rapid development, high yields from in vitro transcription reactions without risk of infection, and insertional mutagenesis. However, one major challenge for effective application of mRNA vaccines lies in the delivery at both the micro and macro levels. mRNA is rapidly degraded by extracellular RNases, and it cannot penetrate cell membranes to be transcribed in the cytosol. Therefore, intracellular delivery is essential to protect it from RNase degradation and facilitate cellular uptake of mRNA. To date, various delivery methods have been developed, including physical delivery methods, cationic peptide protamine, and cationic lipid nanoparticles (LNPs) delivery and ex vivo loading of dendritic cells. Among these, LNPs seem to be the most appealing and commonly used tool (38, 87). Most of the COVID-19 mRNA vaccines developed are based on LNP delivery because LNPs efficiently encapsulate and condense mRNA, promote intracellular delivery of mRNA to the cytosol by increasing cellular uptake and triggering endosomal escape, increase mRNA stability by protecting them from degradation in extracellular spaces, and are composed of biocompatible materials suitable for human use (38) (see Table 12.2).

Pfizer, USA and BioNtech, Germany developed the mRNA-based COVID-19 vaccine candidate BNT162b2 to administer intramuscularly in two doses three weeks (21 days) apart. This mRNA vaccine is delivered in a LNP to express a prefusion-stabilized, membrane-anchored SARS-CoV-2 full-length spike protein (88). A two-dose (30 µg per dose) regimen of BNT162b2 elicited high neutralizing titers and robust, antigen-specific CD4+ and CD8+ T-cell responses against SARS-CoV-2 (89) and conferred 95% protection against COVID-19 from 7 days after the second dose in individuals 16 years of age or older (88). Based on these findings, on December 11, 2020, BNT162b2 received emergency use authorization from the FDA for COVID-19 prevention in persons 16 years of age or older. In the study of adolescents 12 to 15 years of age, BNT162b2 vaccine produced a greater immune response than in young adults, and observed vaccine efficacy against COVID-19 was 100% with an onset of 7 or more days after the second dose. Thus, based on these study outcomes, on May 10, 2021, the emergency use authorization was expanded to include persons 12 years of age or older (90).

Moderna, USA and the US government also developed an mRNA-based vaccine candidate, mRNA-1273 (100 µg), to administer intramuscularly in two doses 28 days apart. The mRNA vaccine is based on a sequence-optimized mRNA encoding the prefusion-stabilized, full-length spike glycoprotein encapsulated in LNPs (91). The mRNA-1273 vaccine elicited significant dose-dependent immune responses (92) and showed 94.1% efficacy in preventing symptomatic COVID-19 at or after 14 days following the second dose in participants 18 years and older (93). The mRNA-1273 vaccine induced binding antibodies and neutralizing antibodies by 28 days after the first dose and increased substantially by 14 days after the second dose to levels higher than those in convalescent serum from COVID-19 patients (92). Binding antibody and neutralizing antibody responses declined slightly over 6 months, but antibody titers remained high, and neutralizing activity persisted over this time (94).

CureVac, Germany developed an mRNA-based vaccine called CVnCoV vaccine (CV07050101) to administer intramuscularly in two doses at 28-day intervals. This mRNA vaccine is delivered in an LNP to express a full-length, prefusion-stabilized spike protein (95). Preclinical results showed that immunization with the CVnCoV vaccine elicits strong humoral responses with high titers of virus-neutralizing antibodies and robust T-cell responses (96). The interim data of a dose-escalation phase 1 study in healthy adults 18 to 60 years old demonstrated that two doses of CVnCoV ranging from 2 μg to 12 μg per dose, administered 28 days apart, were safe, but immune responses 2 weeks after the second dose of 12 μg were comparable with convalescent sera from COVID-19 patients. Seroconversion of virus-neutralizing antibodies 2 weeks after the second dose occurred in all participants who received 12-μg doses (95). On the basis of these outcomes, the 12-μg dose was selected for further clinical investigation in a phase 2b/3 study, the HERALD study. Recently, Curevac announced unsatisfactory results from their phase 2b/3 trial, which demonstrated an interim vaccine efficacy of 47% against COVID-19 disease of any severity, and final results from the phase 2b/3 trial showed an overall vaccine efficacy of 48% (97).

12.6 CHALLENGES IN COVID-19 VACCINE DEVELOPMENT

The outbreak of the COVID-19 pandemic accelerated vaccine development at an unprecedented pace. But there are several challenges with COVID-19 vaccine development, such as limited understanding of the pathophysiology, targeting humoral or mucosal immunity, and poor success of human SARS and MERS-CoV vaccines.

The detailed biological characteristics of SARS-CoV-2 are still unknown, and whether it infects only the respiratory tract or both respiratory and intestinal tracts is yet to be established; furthermore, the route of dissemination of SARS-CoV-2 to the lungs is not clear yet. Elucidation of these biological characteristics is a very crucial factor in the development of potential treatments and preventive strategies. Antibody-dependent enhancement (ADE) of coronavirus infections following vaccination is also a major concern in developing vaccines against COVID-19. Although the mechanism behind ADE is not yet clear, this may occur due to sub-neutralizing antibodies that do not have the capacity to completely neutralize the virus but instead cause enhanced uptake and spread of the viruses by entering Fc receptor–expressing cells (98). Another challenge in the developmental process of COVID-19 vaccines is the lack of suitable animal models to test vaccine efficacy and safety because none of the animal models appropriately mimic human COVID-19 infection and the potential correlates of infection (99). Furthermore, the genetic instability of the virus can result in limited effectiveness of the vaccines against it, which may eventually need an update in the composition of current COVID-19 vaccines to ensure the levels of protection against newly evolved variants. Therefore, it is important to create a secure and reliable vaccine in advance of future outbreaks of SARS-CoV-2 variants (100). Rapid large-scale manufacturing and distribution of billions of doses of COVID-19 vaccines still remains a challenge, with lots of uncertainty to meet the demand of a pandemic.

12.7 COVID-19 VACCINE APPLICATIONS

COVID-19 outbreaks have caused significant global morbidity and mortality; to mitigate the escalating burden of COVID-19, vaccine development has occurred at an unprecedented pace (101). The main aim behind the development of a COVID-19 vaccine was to bring a halt to the current pandemic situation and attain broad protective immunity in the population so as to achieve herd immunity, which can ultimately stop the transmission of the pathogen and control the global public health crisis. It is essential to achieve herd immunity through vaccination globally in order to prevent SARS-CoV-2 from continuing to mutate, becoming more resistant to current vaccines, and causing more periods of mass fatality. Vaccines train our immune system to recognize the targeted virus and create antibodies to fight off the disease without getting the disease itself. After vaccination, the body is ready to fight the virus if it is later exposed to it, thereby preventing serious illness, hospitalizations, and deaths. Thus, COVID-19 vaccination can have a substantial impact on mitigating outbreaks and may be the best hope for ending the pandemic by getting back to a normal way of life.

12.8 CONCLUSION

Previous research experiences with SARS-CoV and MERS-CoV have laid the groundwork for accelerated SARS-CoV-2 vaccine development. Many research groups and companies are undertaking efforts to develop an effective vaccine against SARS-CoV-2 all over the world and speeding up all the usual phases needed to develop and test a vaccine in humans. At present, there are more than 290 vaccine candidates under development, with a number of these already approved for emergency use. These approved vaccine candidates in clinical trials have all shown promising immunogenicity with varying degrees of protective efficacy and an acceptable safety profile, but further investigation on immunization schedules is required. However, these different vaccines have not been studied head-to-head, and thus, comparative efficacy is uncertain. Currently, the vaccine supply is not sufficient to meet worldwide demand; many nations are asking for dose-sparing strategies without impacting effectiveness. Several governments have made up-front payments to secure a number of doses of the vaccines under development. Further development of multiple vaccine candidates using different vaccine delivery systems such as nanoparticles is crucial so that the final vaccine products can be readily produced and formulated for rapid deployment and mass vaccination across the globe. Even though there are still many challenges and unanswered questions regarding anti-SARS-CoV-2 immunity, potential mutations of SARS-CoV-2, and seasonal recurrences, the remarkable breakthroughs in COVID-19 vaccine development have offered hope to return to a pre-pandemic normality.

ACKNOWLEDGMENT

We thank Dr. Aditya S. Abhyankar, dean and head, Department of Technology, SavitribaiPhule Pune University, Pune and Dr. S.D. Lokhande, principal, Sinhgad College of Engineering, SPPU, Pune for support.

REFERENCES

1. COVID-19 vaccine tracker and landscape. https://www.who.int/publications/m/item/draft-landscape-of-covid-19-candidate-vaccines (Accessed on 9 August 2021).
2. COVID-19 vaccine tracker. https://www.raps.org/news-and-articles/news-articles/2020/3/covid-19-vaccine-tracker (Accessed on 9 August 2021).
3. Phan T. Novel coronavirus: From discovery to clinical diagnostics. *Infection, Genetics and Evolution*. 2020 Apr 1;79:104211.
4. Shang J, Wan Y, Luo C, et al. Cell entry mechanisms of SARS-CoV-2. *Proceedings of the National Academy of Sciences*. 2020 May 26;117(21):11727–11734.
5. Salvatori G, Luberto L, Maffei M, et al. SARS-CoV-2 Spike protein: An optimal immunological target for vaccines. *Journal of Translational Medicine*. 2020 Dec;18:1–3.
6. Weston S, Frieman MB. COVID-19: Knowns, unknowns, and questions. *Msphere*. 2020 Mar 18;5(2):e203–e220.
7. Daoust JF. Elderly people and responses to COVID-19 in 27 countries. *PloS One*. 2020 Jul 2;15(7):e0235590.
8. Ko JY, Danielson ML, Town M, et al. Risk factors for COVID-19-associated hospitalization: COVID-19-associated hospitalization surveillance network and behavioral risk factor surveillance system. *medRxiv*. 2020 Jan 1.
9. Tai W, He L, Zhang X, et al. Characterization of the receptor-binding domain (RBD) of 2019 novel coronavirus: Implication for development of RBD protein as a viral attachment inhibitor and vaccine. *Cellular & Molecular Immunology*. 2020 Jun;17(6):613–620.
10. Summary of probable SARS cases with onset of illness from 1 November 2002 to 31 July 2003. https://www.who.int/publications/m/item/summary-of-probable-sars-cases-with-onset-of-illness-from-1-november-2002-to-31-july-2003 (Accessed on 9 August 2021).
11. Li Q, Guan X, Wu P, et al. Early transmission dynamics in Wuhan, China, of novel coronavirus—infected pneumonia. *New England Journal of Medicine*. 2020 Jan 29.
12. Cascella M, Rajnik M, Aleem A, Dulebohn S, Di Napoli R. Features, evaluation, and treatment of coronavirus (COVID-19). *StatPearls*. 2021 Apr 20.
13. Yi Y, Lagniton PN, Ye S, Li E, Xu RH. COVID-19: What has been learned and to be learned about the novel coronavirus disease. *International Journal of Biological Sciences*. 2020;16(10):1753.
14. Lu R, Zhao X, Li J, et al. Genomic characterisation and epidemiology of 2019 novel coronavirus: Implications for virus origins and receptor binding. *The Lancet*. 2020 Feb 22;395(10224):565–574.
15. Wang N, Shang J, Jiang S, Du L. Subunit vaccines against emerging pathogenic human coronaviruses. *Frontiers in Microbiology*. 2020 Feb 28;11:298.
16. Al-Amri SS, Abbas AT, Siddiq LA, et al. Immunogenicity of candidate MERS-CoV DNA vaccines based on the spike protein. *Scientific Reports*. 2017 Mar 23;7(1):1–8.
17. Du L, He Y, Zhou Y, Liu S, Zheng BJ, Jiang S. The spike protein of SARS-CoV—a target for vaccine and therapeutic development. *Nature Reviews Microbiology*. 2009 Mar;7(3):226–236.
18. See RH, Zakhartchouk AN, Petric M, et al. Comparative evaluation of two severe acute respiratory syndrome (SARS) vaccine candidates in mice challenged with SARS coronavirus. *Journal of General Virology*. 2006 Mar 1;87(3):641–650.
19. Zhao J, Li K, Wohlford-Lenane C, et al. Rapid generation of a mouse model for middle East respiratory syndrome. *Proceedings of the National Academy of Sciences*. 2014 Apr 1;111(13):4970–4975.
20. Roper RL, Rehm KE. SARS vaccines: Where are we? *Expert Review of Vaccines*. 2009 Jul 1;8(7):887–898.

21. Li J, Ulitzky L, Silberstein E, Taylor DR, Viscidi R. Immunogenicity and protection efficacy of monomeric and trimeric recombinant SARS coronavirus spike protein subunit vaccine candidates. *Viral Immunology.* 2013 Apr 1;26(2):126–132.
22. Tai W, Zhao G, Sun S, et al. A recombinant receptor-binding domain of MERS-CoV in trimeric form protects human dipeptidyl peptidase 4 (hDPP4) transgenic mice from MERS-CoV infection. *Virology.* 2016 Dec 1;499:375–382.
23. Qiu M, Shi Y, Guo Z, et al. Antibody responses to individual proteins of SARS coronavirus and their neutralization activities. *Microbes and Infection.* 2005 May 1;7(5–6):882–889.
24. Li Y, Wan Y, Liu P, et al. A humanized neutralizing antibody against MERS-CoV targeting the receptor-binding domain of the spike protein. *Cell Research.* 2015 Nov;25(11):1237–1249.
25. van Riel D, de Wit E. Next-generation vaccine platforms for COVID-19. *Nature Materials.* 2020 Aug;19(8):810–812.
26. Hufsky F, Lamkiewicz K, Almeida A, et al. Computational strategies to combat COVID-19: Useful tools to accelerate SARS-CoV-2 and coronavirus research. *Briefings in Bioinformatics.* 2021 Mar;22(2):642–663.
27. Lurie N, Saville M, Hatchett R, Halton J. Developing Covid-19 vaccines at pandemic speed. *New England Journal of Medicine.* 2020 May 21;382(21):1969–1973.
28. Delrue I, Verzele D, Madder A, Nauwynck HJ. Inactivated virus vaccines from chemistry to prophylaxis: Merits, risks and challenges. *Expert Review of Vaccines.* 2012 Jun 1;11(6):695–719.
29. Plotkin S. History of vaccination. *Proceedings of the National Academy of Sciences.* 2014 Aug 26;111(34):12283–12287.
30. Zepp F. Principles of vaccine design—lessons from nature. *Vaccine.* 2010 Aug 31;28:C14–C24.
31. Lauring AS, Jones JO, Andino R. Rationalizing the development of live attenuated virus vaccines. *Nature Biotechnology.* 2010 Jun;28(6):573–579.
32. Lundstrom K. RNA viruses as tools in gene therapy and vaccine development. *Genes.* 2019 Mar;10(3):189.
33. Krause A, Worgall S. Delivery of antigens by viral vectors for vaccination. *Therapeutic Delivery.* 2011 Jan;2(1):51–70.
34. Li L, Petrovsky N. Molecular mechanisms for enhanced DNA vaccine immunogenicity. *Expert Review of Vaccines.* 2016 Mar 3;15(3):313–329.
35. Hobernik D, Bros M. DNA vaccines—how far from clinical use? *International Journal of Molecular Sciences.* 2018 Nov;19(11):3605.
36. Suschak JJ, Williams JA, Schmaljohn CS. Advancements in DNA vaccine vectors, non-mechanical delivery methods, and molecular adjuvants to increase immunogenicity. *Human Vaccines & Immunotherapeutics.* 2017 Dec 2;13(12):2837–2848.
37. Pollard C, Rejman J, De Haes W, et al. Type I IFN counteracts the induction of antigen-specific immune responses by lipid-based delivery of mRNA vaccines. *Molecular Therapy.* 2013 Jan 1;21(1):251–259.
38. Pardi N, Hogan MJ, Porter FW, Weissman D. mRNA vaccines—a new era in vaccinology. *Nature Reviews Drug Discovery.* 2018 Apr;17(4):261–279.
39. Abbasi J. COVID-19 and mRNA vaccines—first large test for a new approach. *Jama.* 2020 Sep 22;324(12):1125–1127.
40. Kamimura K, Suda T, Zhang G, Liu D. Advances in gene delivery systems. *Pharmaceutical Medicine.* 2011 Oct;25(5):293–306.
41. Mali S. Delivery systems for gene therapy. *Indian Journal of Human Genetics.* 2013 Jan;19(1):3.
42. Ramezanpour B, Haan I, Osterhaus A, Claassen E. Vector-based genetically modified vaccines: Exploiting Jenner's legacy. *Vaccine.* 2016 Dec 7;34(50):6436–6448.

43. Escors D, Breckpot K. Lentiviral vectors in gene therapy: Their current status and future potential. *Archivumimmunologiaeettherapiaeexperimentalis*. 2010 Apr;58(2):107–119.
44. Miyazaki M, Obata Y, Abe K, et al. Gene transfer using nonviral delivery systems. *Peritoneal Dialysis International*. 2006 Nov;26(6):633–640.
45. Nelson CE, Duvall CL, Prokop A, Gersbach CA, Davidson JM. Gene delivery into cells and tissues. In *Principles of Tissue Engineering*. 2020 Jan 1 (pp. 519–554). Academic Press.
46. Robert-Guroff M. Replicating and non-replicating viral vectors for vaccine development. *Current Opinion in Biotechnology*. 2007 Dec 1;18(6):546–556.
47. Krammer F. SARS-CoV-2 vaccines in development. *Nature*. 2020 Oct;586(7830):516–527.
48. Poland GA, Ovsyannikova IG, Kennedy RB. SARS-CoV-2 immunity: Review and applications to phase 3 vaccine candidates. *The Lancet*. 2020 Nov 14;396(10262):1595–1606.
49. Zhu FC, Li YH, Guan XH, et al. Safety, tolerability, and immunogenicity of a recombinant adenovirus type-5 vectored COVID-19 vaccine: A dose-escalation, open-label, non-randomised, first-in-human trial. *The Lancet*. 2020 Jun 13;395(10240):1845–1854.
50. Fausther-Bovendo H, Kobinger GP. Pre-existing immunity against Ad vectors: Humoral, cellular, and innate response, what's important? *Human Vaccines & Immunotherapeutics*. 2014 Oct 3;10(10):2875–2884.
51. Humphreys IR, Sebastian S. Novel viral vectors in infectious diseases. *Immunology*. 2018 Jan;153(1):1–9.
52. Case JB, Rothlauf PW, Chen RE, et al. Replication-competent vesicular stomatitis virus vaccine vector protects against SARS-CoV-2-mediated pathogenesis in mice. *Cell Host & Microbe*. 2020 Sep 9;28(3):465–474.
53. Sun W, Leist SR, McCroskery S, et al. Newcastle disease virus (NDV) expressing the spike protein of SARS-CoV-2 as a live virus vaccine candidate. *EBioMedicine*. 2020 Dec 1;62:103132.
54. CanSinoBIO's COVID-19 vaccine 65.7% effective in global trials, Pakistan official says. https://www.reuters.com/article/us-health-coronavirus-vaccine-pakistan/cansinobios-covid-19-vaccine-65-7-effective-in-global-trials-pakistan-official-says-idUSKBN2A81N0 (Accessed on 9 August 2021).
55. Zhu FC, Guan XH, Li YH, et al. Immunogenicity and safety of a recombinant adenovirus type-5-vectored COVID-19 vaccine in healthy adults aged 18 years or older: A randomised, double-blind, placebo-controlled, phase 2 trial. *The Lancet*. 2020 Aug 15;396(10249):479–488.
56. Wu S, Huang J, Zhang Z, et al. Safety, tolerability, and immunogenicity of an aerosolised adenovirus type-5 vector-based COVID-19 vaccine (Ad5-nCoV) in adults: Preliminary report of an open-label and randomised phase 1 clinical trial. *The Lancet Infectious Diseases*. 2021 Dec 1;21(12):1654–1664.
57. Logunov DY, Dolzhikova IV, Zubkova OV, et al. Safety and immunogenicity of an rAd26 and rAd5 vector-based heterologous prime-boost COVID-19 vaccine in two formulations: Two open, non-randomised phase 1/2 studies from Russia. *The Lancet*. 2020 Sep 26;396(10255):887–897.
58. Logunov DY, Dolzhikova IV, Shcheblyakov DV, et al. Safety and efficacy of an rAd26 and rAd5 vector-based heterologous prime-boost COVID-19 vaccine: An interim analysis of a randomised controlled phase 3 trial in Russia. *The Lancet*. 2021 Feb 20;397(10275):671–681.
59. Rossi AH, Ojeda DS, Varese A, et al. Sputnik V vaccine elicits seroconversion and neutralizing capacity to SARS CoV-2 after a single dose. *Cell Reports Medicine*. 2021 Jul 9:100359.
60. Funk CD, Laferrière C, Ardakani A. A snapshot of the global race for vaccines targeting SARS-CoV-2 and the COVID-19 pandemic. *Frontiers in Pharmacology*. 2020 Jun 19;11:937.

61. Sadoff J, Le Gars M, Shukarev G, et al. Interim results of a phase 1–2a trial of Ad26. COV2. S Covid-19 vaccine. *New England Journal of Medicine.* 2021 May 13;384(19):1824–1835.
62. Stephenson KE, Le Gars M, Sadoff J, et al. Immunogenicity of the Ad26. COV2. S Vaccine for COVID-19. *Jama.* 2021 Apr 20;325(15):1535–1544.
63. Barouch DH, Stephenson KE, Sadoff J, et al. Durable humoral and cellular immune responses 8 months after Ad26. COV2. S vaccination. *New England Journal of Medicine.* 2021 Sep 2;385(10):951–953.
64. Sadoff J, Gray G, Vandebosch A, et al. Safety and efficacy of single-dose Ad26. COV2. S vaccine against Covid-19. *New England Journal of Medicine.* 2021 Jun 10;384(23):2187–2201.
65. Folegatti PM, Ewer KJ, Aley PK, et al. Safety and immunogenicity of the ChAdOx1 nCoV-19 vaccine against SARS-CoV-2: A preliminary report of a phase 1/2, single-blind, randomised controlled trial. *The Lancet.* 2020 Aug 15;396(10249):467–478.
66. Ramasamy MN, Minassian AM, Ewer KJ, et al. Safety and immunogenicity of ChAdOx1 nCoV-19 vaccine administered in a prime-boost regimen in young and old adults (COV002): A single-blind, randomised, controlled, phase 2/3 trial. *The Lancet.* 2020 Dec 19;396(10267):1979–1993.
67. Voysey M, Clemens SA, Madhi SA, et al. Safety and efficacy of the ChAdOx1 nCoV-19 vaccine (AZD1222) against SARS-CoV-2: An interim analysis of four randomised controlled trials in Brazil, South Africa, and the UK. *The Lancet.* 2021 Jan 9;397(10269):99–111.
68. Voysey M, Clemens SA, Madhi SA, et al. Single-dose administration and the influence of the timing of the booster dose on immunogenicity and efficacy of ChAdOx1 nCoV-19 (AZD1222) vaccine: A pooled analysis of four randomised trials. *The Lancet.* 2021 Mar 6;397(10277):881–891.
69. AZD1222 US Phase III primary analysis confirms safety and efficacy. https://www.astrazeneca.com/content/astraz/media-centre/press-releases/2021/azd1222-us-phase-iii-primary-analysis-confirms-safety-and-efficacy.html (Accessed on 9 August 2021).
70. Flaxman A, Marchevsky NG, Jenkin D, et al. Reactogenicity and immunogenicity after a late second dose or a third dose of ChAdOx1 nCoV-19 in the UK: A substudy of two randomised controlled trials (COV001 and COV002). *The Lancet.* 2021 Sep 11;398(10304):981–990.
71. Yu J, Tostanoski LH, Peter L, et al. DNA vaccine protection against SARS-CoV-2 in rhesus macaques. *Science.* 2020 Aug 14;369(6505):806–811.
72. Jorritsma SH, Gowans EJ, Grubor-Bauk B, Wijesundara DK. Delivery methods to increase cellular uptake and immunogenicity of DNA vaccines. *Vaccine.* 2016 Nov 4;34(46):5488–5494.
73. Smith TR, Patel A, Ramos S, et al. Immunogenicity of a DNA vaccine candidate for COVID-19. *Nature Communications.* 2020 May 20;11(1):1–3.
74. Tebas P, Yang S, Boyer JD, et al. Safety and immunogenicity of INO-4800 DNA vaccine against SARS-CoV-2: A preliminary report of an open-label, Phase 1 clinical trial. *EClinicalMedicine.* 2021 Jan 1;31:100689.
75. Mammen MP, Tebas P, Agnes J, et al. Safety and immunogenicity of INO-4800 DNA vaccine against SARS-CoV-2: A preliminary report of a randomized, blinded, placebo-controlled, Phase 2 clinical trial in adults at high risk of viral exposurre. *medRxiv.* 2021 Jan 1; 2021.05.07.21256652.
76. INOVIO expands partnership with advaccine to conduct global phase 3 efficacy trial of COVID-19 DNA vaccine candidate, INO-4800. https://ir.inovio.com/news-releases/news-releases-details/2021/INOVIO-Expands-Partnership-with-Advaccine-to-Conduct-Global-Phase-3-Efficacy-Trial-of-COVID-19-DNA-Vaccine-Candidate-INO-4800/default.aspx (Accessed on 9 August 2021).

77. Alturki SO, Alturki SO, Connors J, et al. The 2020 pandemic: Current SARS-CoV-2 vaccine development. *Frontiers in Immunology*. 2020 Aug 19;11:1880.
78. Nucleus networks initiates first-in-human trial of Symvivo's oral COVID-19 vaccine candidate, bacTRL-Spike™. https://www.einnews.com/pr_news/528699687/nucleus-networks-initiates-first-in-human-trial-of-symvivo-s-oral-covid-19-vaccine-candidate-bactrl-spike (Accessed on 9 August 2021).
79. Safety and immunogenicity of GX-19N, a COVID-19 preventive DNA vaccine in elderly individuals. https://clinicaltrials.gov/ct2/show/NCT04915989 (Accessed on 9 August 2021).
80. Seo YB, Suh YS, Ryu JI, et al. Soluble spike DNA vaccine provides long-term protective immunity against SARS-CoV-2 in mice and nonhuman primates. *Vaccines*. 2021 Apr;9(4):307.
81. Ahn JY, Lee J, Suh YS, et al. Safety and immunogenicity of a recombinant DNA COVID-19 vaccine containing the coding regions of the spike and nucleocapsid proteins: Preliminary results from an open-label, phase 1 trial in healthy adults aged 19–55 years. *medRxiv*. 2021 Jan 1; 2021.05.26.21257700.
82. Anges starts Japan's 1st COVID-19 vaccine clinical trial on humans. https://english.kyodonews.net/news/2020/06/0b4d42d1c638-update1-anges-starts-japans-1st-covid-19-vaccine-clinical-test-on-humans.html (Accessed on 9 August 2021).
83. Study of COVID-19 DNA vaccine (AG0301-COVID19). https://clinicaltrials.gov/ct2/show/NCT04463472 (Accessed on 9 August 2021).
84. Race for COVID-19 vaccine: Covaxin and ZyCoV-D begin human trials in India, Moderna publishes preliminary data from phase 1. https://www.firstpost.com/health/race-for-covid-19-vaccine-covaxin-and-zycov-d-begin-human-trials-in-india-moderna-publishes-preliminary-data-from-phase-1–8600211.html (Accessed on 9 August 2021).
85. Momin T, Kansagra K, Patel H, et al. Safety and Immunogenicity of a DNA SARS-CoV-2 vaccine (ZyCoV-D): Results of an open-label, non-randomized phase I part of phase I/II clinical study by intradermal route in healthy subjects in India. *EClinicalMedicine*. 2021 Aug 1;38:101020.
86. India's ZydusCadila applies for emergency use nod for COVID-19 vaccine. https://economictimes.indiatimes.com/industry/healthcare/biotech/pharmaceuticals/indias-zydus-cadila-applies-for-emergency-use-nod-for-covid-19-vaccine/articleshow/84008502.cms (Accessed on 9 August 2021).
87. Tan L, Sun X. Recent advances in mRNA vaccine delivery. *Nano Research*. 2018 Oct;11(10):5338–5354.
88. Polack FP, Thomas SJ, Kitchin N, et al. Safety and efficacy of the BNT162b2 mRNA Covid-19 vaccine. *New England Journal of Medicine*. 2020 Dec 31; 383:2603–2615.
89. Walsh EE, FrenckJr RW, Falsey AR, et al. Safety and immunogenicity of two RNA-based Covid-19 vaccine candidates. *New England Journal of Medicine*. 2020 Dec 17;383(25):2439–2450.
90. FrenckJr RW, Klein NP, Kitchin N, et al. Safety, immunogenicity, and efficacy of the BNT162b2 Covid-19 vaccine in adolescents. *New England Journal of Medicine*. 2021 Jul 15;385(3):239–250.
91. Jackson LA, Anderson EJ, Rouphael NG, et al. An mRNA vaccine against SARS-CoV-2—preliminary report. *New England Journal of Medicine*. 2020 Nov 12; 383:1920–1931.
92. Chu L, McPhee R, Huang W, et al. A preliminary report of a randomized controlled phase 2 trial of the safety and immunogenicity of mRNA-1273 SARS-CoV-2 vaccine. *Vaccine*. 2021 May 12;39(20):2791–2799.
93. Baden LR, El Sahly HM, Essink B et al. Efficacy and safety of the mRNA-1273 SARS-CoV-2 vaccine. *New England Journal of Medicine*. 2021 Feb 4;384(5):403–416.

94. Doria-Rose N, Suthar MS, Makowski M, et al. Antibody persistence through 6 months after the second dose of mRNA-1273 vaccine for Covid-19. *New England Journal of Medicine.* 2021 Jun 10;384(23):2259–2261.
95. Kremsner PG, Mann P, Kroidl A, et al. Safety and immunogenicity of an mRNA-lipid nanoparticle vaccine candidate against SARS-CoV-2. *Wiener klinische Wochenschrift.* 2021 Sep;133(17):931–941.
96. Rauch S, Roth N, Schwendt K, Fotin-Mleczek M, Mueller SO, Petsch B. mRNA-based SARS-CoV-2 vaccine candidate CVnCoV induces high levels of virus-neutralising antibodies and mediates protection in rodents. *NPJ Vaccines.* 2021 Apr 16;6(1):1–9.
97. CureVac provides update on phase 2b/3 trial of first-generation COVID-19 vaccine candidate, CVnCoV. https://www.curevac.com/en/2021/06/16/curevac-provides-update-on-phase-2b-3-trial-of-first-generation-covid-19-vaccine-candidate-cvncov/ (Accessed on 9 August 2021).
98. Wan Y, Shang J, Sun S, et al. Molecular mechanism for antibody-dependent enhancement of coronavirus entry. *Journal of Virology.* 2020 Mar 1;94(5):e02015–e02019.
99. Saif LJ. Vaccines for COVID-19: Perspectives, prospects, and challenges based on candidate SARS, MERS, and animal coronavirus vaccines. *Euro Med J.* 2020 Mar 24;200324(10.33590).
100. Malik YS, Sircar S, Bhat S, et al. Emerging novel coronavirus (2019-nCoV)—current scenario, evolutionary perspective based on genome analysis and recent developments. *Veterinary Quarterly.* 2020 Jan 1;40(1):68–76.
101. Le TT, Andreadakis Z, Kumar A, et al. The COVID-19 vaccine development landscape. *Nat Rev Drug Discov.* 2020 May;19(5):305–306.

13 In Vivo Gene Therapy
AAV2 Vectors

Vandit Shah and Jigna Shah

CONTENTS

13.1 INTRODUCTION

The discovery of DNA as an agent for inheritance and disease has led to the development of novel therapies for genetic diseases. With the application of next-generation sequencing, various genes involved in disease conditions have been identified. This led to a simple hypothesis that fixing a mutant gene or normalizing an overexpressed/underexpressed gene can cure the disease. However, this seemingly simple goal required 40 years of research and technology development to safely transport the nucleic acid inside the target cells. Viruses have evolved to specifically target and deliver nucleic acids in the host cell for replication. On the other hand, the ability of viral vectors to cause immune reactions, cancer and other clinically severe side effects has resulted in their limited therapeutic application. Adeno-associated viruses (AAVs) were found to be replicative defective and were immunologically distinct from adenoviruses (Atchison, Casto, and Hammon 1965). Furthermore, the non-pathogenicity of the AAV was validated by Hoggan and colleagues in 1966 (Hoggan, Blacklow, and Rowe 1966). For the generation of gene therapeutics, recombinant AAV (rAAV) that lacks viral DNA is used to transduce the cell and deliver the DNA cargo into the nucleus. The transgene flanked on both side by inverted terminal repeats (ITR) forms circular concatemers that remain as episomes in the nucleus (Choi, McCarty, and Samulski 2006). Furthermore, episomal DNA does not integrate into host genomes,

DOI: 10.1201/9781003186069-13

decreasing the chances of cancer. Also, it gets diluted with repeated rounds of replication, making it an ideal candidate for gene therapy applications. Recently, an understanding of viral biology, molecular recombination techniques, vector engineering and base editing methods have enabled several AAV-based gene therapy candidates to be developed in the clinical stage (Balakrishnan and R. Jayandharan 2014). Thus, the AAV vector is destined to overcome all the current limitations associated with gene therapy and expand the applications to several genetic diseases.

13.2 ADENO-ASSOCIATED VIRUS

AAV was discovered in 1965 as a contaminant in the adenovirus stock and is a helper-dependent virus (Atchison, Casto, and Hammon 1965). AAV belongs to the *Dependovirus* genus of the Parvoviridae family, which has been known to infect various mammalian species (Nóbrega, Mendonça, and Matos 2020). However, no superinfection-associated immunity was observed with AAV vectors (Lebkowski et al. 1988). AAVs are small viruses of 18 to 25 nm in size, protected by a capsid protein (Weitzman and Linden 2012). It has a single-stranded DNA genome of ~ 4.7 kb, consisting of two open reading frames (ORFs), cap and rep. On both sides of its genome, it is flanked by ITRs with a hairpin-like structure, which is essential for replication and packaging of the virus. The use of alternative translational sites, three promoters (p5, p19 and p40) and differential splicing gives rise to at least nine gene products. The Rep gene encodes four different proteins such as Rep40, Rep52, Rep68 and Rep78 that are essential for viral packaging and replication (Weitzman and Linden 2012; R. Jude Samulski and Muzyczka 2014). Cap expression forms the viral capsid proteins VP1, VP2 and VP3 that are involved in outer capsid shell formation, cell binding and internalization. It collectively forms an icosahedral viral coat with about 60 capsid proteins in the molar ratio of VP1:VP2:VP3 (1:1:10) (R. Jude Samulski and Muzyczka 2014). About 12 different AAV serotypes have been identified and isolated over the years (Table 13.1). Furthermore, 100 variants have been isolated from different sources such as primates and humans. The capsid protein motifs provide unique viral features like cell/tissue specificity or main receptors to adhere and enter the cells (Saraiva, Nobre, and Pereira de Almeida 2016). The genome organization of different AAV serotypes is conserved; however, the transcriptional profiles have several differences (Weitzman and Linden 2012). This imparts a unique property to each serotype, enabling it to bind specifically with certain receptors in the target organ (Table 13.1). The capsid surface of the AAV serotype is essential for specific binding and internalization of a target cell, thereby achieving target organ and cell specificity and increased level and duration of transgene expression. AAV serotype–specific antibodies have been identified in primates as a consequence of natural infection. However, no clinical abnormalities have been associated with AAV serotypes recently (Neil R. Blacklow, Hoggan, and Rowe 1968; N R Blacklow, Hoggan, and Rowe 1967; Blacklow et al. 1968).

13.3 INTRODUCTION TO AAV2

In the human population, AAV2 is the most serologically prevalent AAV (Chirmule et al. 1999). Samulski and colleagues in 1983 for the first time isolated and cloned

TABLE 13.1
AAV Serotypes and Their Receptors

AAV Serotype	Receptor	Target Organ	Expression Level	Origin/Host	Neutralizing Antibody (%)
AAV1	2,3N/2,6N Sialic Acid	Liver, Muscle, CNS	Medium	Non-Human Primates	67
AAV2	Heparan Sulfate Proteoglycans (HSPG)	Liver, CNS	Low	Human	72
AAV3	Heparan Sulfate Proteoglycans (HSPG)	Liver (Cancer Cell)	Low	Non-Human Primates	Not Known
AAV4	2,3O-Sialic Acid	Ependymal Cells, Lung	Low	Non-Human Primates	10
AAV5	2,3N-Sialic Acid	Retina, Liver, Muscle, CNS	Medium	Human	40
AAV6	2,3N/2,6N Sialic Acid	Spinal Cord, Muscle, Liver	Medium	AAV1 × AAV2	46
AAV7	N-Sialic Acid	Liver, Muscle	High	Non-Human Primates	Not Known
AAV8	Not Known	Retina, Muscle, Liver	High	Non-Human Primates	38
AAV9	N-Galactose	Muscle, CNS, Heart, Liver	High	Human	47
AAV10	Not Known	Liver, CNS, Muscle	Medium	Monkey	Not known
AAV11	Not Known	Spleen	Not Known	Monkey	Not known
AAV12	Not Known	Submandibular Glands	Not Known	Monkey	Not known

Source: Nóbrega, Mendonça, and Matos 2020; Asokan, Schaffer, and Samulski 2012; Schmidt et al. 2008; Guo et al. 2015; Miyake et al. 2012; Gao, Vandenberghe, and Wilson 2005.

AAV2, thereby establishing its application as a vector for somatic gene transfer (Richard J. Samulski et al. 1983). The gene therapy vectors derived from AAV2 are produced by recombinant AAV genomes and lack viral ORF but harbor a transgene cassette that is flanked between 5' and 3' ITRs. Also, AAV vector production requires rep/cap and the adenohelper cassette in trans to the recombinant AAV. The earliest application of an AAV2-based vector in several animal models showed prolonged expression of the transgene in various tissues like muscle, eyes and central nervous system (CNS). Furthermore, in these studies no host immune response and vector related toxicity were observed (Grimm and Kay 2005; Rabinowitz and Samulski 1998; Kotin 2008).

These studies established the application of AAV2-based vector systems as a gene delivery vehicle for a variety of genetically inherited disorders. However, to establish clinical application of AAV-based vectors for gene therapy, challenges need to be overcome, like the low efficiency of gene transfer, restricted tissue tropism, preexisting and highly prevalent immunity in humans and delayed onset of gene expression. New approaches to improve AAV vector–based gene delivery and engineer transgenes for cell type–specific expression have enabled us to improve and overcome the aforementioned barriers. Additionally, integrating the knowledge of disease pathology and genetics with the delivery system can bring a breakthrough medical revolution for monogenic disorders. This is evident from the recent success in the treatment of genetic diseases like RPE65 deficiency (Bainbridge et al. 2009), spinal muscular atrophy (Mendell et al. 2017) and hemophilia B (George et al. 2017). Also, there has been a significant increase in the number of phase I to III clinical trials with AAV-based vectors (Table 13.2).

AAV2 serotype–based studies show higher safety and efficacy in terms of their application as compared to other serotypes (Kuzmin et al. 2021). Of these, a number of trials used tissue-specific strong promoters like albumin in order to achieve tissue-specific expression. Second, improvement in the cassette design has contributed towards trials with no serious side effects. Furthermore, animal studies for synthetic promoters designed to target functionally or genetically defined subsets of the cell are promising, but no clinical data for these agents are available.

13.4 EMERGING ISSUES IN AAV2-BASED IN VIVO GENE THERAPY

13.4.1 Cellular Barriers

It is well recognized that cellular barriers and intracellular trafficking are rate-limiting steps for AAV-based gene therapy. The surface of the target cell might lack receptors for AAV vector binding and internalization, thus limiting its infection capacity. The post-internalization cellular ubiquitin-proteosomal system degrades the capsid protein (Yan et al. 2002). Furthermore, endosomal escape, nuclear entry and vector unpackaging are concerns that need to be answered by a variety of pharmacological and capsid engineering techniques.

13.4.2 Transport to Target Cells

The liver is the primary target for systematically delivered viruses, thus limiting targeted application to other organs. To penetrate the tissues, it must bypass physical barriers like the blood–brain barrier. Direct delivery into an organ leads to many transport barriers like cell bodies and the extracellular matrix such as heparan sulphate onto which many AAV serotypes attach (Dalkara et al. 2009; Summerford and Samulski 1998), thereby limiting the gene transfer to the target cell type.

13.4.3 Packaging Capacity

AAV packaging capacity is about 4.7 kb. However, packaging of up to 5 kb can be achieved with normal titer and infectivity values. Packaging of genomes >5 kb in size shows remarkable decrease in viral packaging, g and 5' truncated genomes are encapsidated (Wu, Yang, and Colosi 2010; Ghosh and Duan 2007).

TABLE 13.2
AAV2 Vector–Based Gene Therapy Trials (https://clinicaltrials.gov)

Sr. No.	NCT Number	Title	Status	Disease	Interventions	Phases	No. of Patients	Primary Completion Date
Phase I	NCT03533673	"AAV2/8-LSPhGAA in Late-Onset Pompe Disease"	Recruiting	Pompe Disease	AAV2/8LSPhGAA	Phase 1| Phase 2	8	Dec-22
Phase II	NCT01395641	"A Phase I/II Clinical Trial for Treatment of Aromatic L-amino Acid Decarboxylase (AADC) Deficiency Using AAV2-hAADC"	Active, not recruiting	Aromatic L-amino Acid Decarboxylase (AADC) Deficiency	AADC	Phase 1| Phase 2	10	31-Dec-20
Phase III	NCT01621581	"AAV2-GDNF for Advanced Parkinson s Disease"	Active, not recruiting	Parkinson's Disease	AAV2-GDNF	Phase 1	25	01-Feb-22
Phase IV	NCT04046224	"Dose-Ranging Study of ST-920, an AAV2/6 Human Alpha Galactosidase A Gene Therapy in Subjects With Fabry Disease"	Recruiting	Fabry Disease	ST-920	Phase 1| Phase 2	48	Dec-23
Phase V	NCT03602820	"Long-term Follow-up Study in Subjects Who Received Voretigene Neparvovec-rzyl (AAV2-hRPE65v2)"	Active, not recruiting	Inherited Retinal Dystrophy Due to RPE65 Mutations	AAV2-hRPE65v2	Not Available	41	Mar-30
Phase VI	NCT02926066	"A Clinical Trial for Treatment of Aromatic L-amino Acid Decarboxylase (AADC) Deficiency Using AAV2-hAADC—An Expansion"	Active, not recruiting	Aromatic Amino Acid Decarboxylase Deficiency	AAV2-hAADC	Phase 2	12	Jan-22

(Continued)

TABLE 13.2 (Continued)

<table>
<tr><th>Sr. No.</th><th>NCT Number</th><th>Title</th><th>Status</th><th>Disease</th><th>Interventions</th><th>Phases</th><th>No. of Patients</th><th>Primary Completion Date</th></tr>
<tr><td>Phase VII</td><td>NCT03061201</td><td>“A Study of Recombinant AAV2/6 Human Factor 8 Gene Therapy SB-525 (PF-07055480) in Subjects With Severe Hemophilia A”</td><td>Active, not recruiting</td><td>Hemophilia A</td><td>SB-525 (PF-07055480)</td><td>Phase 2</td><td>11</td><td>23-Jul-24</td></tr>
<tr><td>Phase VIII</td><td>NCT04043104</td><td>“A Phase 1 Open-Label, Dose Escalation Study to Determine the Optimal Dose, Safety, and Activity of AAV2hAQP1 in Subjects With Radiation-Induced Parotid Gland Hypofunction and Xerostomia”</td><td>Recruiting</td><td>Radiation-Induced Parotid Gland Hypofunction| Xerostomia Due to Radiotherapy |Head and Neck Cancer</td><td>AAV2hAQP1</td><td>Phase 1</td><td>30</td><td>Dec-21</td></tr>
<tr><td>Phase IX</td><td>NCT02341807</td><td>“Safety and Dose Escalation Study of AAV2-hCHM in Subjects With CHM (Choroideremia) Gene Mutations”</td><td>Active, not recruiting</td><td>Choroideremia| CHM (Choroideremia) Gene Mutations</td><td>AAV2-hCHM</td><td>Phase 1| Phase 2</td><td>15</td><td>Oct-22</td></tr>
<tr><td>Phase X</td><td>NCT01024998</td><td>“Safety and Tolerability Study of AAV2-sFLT01 in Patients With Neovascular Age-Related Macular Degeneration (AMD)”</td><td>Completed</td><td>Macular Degeneration| Age-Related Maculopathies| Age-Related Maculopathy| Maculopathies, Age-Related| Maculopathy, Age-Related| Retinal</td><td>AAV2-sFLT01</td><td>Phase 1</td><td>19</td><td>Jul-14</td></tr>
</table>

				Degenerationl Retinal Neovascularizationl Gene Therapyl Therapy, Genel Eye Diseases				
Phase XI	NCT01208389	"Phase 1 Follow-on Study of AAV2-hRPE65v2 Vector in Subjects With Leber Congenital Amaurosis (LCA) 2"	Active, not recruiting	Leber Congenital Amaurosis	rzyl	Phase 1l Phase 2	12	Mar-30
Phase XII	NCT00252850	"Safety of CERE-120 (AAV2-NTN) in Subjects With Idiopathic Parkinson's Disease"	Completed	Parkinson's Disease	CERE-120 AAV2-NTN	Phase 1	12	Mar-07
Phase XIII	NCT02446249	"Safety of a Single Administration of AAV2hAQP1, an Adeno-Associated Viral Vector Encoding Human Aquaporin-1 to One Parotid Salivary Gland in People With Irradiation-Induced Parotid Salivary Hypofunction"	Recruiting	Squamous Cell Head and Neck Cancerl Radiation Induced Xerostomial Salivary Hypofunction	AAV2hAQP1	Phase 1	50	01-Nov-22
Phase XIV	NCT04167540	"GDNF Gene Therapy for Parkinson's Disease"	Recruiting	Parkinson's Disease	AAV2-GDNF	Phase 1	12	Dec-22
Phase XV	NCT04680065	"GDNF Gene Therapy for Multiple System Atrophy"	Not yet recruiting	Multiple System Atrophy	AAV2-GDNF	Phase 1	9	Apr-22
Phase XVI	NCT02553135	"Choroideremia Gene Therapy Clinical Trial"	Completed	Choroideremia	AAV2-REP1	Phase 2	6	Feb-18

(Continued)

TABLE 13.2 (Continued)

Sr. No.	NCT Number	Title	Status	Disease	Interventions	Phases	No. of Patients	Primary Completion Date
Phase XVII	NCT03507686	"A Safety Study of Retinal Gene Therapy for Choroideremia With Administration of BIIB111"	Active, not recruiting	Choroideremia	BIIB111	Phase 2	60	28-Feb-22
Phase XVIII	NCT02671539	"THOR—TÃ¼bingen Choroideremia Gene Therapy Trial"	Completed	Choroideremia	rAAV2.REP1	Phase 2	6	Feb-18
Phase XIX	NCT02407678	"REP1 Gene Replacement Therapy for Choroideremia"	Active, not recruiting	Choroideremia	AAV-REP1	Phase 2	30	Aug-21
Phase XX	NCT02077361	"An Open Label Clinical Trial of Retinal Gene Therapy for Choroideremia"	Active, not recruiting	Choroideremia	rAAV2.REP1 vector	Phase 1| Phase 2	6	30-Aug-17
Phase XXI	NCT04370054	"Study to Evaluate the Efficacy and Safety of PF-07055480 / Giroctocogene Fitelparvovec Gene Therapy in Moderately Severe to Severe Hemophilia A Adults"	Recruiting	Hemophilia A	PF-07055480 Human Factor VIII	Phase 3	63	10-Sep-22
Phase XXII	NCT03758404	"Gene Therapy for Achromatopsia (CNGA3)"	Completed	Achromatopsia	AAV-CNGA3	Phase 1| Phase 2	11	10-Jun-21
Phase XXIII	NCT03001310	"Gene Therapy for Achromatopsia (CNGB3)"	Completed	Achromatopsia	AAV—CNGB3	Phase 1| Phase 2	23	25-Oct-19
Phase XXIV	NCT03496012	"Efficacy and Safety of BIIB111 for the Treatment of Choroideremia"	Completed	Choroideremia	BIIB111	Phase 3	170	01-Dec-20

Phase XXV	NCT02695160	"Ascending Dose Study of Genome Editing by Zinc Finger Nuclease Therapeutic SB-FIX in Subjects With Severe Hemophilia B"	Terminated	Hemophilia B	SB-FIX	Phase 1	1	19-Apr-21
Phase XXVI	NCT01461213	"Gene Therapy for Blindness Caused by Choroideremia"	Completed	Choroideremia	rAAV2.REP1	Phase 1| Phase 2	14	Oct-17
Phase XXVII	NCT03252847	"Gene Therapy for X-linked Retinitis Pigmentosa (XLRP) Retinitis Pigmentosa GTPase Regulator (RPGR)"	Active, not recruiting	X-Linked Retinitis Pigmentosa	AAV2/5-RPGR	Phase 1| Phase 2	46	Nov-20
Phase XXVIII	NCT00643747	"Safety Study of RPE65 Gene Therapy to Treat Leber Congenital Amaurosis"	Completed	Retinal Degeneration	tgAAG76 (rAAV 2/2.hRPE65p. hRPE65)	Phase 1| Phase 2	12	Dec-14
Phase XXIX	NCT04312672	"Long Term Follow-Up Gene Therapy Study for XLRP RPGR"	Recruiting	X-Linked Retinitis Pigmentosa	AAV-RPGR	Not Available	36	Jun-23
Phase XXX	NCT02946879	"Long-Term Follow-Up Gene Therapy Study for Leber Congenital Amaurosis OPTIRPE65 (Retinal Dystrophy Associated With Defects in RPE65)"	Recruiting	Leber Congenital Amaurosis (LCA)|Eye Diseases| Eye Diseases, Hereditary| Retinal Diseases	AAV OPTIRPE65	Not Available	27	Apr-23
Phase XXXI	NCT03278873	"Long-Term Follow-Up Gene Therapy Study for Achromatopsia CNGB3 and CNGA3"	Recruiting	Achromatopsia	either AAV—CNGB3 or AAV—CNGA3	Phase 1| Phase 2	72	10-Jul-24

(Continued)

TABLE 13.2 (Continued)

Sr. No.	NCT Number	Title	Status	Disease	Interventions	Phases	No. of Patients	Primary Completion Date
Phase XXXII	NCT00999609	"Safety and Efficacy Study in Subjects With Leber Congenital Amaurosis"	Active, not recruiting	Inherited Retinal Dystrophy Due to RPE65 Mutations| Leber Congenital Amaurosis	AAV2-hRPE65v2, rzyl	Phase 3	31	Jul-15
Phase XXXIII	NCT03584165	"Long-term Safety and Efficacy Follow-up of BIIB111 for the Treatment of Choroideremia and BIIB112 for the Treatment of X-Linked Retinitis Pigmentosa"	Enrolling by invitation	Choroideremia| X-Linked Retinitis Pigmentosa	BIIB111| BIIB112	Not Available	440	23-Mar-27
Phase XXXIV	NCT00985517	"Safety and Efficacy of CERE-120 in Subjects With Parkinson's Disease"	Completed	Idiopathic Parkinson's Disease	CERE-120	Phase 1| Phase 2	57	09-Nov-14
Phase XXXV	NCT00516477	"Safety Study in Subjects With Leber Congenital Amaurosis"	Completed	Leber Congenital Amaurosis	rzyl	Phase 1	12	20-Mar-18
Phase XXXVI	NCT00400634	"Double-Blind, Multicenter, Sham Surgery Controlled Study of CERE-120 in Subjects With Idiopathic Parkinson's Disease"	Completed	Idiopathic Parkinson's Disease	CERE-120 -Neurturin (NTN)	Phase 2	58	Nov-08
Phase XXXVII	NCT02161380	"Safety Study of an Adeno-associated Virus Vector for Gene Therapy of Leber's Hereditary Optic Neuropathy"	Active, not recruiting	Leber's Hereditary Optic Neuropathy	scAAV2-P1ND4v2	Phase 1	28	Mar-23

Phase XXXVIII	NCT03065192	"Safety and Efficacy Study of VY-AADC01 for Advanced Parkinson's Disease"	Active, not recruiting	Idiopathic Parkinson's Disease| Parkinson's Disease| Basal Ganglia Disease| Brain Diseases| Central Nervous System Diseases| Movement Disorders| Nervous System Diseases| Neurodegenerative Diseases| Parkinsonian Disorders	VY-AADC01	Phase 1	16	Dec-21
Phase XXXIX	NCT01973543	"Safety Study of AADC Gene Therapy (VY-AADC01) for Parkinson's Disease"	Completed	Parkinson's Disease	VY-AADC01	Phase 1	15	24-Jan-20
Phase XXXX	NCT03562494	"VY-AADC02 for Parkinson's Disease With Motor Fluctuations (RESTORE-1)"	Active, not recruiting	Parkinson's Disease	VY-AADC02	Phase 2	85	Dec-22
Phase XXXXI	NCT03733496	"Observational, Long-term Extension Study for Participants of Prior VY-AADC01 Studies"	Enrolling by invitation	Parkinson's Disease	Not available	Not Available	23	Apr-26
Phase XXXXII	NCT03406104	"RESCUE and REVERSE Long-term Follow-up"	Active, not recruiting	Leber Hereditary Optic Neuropathy	GS010	Phase 3	61	Jul-22
Phase XXXXIII	NCT03293524	"Efficacy & Safety Study of Bilateral IVT Injection of GS010 in LHON Subjects Due to the ND4 Mutation for up to 1 Year"	Active, not recruiting	Leber Hereditary Optic Neuropathy	GS010	Phase 3	90	30-Jun-24

(Continued)

TABLE 13.2 (Continued)

Sr. No.	NCT Number	Title	Status	Disease	Interventions	Phases	No. of Patients	Primary Completion Date
Phase XXXXIV	NCT02652780	"Efficacy Study of GS010 for Treatment of Vision Loss From 7 Months to 1 Year From Onset in LHON Due to the ND4 Mutation (REVERSE)"	Completed	Optic, Atrophy, Hereditary, Leber	GS010	Phase 3	37	Jan-18
Phase XXXXV	NCT02652767	"Efficacy Study of GS010 for the Treatment of Vision Loss up to 6 Months From Onset in LHON Due to the ND4 Mutation"	Completed	Optic, Atrophy, Hereditary, Leber	GS010	Phase 3	39	07-Aug-18
Phase XXXXVI	NCT02418598	"AADC Gene Therapy for Parkinson's Disease"	Terminated	Parkinson Disease	Not available	Phase 1| Phase 2	2	31-Mar-18

13.4.4 Immune Interaction

The immune system is very effective in eliminating foreign nucleic materials. Also, most of the human population has been infected with AAVs. Since the sequence of natural and other AAV serotypes are identical (Lisowski et al. 2013), neutralizing antibodies against the capsids are seen in the blood and other body fluids (Boutin et al. 2010). These properties limit the application of the natural AAV-based gene transfer. Post transduction, the AAV capsid epitope gets cross-presented on the major histocompatibility complex (MHC) class I molecule. Thus, it is eliminated by capsid-specific cytotoxic T lymphocytes. Many $CD8^+$ and $CD4^+$ T-cell epitopes for the AAV capsid have been identified (Madsen et al. 2009; Mingozzi et al. 2007; Manno et al. 2006). AAV vectors with deleted CpG motifs have been shown to reduce immunogenicity (Faust et al. 2013). Thus, it is necessary to design vectors that evade all the MHC combinations and transporters associated with antigen-processing proteins.

13.5 DESIGNER AAV2 VECTOR CAPSIDS

Natural AAV-based viral infection in human populations has not evolved for medical applications. With the help of vector engineering, it is now possible to imbibe biomedically important phenotypes. AAV structural analysis, in addition to the knowledge of its infection cycle, can increase the efficacy of the vector (DiMattia et al. 2012; Govindasamy et al. 2013). For instance, AAV vectors undergo ubiquitylation and proteasomal degradation by replacing tyrosine residues in capsids with phenylalanine. This change leads to increased transgene expression of about 30-fold in vivo (Zhong et al. 2008). Additionally, cytotoxic T-lymphocyte reactions against AAV are a key limitation of clinical application of AAV-based gene therapy. MHC class I is thought to underlie this cytotoxic reaction by presentation of an AAV capsid epitope. Recently, tyrosine to phenylalanine was tested to decrease this immune response, as it targets the proteosomal degradation of cytosolic proteins (Martino et al. 2013).

To restrict and redirect viral tropism, high-affinity ligands are incorporated into the AAV capsid for binding to an alternative cell surface receptor. For instance, insertion of ankyrin repeat proteins at the N-terminus of the VP2 region of AAV2 capsid showed specificity to human epidermal growth factor receptor 2 (HER2). This strategy helped in increasing the specificity towards tumor cells by about 20fold in vivo (Münch et al. 2013). Furthermore, redirection of AAV tropism can be achieved by incorporating amino acids responsible for binding to galactose residue from AAV9 to its corresponding site in the AAV2 capsid, thereby producing an AAV vector that uses both galactose and heparin sulphate for cell entry, ultimately resulting in a vector system with significantly higher infectivity and specificity towards the liver (Shen et al. 2013). The strategies used for tackling the challenges of preexisting neutralizing antibodies are to discover and mutate the epitope that is responsible for the development of capsid-specific antibody binding. In the last few years, efforts at mapping conformational and linear AAV epitopes have increased to understand its docking sites with neutralizing antibodies (Moskalenko et al. 2000; Wobus et al. 2000). For example, potential target sites to develop variants were identified by in silico docking of IgG2a with AAV2. The developed variants showed lower neutralization by human and mouse antibodies (Lochrie et al. 2006).

A newer approach applied to progressively enhance the function of AAV vectors is the use of directed evolution strategies. To achieve this, a large genetic library of viral particles with diversified AAV capsids was generated. The initial directed evolution strategies were aimed at overcoming the problem of neutralizing antibodies. These studies showed that AAV2 variants were able to endure significantly high levels of neutralizing antibodies in both in vivo (Maheshri et al. 2006) and in vitro (Perabo et al. 2006). AAV variants generated by mutations in amino acids, which is crucial for antibody binding, required about a 35-fold higher concentration of pooled human antibodies as compared to wild-type AAV2 (Bartel et al. 2012). The variant also showed an increased level of transduction in muscle, liver and heart as compared to AAV2 in mice. Using vector engineering, a variant AAV capsid has been designed for specific and efficient infection of target cell types. For example, vectors generated to target neural stem cells showed a 50-fold increase in transduction (Jang et al. 2011); similarly, a 100-fold increase was observed in human epithelial cells (Excoffon et al. 2009).

Tissue transport is a barrier to viral vector delivery, as many target cell types are present inside a dense tissue structure. For example, retinal pigment epithelial cells and photoreceptor cells are inside a highly dense tissue structure. An AAV vector generated using direct evolution was able to deliver genetic material directly into the photoreceptor cells and cross the retina after intravitreal delivery (Dalkara et al. 2013). Significantly higher gene expression was observed as compared to wild-type AAV2, rescuing Leber's congenital amaurosis type 2 and X-linked retinoschisis in a murine model (Dalkara et al. 2013) and thus making it a promising platform for cell-targeted gene delivery.

The application of rational vector engineering and a direct evolution method has overcome several challenges offered by gene therapy. Combining this knowledge with gene cassette designing will pave the way for targeted genetic material delivery.

13.6 STRATEGIES TO IMPROVE GENE THERAPY BY AAV2 GENETIC PAYLOAD ENGINEERING

The AAV vector has a limited packaging capacity of about 4.7 kb, which is quite small as compared to a dysfunctional disease gene. Furthermore, gene therapy for autosomal dominant genetic diseases requires an allele to be removed. To address such challenges, it is required to alter and design a gene cassette other than the capsid. The use of genome editing techniques like lustered regularly interspaced short palindromic repeat–CRISPR-associated protein (CRISPR-Cas) system, zinc-finger nucleases (ZFNs) and transcription activator–like effector nucleases (TALENs) offers a platform to resolve these problems. Application of sequence-specific endonucleases like CRISPR-Cas has effectively led to homologous recombination of donor DNA and its corresponding defective allele (Russell and Hirata 1998). Additionally, these gene correction cassettes are smaller in size and can be easily packed in AAV vectors. Therefore, this can be a promising candidate for the treatment of Duchenne muscular dystrophy (DMD) and the Usher syndrome 2A (USH2A) gene. RNA interference

(RNAi) has been implemented for specific knockdown of the pathological alleles (McBride et al. 2011). To increase the packaging capacity of the AAV vectors, dual-vector systems are being tested. To achieve transgene expression of >4.7 kb size, the gene cassette is split in two and the halves are independently packed in the AAV vector. Post transduction of the target cell type by both vectors, full-length transgene expression can be achieved by homologous recombination or ITR-mediated recombination (Zhang et al. 2013; Trapani et al. 2014; Colella et al. 2014). However, dual-vector transduction efficiency is not consistent across the species, suggesting further investigation prior to its clinical application is needed. Hence, by combining the knowledge of vector engineering and gene cassette design, gene therapy is destined to extend its clinical application.

13.7 CONCLUSION

Fifty years since the discovery of AAV vectors as a contaminant in culture has led to the development of the most promising gene therapy vectors. Recent success with AAV-based clinical trials for several monogenic disorders has provided a strong momentum. Nonetheless, to establish the AAV vector as a promising candidate, several challenges need to be overcome in both payload and targeted delivery. The advent of vector engineering and development of gene cassettes, especially site-specific endonucleases, have provided an opportunity to target previously untreatable diseases like dominant genetic disorders. Additionally, the knowledge of AAV–host interactions will enable us to overcome the barriers to successful transduction to target cells and thereby extend the clinical landscape of AAV-mediated gene therapy.

REFERENCES

Asokan, Aravind, David V. Schaffer, and R. Jude Samulski. 2012. "The AAV Vector Toolkit: Poised at the Clinical Crossroads." *Molecular Therapy* 20 (4). Cell Press: 699–708. doi:10.1038/MT.2011.287.

Atchison, Robert W., Bruce C. Casto, and William McD Hammon. 1965. "Adenovirus-Associated Defective Virus Particles." *Science* 149 (3685). American Association for the Advancement of Science: 754–755. doi:10.1126/SCIENCE.149.3685.754.

Bainbridge, James W. B., Alexander J. Smith, Susie S. Barker, Scott Robbie, Robert Henderson, Kamaljit Balaggan, Ananth Viswanathan, et al. 2009. "Effect of Gene Therapy on Visual Function in Leber's Congenital Amaurosis." 358 (21). Massachusetts Medical Society: 2231–2239. doi:10.1056/NEJMOA0802268.

Balakrishnan, Balaji, and Giridhara R. Jayandharan. 2014. "Basic Biology of Adeno-Associated Virus (AAV) Vectors Used in Gene Therapy." *Current Gene Therapy* 14 (2). Bentham Science Publishers: 86–100.

Bartel, Melissa A., Bum-Yeol Hwang, Daniel Stone, James T. Koerber, Linda Couto, Federico Mingozzi, Katherine A. High, and David V. Schaffer. 2012. "Directed Evolution of AAV for Enhanced Evasion of Human Neutralizing Antibodies." *Molecular Therapy* 20 (May). Elsevier: S140. doi:10.1016/S1525-0016(16)36162-7.

Blacklow, Neil R., M. David Hoggan, Albert Z. Kapikian, Joan B. Austin, and Wallace P. Rowe. 1968. "Epidemiology of Adenovirus-Associated Virus Infection in a Nursery Population." *American Journal Of Epidemiology* 88 (3). Oxford Academic: 368–378. doi:10.1093/Oxfordjournals.Aje.A120897.

Blacklow, N. R., M. D. Hoggan, and W. P. Rowe. 1967. "Isolation of Adenovirus-Associated Viruses from Man." *Proceedings of the National Academy of Sciences of the United States of America* 58 (4). National Academy of Sciences: 1410–1415. doi:10.1073/PNAS.58.4.1410.

Blacklow, Neil R., M. David Hoggan, and Wallace P. Rowe. 1968. "Serologic Evidence for Human Infection with Adenovirus-Associated Viruses." *JNCI: Journal of the National Cancer Institute* 40 (2). Oxford Academic: 319–327. doi:10.1093/JNCI/40.2.319.

Boutin, Sylvie, Virginie Monteilhet, Philippe Veron, Christian Leborgne, Olivier Benveniste, Marie Françoise Montus, and Carole Masurier. 2010. "Prevalence of Serum IgG and Neutralizing Factors Against Adeno-Associated Virus (AAV) Types 1, 2, 5, 6, 8, and 9 in the Healthy Population: Implications for Gene Therapy Using AAV Vectors." *Https://Home.Liebertpub.Com/Hum* 21 (6). Mary Ann Liebert, Inc. 140 Huguenot Street, 3rd Floor New Rochelle, NY 10801 USA: 704–712. doi:10.1089/HUM.2009.182.

Chirmule, N., K. J. Propert, S. A. Magosin, Y. Qian, R. Qian, and J. M. Wilson. 1999. "Immune Responses to Adenovirus and Adeno-Associated Virus in Humans." *Gene Therapy 1999 6:9* 6 (9). Nature Publishing Group: 1574–1583. doi:10.1038/sj.gt.3300994.

Choi, Vivian W., Douglas M. McCarty, and R. Jude Samulski. 2006. "Host Cell DNA Repair Pathways in Adeno-Associated Viral Genome Processing." *Journal of Virology* 80 (21). American Society for Microbiology: 10346–10356. doi:10.1128/JVI.00841-06.

Colella, P., I. Trapani, G. Cesi, A. Sommella, A. Manfredi, A. Puppo, C. Iodice, et al. 2014. "Efficient Gene Delivery to the Cone-Enriched Pig Retina by Dual AAV Vectors." *Gene Therapy 2014 21:4* 21 (4). Nature Publishing Group: 450–456. doi:10.1038/gt.2014.8.

Dalkara, Deniz, Leah C. Byrne, Ryan R. Klimczak, Meike Visel, Lu Yin, William H. Merigan, John G. Flannery, and David V. Schaffer. 2013. "In Vivo—Directed Evolution of a New Adeno-Associated Virus for Therapeutic Outer Retinal Gene Delivery from the Vitreous." *Science Translational Medicine* 5 (189). American Association for the Advancement of Science: 189ra76–189ra76. doi:10.1126/SCITRANSLMED.3005708.

Dalkara, Deniz, Kathleen D. Kolstad, Natalia Caporale, Meike Visel, Ryan R. Klimczak, David V. Schaffer, and John G. Flannery. 2009. "Inner Limiting Membrane Barriers to AAV-Mediated Retinal Transduction from the Vitreous." *Molecular Therapy* 17 (12). Cell Press: 2096–2102. doi:10.1038/MT.2009.181.

DiMattia, Michael A., Hyun-Joo Nam, Kim Van Vliet, Matthew Mitchell, Antonette Bennett, Brittney L. Gurda, Robert McKenna, et al. 2012. "Structural Insight into the Unique Properties of Adeno-Associated Virus Serotype 9." *Journal of Virology* 86 (12). American Society for Microbiology: 6947–6958. doi:10.1128/JVI.07232-11.

Excoffon, Katherine J. D. A., James T. Koerber, David D. Dickey, Matthew Murtha, Shaf Keshavjee, Brian K. Kaspar, Joseph Zabner, and David V. Schaffer. 2009. "Directed Evolution of Adeno-Associated Virus to an Infectious Respiratory Virus." *Proceedings of the National Academy of Sciences* 106 (10). National Academy of Sciences: 3865–3870. doi:10.1073/PNAS.0813365106.

Faust, Susan M., Peter Bell, Benjamin J. Cutler, Scott N. Ashley, Yanqing Zhu, Joseph E. Rabinowitz, and James M. Wilson. 2013. "CpG-Depleted Adeno-Associated Virus Vectors Evade Immune Detection." *The Journal of Clinical Investigation* 123 (7). American Society for Clinical Investigation: 2994–3001. doi:10.1172/JCI68205.

Gao, Guangping, Luk Vandenberghe, and James Wilson. 2005. "New Recombinant Serotypes of AAV Vectors." *Current Gene Therapy* 5 (3). Bentham Science Publishers Ltd.: 285–297. doi:10.2174/1566523054065057.

George, Lindsey A., Spencer K. Sullivan, Adam Giermasz, John E. J. Rasko, Benjamin J. Samelson-Jones, Jonathan Ducore, Adam Cuker, et al. 2017. "Hemophilia B Gene Therapy with a High-Specific-Activity Factor IX Variant." 377 (23). Massachusetts Medical Society: 2215–2227. doi:10.1056/NEJMOA1708538.

Ghosh, Arkasubhra, and Dongsheng Duan. 2007. "Biotechnology and Genetic Engineering Reviews Expanding Adeno-Associated Viral Vector Capacity: A Tale of Two Vectors." *Biotechnology and Genetic Engineering Reviews* 24 (1): 165–178. doi:10.1080/02648725.2007.10648098.

Govindasamy, Lakshmanan, Michael A. DiMattia, Brittney L. Gurda, Sujata Halder, Robert McKenna, John A. Chiorini, Nicholas Muzyczka, Sergei Zolotukhin, and Mavis Agbandje-McKenna. 2013. "Structural Insights into Adeno-Associated Virus Serotype 5." *Journal of Virology* 87 (20). American Society for Microbiology: 11187–11199. doi:10.1128/JVI.00867-13.

Grimm, D., and M. Kay. 2005. "From Virus Evolution to Vector Revolution: Use of Naturally Occurring Serotypes of Adeno-Associated Virus (AAV) as Novel Vectors for Human Gene Therapy." *Current Gene Therapy* 3 (4). Bentham Science Publishers Ltd.: 281–304. doi:10.2174/1566523034578285.

Guo, Yansu, Dan Wang, Tao Qiao, Chunxing Yang, Qin Su, Guangping Gao, and Zuoshang Xu. 2015. "A Single Injection of Recombinant Adeno-Associated Virus into the Lumbar Cistern Delivers Transgene Expression Throughout the Whole Spinal Cord." *Molecular Neurobiology 2015 53:5* 53 (5). Springer: 3235–3248. doi:10.1007/S12035-015-9223-1.

Hoggan, M. D., N. R. Blacklow, and W. P. Rowe. 1966. "Studies of Small DNA Viruses Found in Various Adenovirus Preparations: Physical, Biological, and Immunological Characteristics." *Proceedings of the National Academy of Sciences of the United States of America* 55 (6). National Academy of Sciences: 1474. doi:10.1073/PNAS.55.6.1467.

Jang, Jae Hyung, James T. Koerber, Jung Suk Kim, Prashanth Asuri, Tandis Vazin, Melissa Bartel, Albert Keung, Inchan Kwon, Kook In Park, and David V. Schaffer. 2011. "An Evolved Adeno-Associated Viral Variant Enhances Gene Delivery and Gene Targeting in Neural Stem Cells." *Molecular Therapy* 19 (4). Cell Press: 667–675. doi:10.1038/MT.2010.287.

Kotin, Robert M. 2008. "Prospects for the Use of Adeno-Associated Virus as a Vector for Human Gene Therapy." *Https://Home.Liebertpub.Com/Hum* 5 (7). Mary Ann Liebert, Inc. 2 Madison Avenue Larchmont, NY 10538 USA: 793–801. doi:10.1089/HUM.1994.5.7-793.

Kuzmin, D. A., Shutova, M. V., Johnston, N. R., Smith, O. P., Fedorin, V. V., Kukushkin, Y. S., van der Loo, J. C. M., and Johnstone, E. C. 2021. "The Clinical Landscape for AAV Gene Therapies." *Nature Reviews. Drug Discovery* 20 (3). NLM (Medline): 173–174. doi:10.1038/D41573-021-00017-7.

Lebkowski, J. S., M. M. McNally, T. B. Okarma, and L. B. Lerch. 1988. "Adeno-Associated Virus: A Vector System for Efficient Introduction and Integration of DNA into a Variety of Mammalian Cell Types." *Molecular and Cellular Biology* 8 (10). American Society for Microbiology: 3988–3996. doi:10.1128/MCB.8.10.3988-3996.1988.

Lisowski, Leszek, Allison P. Dane, Kirk Chu, Yue Zhang, Sharon C. Cunningham, Elizabeth M. Wilson, Sean Nygaard, Markus Grompe, Ian E. Alexander, and Mark A. Kay. 2013. "Selection and Evaluation of Clinically Relevant AAV Variants in a Xenograft Liver Model." *Nature 2013 506:7488* 506 (7488). Nature Publishing Group: 382–386. doi:10.1038/nature12875.

Lochrie, Michael A., Gwen P. Tatsuno, Brian Christie, Jennifer Wellman McDonnell, Shangzhen Zhou, Richard Surosky, Glenn F. Pierce, and Peter Colosi. 2006. "Mutations on the External Surfaces of Adeno-AssociatedVirus Type 2 Capsids That Affect Transduction AndNeutralization." *Journal of Virology* 80 (2). American Society for Microbiology: 821–834. doi:10.1128/JVI.80.2.821-834.2006.

Madsen, Declan, Emma R. Cantwell, Timothy O'Brien, Patricia A. Johnson, and Bernard P. Mahon. 2009. "Adeno-Associated Virus Serotype 2 Induces Cell-Mediated Immune Responses Directed Against Multiple Epitopes of the Capsid Protein VP1." *The Journal of General Virology* 90 (Pt 11). Microbiology Society: 2622–2633. doi:10.1099/VIR.0.014175-0.

Maheshri, Narendra, James T. Koerber, Brian K. Kaspar, and David V. Schaffer. 2006. "Directed Evolution of Adeno-Associated Virus Yields Enhanced Gene Delivery Vectors." *Nature Biotechnology 2006 24:2* 24 (2). Nature Publishing Group: 198–204. doi:10.1038/nbt1182.

Manno, Catherine S., Glenn F. Pierce, Valder R. Arruda, Bertil Glader, Margaret Ragni, John J. E. Rasko, Margareth C. Ozelo, et al. 2006. "Successful Transduction of Liver in Hemophilia by AAV-Factor IX and Limitations Imposed by the Host Immune Response." *Nature Medicine 2006 12:3* 12 (3). Nature Publishing Group: 342–347. doi:10.1038/nm1358.

Martino, Ashley T., Etiena Basner-Tschakarjan, David M. Markusic, Jonathan D. Finn, Christian Hinderer, Shangzhen Zhou, David A. Ostrov, et al. 2013. "Engineered AAV Vector Minimizes in Vivo Targeting of Transduced Hepatocytes by Capsid-Specific CD8+ T Cells." *Blood* 121 (12). American Society of Hematology: 2224–2233. doi:10.1182/BLOOD-2012-10-460733.

McBride, Jodi L., Mark R. Pitzer, Ryan L. Boudreau, Brett Dufour, Theodore Hobbs, Sergio R. Ojeda, and Beverly L. Davidson. 2011. "Preclinical Safety of RNAi-Mediated HTT Suppression in the Rhesus Macaque as a Potential Therapy for Huntington's Disease." *Molecular Therapy* 19 (12). Cell Press: 2152–2162. doi:10.1038/MT.2011.219.

Mendell, Jerry R., Samiah Al-Zaidy, Richard Shell, W. Dave Arnold, Louise R. Rodino-Klapac, Thomas W. Prior, Linda Lowes, et al. 2017. "Single-Dose Gene-Replacement Therapy for Spinal Muscular Atrophy." 377 (18). Massachusetts Medical Society: 1713–1722. doi:10.1056/NEJMOA1706198.

Mingozzi, Federico, Marcela V. Maus, Daniel J. Hui, Denise E. Sabatino, Samuel L. Murphy, John E. J. Rasko, Margaret V. Ragni, et al. 2007. "CD8 + T-Cell Responses to Adeno-Associated Virus Capsid in Humans." *Nature Medicine 2007 13:4* 13 (4). Nature Publishing Group: 419–422. doi:10.1038/nm1549.

Miyake, Koichi, Noriko Miyake, Yoshiyuki Yamazaki, Takashi Shimada, and Yukihiko Hirai. 2012. "Serotype-Independent Method of Recombinant Adeno-Associated Virus (AAV) Vector Production and Purification." *Journal of Nippon Medical School* 79 (6). The Medical Association of Nippon Medical School: 394–402. doi:10.1272/JNMS.79.394.

Moskalenko, Marina, Lili Chen, Melinda van Roey, Brian A. Donahue, Richard O. Snyder, James G. McArthur, and Salil D. Patel. 2000. "Epitope Mapping of Human Anti-Adeno-Associated Virus Type 2 Neutralizing Antibodies: Implications for Gene Therapy and Virus Structure." *Journal of Virology* 74 (4). American Society for Microbiology: 1761–1766. doi:10.1128/JVI.74.4.1761-1766.2000.

Münch, Robert C., Hanna Janicki, Iris Völker, Anke Rasbach, Michael Hallek, Hildegard Büning, and Christian J. Buchholz. 2013. "Displaying High-Affinity Ligands on Adeno-Associated Viral Vectors Enables Tumor Cell-Specific and Safe Gene Transfer." *Molecular Therapy* 21 (1). Cell Press: 109–118. doi:10.1038/MT.2012.186.

Nóbrega, Clévio, Liliana Mendonça, and Carlos A. Matos. 2020. "Viral Vectors for Gene Therapy." *A Handbook of Gene and Cell Therapy*. Springer, Cham, 39–90. doi:10.1007/978-3-030-41333-0_3.

Perabo, Luca, Jan Endell, Susan King, Kerstin Lux, Daniela Goldnau, Michael Hallek, and Hildegard Büning. 2006. "Combinatorial Engineering of a Gene Therapy Vector: Directed Evolution of Adeno-Associated Virus." *The Journal of Gene Medicine* 8 (2). John Wiley & Sons, Ltd: 155–162. doi:10.1002/JGM.849.

Rabinowitz, Joseph E., and Jude Samulski. 1998. "Adeno-Associated Virus Expression Systems for Gene Transfer." *Current Opinion in Biotechnology* 9 (5). Elsevier Current Trends: 470–475. doi:10.1016/S0958-1669(98)80031-1.

Russell, David W., and Roll K. Hirata. 1998. "Human Gene Targeting by Viral Vectors." *Nature Genetics 1998 18:4* 18 (4). Nature Publishing Group: 325–330. doi:10.1038/ng0498-325.

Samulski, R. Jude, and Nicholas Muzyczka. 2014. "AAV-Mediated Gene Therapy for Research and Therapeutic Purposes." 1 (1). Annual Reviews: 427–451. doi:10.1146/ANNUREV-VIROLOGY-031413-085355.

Samulski, Richard J., Arun Srivastava, Kenneth I. Berns, and Nicholas Muzyczka. 1983. “Rescue of Adeno-Associated Virus from Recombinant Plasmids: Gene Correction Within the Terminal Repeats of AAV.” *Cell* 33 (1). Cell Press: 135–143. doi:10.1016/0092-8674(83)90342-2.

Saraiva, Joana, Rui Jorge Nobre, and Luis Pereira de Almeida. 2016. “Gene Therapy for the CNS Using AAVs: The Impact of Systemic Delivery by AAV9.” *Journal of Controlled Release* 241 (November). Elsevier: 94–109. doi:10.1016/J.JCONREL.2016.09.011.

Schmidt, Michael, Antonis Voutetakis, Sandra Afione, Changyu Zheng, Danielle Mandikian, and John A. Chiorini. 2008. “Adeno-Associated Virus Type 12 (AAV12): A Novel AAV Serotype with Sialic Acid- and Heparan Sulfate Proteoglycan-Independent Transduction Activity.” *Journal of Virology* 82 (3). American Society for Microbiology: 1399–1406. doi:10.1128/JVI.02012-07.

Shen, Shen, Eric D. Horowitz, Andrew N. Troupes, Sarah M. Brown, Nagesh Pulicherla, Richard J. Samulski, Mavis Agbandje-McKenna, and Aravind Asokan. 2013. “Engraftment of a Galactose Receptor Footprint onto Adeno-Associated Viral Capsids Improves Transduction Efficiency *.” *Journal of Biological Chemistry* 288 (40). Elsevier: 28814–28823. doi:10.1074/JBC.M113.482380.

Summerford, Candace, and Richard Jude Samulski. 1998. “Membrane-Associated Heparan Sulfate Proteoglycan Is a Receptor for Adeno-Associated Virus Type 2 Virions.” *Journal of Virology* 72 (2). American Society for Microbiology: 1438–1445. doi:10.1128/JVI.72.2.1438-1445.1998.

Trapani, Ivana, Pasqualina Colella, Andrea Sommella, Carolina Iodice, Giulia Cesi, Sonia de Simone, Elena Marrocco, et al. 2014. “Effective Delivery of Large Genes to the Retina by Dual AAV Vectors.” *EMBO Molecular Medicine* 6 (2). John Wiley & Sons, Ltd: 194–211. doi:10.1002/EMMM.201302948.

Weitzman, Matthew D., and R. Michael Linden. 2012. “Adeno-Associated Virus Biology.” *Methods in Molecular Biology* 807. Humana Press: 1–23. doi:10.1007/978-1-61779-370-7_1.

Wobus, Christiane E., Barbara Hügle-Dörr, Anne Girod, Gabriele Petersen, Michael Hallek, and Jürgen A. Kleinschmidt. 2000. “Monoclonal Antibodies Against the Adeno-Associated Virus Type 2 (AAV-2) Capsid: Epitope Mapping and Identification of Capsid Domains Involved in AAV-2—Cell Interaction and Neutralization of AAV-2 Infection.” *Journal of Virology* 74 (19). American Society for Microbiology (ASM): 9281–9293. doi:10.1128/jvi.74.19.9281-9293.2000.

Wu, Zhijian, Hongyan Yang, and Peter Colosi. 2010. “Effect of Genome Size on AAV Vector Packaging.” *Molecular Therapy* 18 (1). Cell Press: 80–86. doi:10.1038/MT.2009.255.

Yan, Ziying, Roman Zak, G. W. Gant Luxton, Teresa C. Ritchie, Ursula Bantel-Schaal, and John F. Engelhardt. 2002. “Ubiquitination of Both Adeno-Associated Virus Type 2 and 5 Capsid Proteins Affects the Transduction Efficiency of Recombinant Vectors.” *Journal of Virology* 76 (5). American Society for Microbiology: 2043–2053. doi:10.1128/JVI.76.5.2043-2053.2002.

Zhang, Yadong, Yongping Yue, Liang Li, Chady H. Hakim, Keqing Zhang, Gail D. Thomas, and Dongsheng Duan. 2013. “Dual AAV Therapy Ameliorates Exercise-Induced Muscle Injury and Functional Ischemia in Murine Models of Duchenne Muscular Dystrophy.” *Human Molecular Genetics* 22 (18). Oxford Academic: 3720–3729. doi:10.1093/HMG/DDT224.

Zhong, Li, Baozheng Li, Cathryn S. Mah, Lakshmanan Govindasamy, Mavis Agbandje-McKenna, Mario Cooper, Roland W. Herzog, et al. 2008. “Next Generation of Adeno-Associated Virus 2 Vectors: Point Mutations in Tyrosines Lead to High-Efficiency Transduction at Lower Doses.” *Proceedings of the National Academy of Sciences* 105 (22). National Academy of Sciences: 7827–7832. doi:10.1073/PNAS.0802866105.

14 Gene Therapy for Acquired Tissue Damage

Scope, Quality, Non-Clinical and Clinical Guidelines of Gene Therapy Medical Products

Rakesh Sharma, Robert Moffatt, Yuvraj Singh Negi and Shashi Prabha Singh

CONTENTS

DOI: 10.1201/9781003186069-14

14.1 BACKGROUND

Gene therapy by geno-ceutical medical products (GTMPs) can be coined as 'orphan drugs' due to less known drug-like nature of therapeutic nucleotides in metabolic intervention. FDA also approved recently this terminology. FDA approved vector for a gene delivery formulation/system containing a genetic construct engineered to express a specific transgene 'gene therapy sequence' for the regulation, repair, replacement, addition or deletion of a genetic sequence (in acquired tissues)(0). The active substance in 'orphan drug-like geno-ceutical' are the nucleic acid sequences or genetically modified microorganisms, viruses or cells. The active substance may be composed of multiple elements. By delivery of such gene therapy constructs or vectors (so-called gene delivery vectors), in vivo genetic regulation or genetic modification of somatic cells can be achieved. Fortunately, genetic modification or geno-ceutical 'orphan drug' products may offer great therapeutic value. In fact, vectors used in GTMPs can be engineered to target specific diseased tissues or tumor cells or to ensure the safety of the GTMP (deletion of genes associated with virulence, pathogenicity, immunotoxicity or replication-competence). Chapter 8 in this book describes a detailed application of virus therapy applications using adenovirus, herpes simplex, measles and other viruses currently in use. Continued efforts on development of gene therapy by using geno-ceutical orphan drug clinical trials over a half-century, now regulatory government authorities force scientists and industries to follow guidelines and fulfill requirements in terms of compliance to avoid futile attempts and saving time.

In the present chapter, the authors focus from on legal guidelines addressing the requirement for a marketing authorization application (MAA) of gene therapy in terms of non-cell-based gene delivery GTMPs from a biological origin, which fall broadly into three groups: (1) viral vectors; (2) DNA vectors (e.g., plasmid DNA, chromosome-based vectors, iBAC, S/MAR and transposon vectors; and (3) bacterial vectors (e.g., modified *Lactococcus* spp., *Listeria* spp. and *Streptococcus* spp.). However, the most common vector systems used for gene therapy are viral vectors and plasmid DNA vectors. Viral vectors may be replication-defective, replication-competent or replication-conditional types. Plasmid DNA vectors may be administered either in a simple salt solution ('naked' DNA) or may be complexed with a carrier or in a delivery formulation. These vectors can be used to manufacture genetically modified cells. For it, lot of vector details are required to mention them as controlled or safe materials in gene delivery.

Historically many gene therapy approaches have been based on gene expression of a transgene (transgene delivery) encoding a functional protein (i.e., the transgene GTMP product). Today, nucleic acid sequences such as microRNA; RNA interference (RNAi) via short hairpin RNAs (shRNA); molecular scissors and gene editing approaches such as CRISPR-Cas, zinc finger nucleases (ZFNs) or transcription activator–like effector nucleases (TALENs) are used for gene delivery to repair, add or delete a genetic sequence via gene silencing, exon skipping, gene regulation, gene knockdown and nucleotide changes. The term 'gene therapy sequence' refers to nucleic acid sequences that may be delivered and used in gene therapy.

In present time, no clear unanimous guidelines and regulations exist for experimental, non-clinical, pre-clinical and clinical use of viruses, bacteria and nucleic acids as GTMPs to end-user manufacturing industries. The chapter presents pieces of newly proposed updated guidelines on minimal requirements to serve as a road map to dedicated scientists, researchers and corporate industries and clinical medical teams to propose new test protocols using available GTMPs and advanced therapy medicinal products (ATMPs) in their own gene therapy trials. By keeping in mind ethical, scientific, legal, commercial and technical requirements in terms of compliance by manufacturing industries, the components of these guidelines are defined to minimize differences and avoid the weakness in new proposals of a sound and effective use of GTMPs or therapeutic vectors for specific clinical gene therapy applications. It is necessary to fulfill requirements of gene delivery minimum norms before approval of GTMPs can undergo MAA for gene therapy (1).

14.2 SCOPE

The geno-ceutical 'orphan drug' or GTMPs contain recombinant nucleic acid sequences (e.g., DNA vectors) or genetically modified micro-organisms or viruses and recombinant elements for example, gene delivery vectors. ATMPs include GTMPs, somatic cell therapy. Tissue engineered medicinal products combined with ATMPs are used in human use for treatment of cancers of the prostate, breast, colon, pancreas, and liver; meningioma; melanoma; glioma; polio; measles; and many more. All these need guidelines for gene editing and delivery tools. However, the Food and Drug Administration (FDA) and European Commission (EC) have set separate requirements for the environmental risk assessment (ERA) for genetically modified organisms, including genetically modified cells (allogeneic or autologous somatic cells modified ex vivo or in vitro with a gene therapy vector prior to gene delivery in the human subject (2). Hence, they are also described separately in terms of quality, non-clinical and clinical aspects for manufacturing industries with marketing authorization.

The principles outlined here apply to the vectors used in gene delivery of geno-ceuticals, modification or gene editing in such cells. Guidelines are presented on gene editing in such cells. Guidelines are presented on gene editing approaches for GTMP, design and safety of GTMP relevant to the geno-ceutical products for industries. The same applies to chemically synthesize the therapeutic nucleotide sequences for human use. Major difference is that pharma drug action is at pin-pointed metabolic step while geno-ceutical action is like 'orphan' with uncertainty of specific metabolic protein(s) synthesized for need.

14.3 LEGAL AUTHORITIES TO APPROVE GTMPS FOR GENE DELIVERY

The two EC and FDA guidelines from European Commission and United States of America are well established. However, each country follows own specific guidelines, reflection papers. International Conference of Harmonization (ICH) guidelines are applicable to GTMPs, ATMPs and pharmacopoeia requirements (see Table 14.1). ATMPs are regulated by bodies such as EC 1394/2007 for human use. Part IV of the Annex I to Directive 2001/83/EC, as amended by Commission Directive 2009/120/EC, includes the definition of a GTMP, the technical requirements for GTMPs with definitions of starting materials and the principle of a risk-based approach to determine quality, non-clinical and clinical data for MAA (1). The FDA recommends stringent requirements for manufacturing industries (FDA CMC 2020 guidelines) to comply with six guidelines when using replication-competent retrovirus in humans (see Table 14.1) (3–6). The definition of geno-ceutical, orphan drug, geno-ceutical action and GTMPs are not well presented. The technical requirements for GTMPs with definitions of starting materials, quality attributes, manufacturing processes, process controls, control of critical steps and intermediates, pharmaceutical development and purity testing with a principle of risk-based approach are described by FDA to determine the high quality of non-clinical and clinical data output for MAA. Major focus is urgent marketing authorization due to available several products in market without much research.

The following description of requirements and compliance for scientists and manufacturers is based on several references and regulatory guidelines as compiled in Table 14.1.

14.4 QUALITY CONTROL DETAILS: WHAT INFORMATION SHOULD BE DISCLOSED?

For MAA of geno-ceutical GTMPs and ATMPs, a quality control dossier demands details in geno-ceutical orphan substance and orphan product format (7–8, 24). Most of the GTMPs and ATMPs are controlled materials taken from a pooled supply from regulated gene banks. The genoceutical section demands only a probable formulation step, while the major focus is on delivery and manufacturing ensures successful gene therapy.

14.4.1 General Information on the GTMP

The drug-like geno-ceutical substance nature as per the World Health Organization (WHO) international is non-proprietary 'orphan drug' or its trade name proposed for the product. A full description of the geno-ceutical action of GTMP should be disclosed. The clinical indication for the drug-like GTMP/ATMP product behavior

TABLE 14.1
Guidelines on Gene Delivery Medical Products for Gene Therapy

Guidelines	Human Use	Reference
EMA/CAT/686637/2011(part IV)	Risk-based approach applied to GTMPs	1
EMEA/ CHMP/ GTWP/125491/2006	Environment risk assessment	2
MEA/CHMP/GTWP/60436/2007	Retrovirus-based human gene therapy	3
FDA CMC 2020(Part I)	Investigational new GTMP	4a
FDA CMC 2020 (Part II)	Testing of retroviral vector–based gene delivery for RCR manufacturing	4b
FDA CMC 2020 (Part III) [21CFR316.3(b)12]	Long-term follow-up after administration of human gene therapy	4c
FDA CMC 2020 (Part IV)	Gene therapy for rare diseases, retinal disorders, hemophilia	5
FDA CMC2020 Part V	Sameness of GTMPs vs. drugs orphan drug regulations (ODA)	6
EMEA/CHMP/ GTWP/671639/2008	Quality, non-clinical and clinical uses of GTMPs	7
EMEA/EMA/410/01 rev.3	Risk of transmitting animal spongiform encephalopathy in GTMPs	8
EMA/CHMP/BWP/814397/2011	Use of porcine trypsin in manufacturing GTMPs	9
EMEA/CHMP/QWP/396951/2006	Excipients in dossier for MAA for marketing GTMPs	10
EMEA/CHMP/ GTWP/587488/2007	Quality, non-clinical and clinical use of viral vector delivery system	11
EMA/CAT/GTWP/44236/2009	Design modifications of gene therapy medicinal products	12
EMEA/CHMP/ICH/607698/08	Considerations on oncolytic viruses in gene delivery	13
EMEA/CHMP/ICH/449035/09	General principles to address virus and vector shedding	14
EMEA/CPMP/ICH/295/95	ICH-Q5A(R1) for viral safety evaluation of biotechnology GTMPs	15
EMEA/CPMP/ICH/138/95	ICH-Q5C for on stability testing of biotechnological/ biological products	16
EMEA/CPMP/ICH/294/95	ICH-Q5D on derivation and characterization of cell substrates for GTMPs	17
EMEA/CPMP/ICH/5721/03	ICH-Q5E on comparability of biotechnological/ biological products	18
EMEA/CPMP/ICH/365/96	ICH-Q6B on specifications, test procedures and acceptance of GTMPs	19
EMA/CHMP/ICH/425213/2011	ICH-Q11 on development and manufacture of drug/ biotech GTMPs	20

needs with in vivo mode of action, design of the vector, individual components and the therapeutic geno-ceutical sequences, junction regions and regulatory elements should be described. Other information to ensure delivery, regulation, expression or safety of the GTMP constructs.

14.4.1.1 Vector Design for Geno-ceutical Use

The vector design includes its clinical indication, mechanism of geno-ceutical action, method and frequency of administration (i.e., potential need for retreatment), selectivity and transduction/transfection efficiency of the vector for the target somatic cells, and expression and functional activity of the therapeutic sequences. Gene therapy vector design includes: vector uptake by the target cells, transport and its uncoating, vector or sequence persistence, sustained transcription/expression of the transgene, tissue-specific transcription or expression, preexisting or induced immunity to vectors and protein expressed from the transgene (action of geno-ceuticals) and scalability of the vector system.

For geno-ceutical GTMP product actions based on viral or bacterial vectors need following details of the vector design:

i) Pathogenicity and virulence in man and in other animal species of the parental organism and the vector components and the deletion of virulent determinants;
ii) The minimization of non-essential accessory vector components or engineering of viral proteins and replication defective virus vector;
iii) The use of production and packaging cell lines with no or minimal sequence homology with the vector;
iv) The minimization of vector sequence homology with any human pathogens or endogenous viruses, thus reducing the risk of generating a novel infectious agent or replication-competent virus (RCV);
v) Tissue tropism;
vi) Transduction efficiency in the target cell population or cell type g., whether the cells are dividing or terminally differentiated or are expressing the appropriate viral receptor for internalization;
vii) The presence and persistence of the viral gene sequences necessary for antiviral chemotherapy of the wild-type virus;
viii) The tissue specificity of replication;
ix) Germ line transmission;
x) For gene integrating vectors, details on the risk of insertion mutagenesis;
xi) For replication-deficient viral vectors, highlight the viral vector replication incompetent;
xii) The possibility of any recombination events leading to RCV or replication via trans regulation should be discussed before geno-ceutical packaging/ producer cell lines. At the stage of geno-ceutical production, RCV screening and testing are mandatory.

For RCV vectors or replication-conditional viral vectors, a clear rationale for the construct and the individual genetic elements to control replication should be provided with regard to its safe use for the proposed clinical indications. Consideration should be given to the following factors with regard to the acceptability of using an RCV as a GTMP:

i) That replication competence is required for the efficacy of the medicinal product;

ii) That the vector does not contain any element(s) known to induce oncogenicity/tumorigenicity in humans;
iii) That the parental viral strain is a known pathogen,
iv) infectivity, virulence and pathogenicity of the RCV after the desired genetic manipulations;
v) The tissue specificity of replication.

For viral vectors which are selected on the basis of their organ/tissue tropism, evidence should be provided on the selective transduction/expression of the inserted gene or an appropriate reporter gene at the desired site. This should inform the design and development of bio-distribution studies.

14.4.1.2 Developmental Genetic Concerns

For all vectors, either virus or bacteria, its origin, history and biological characteristics with any lacuna in known risk are mandatory with the following details:

- All geno-ceutical GTMP is aimed at therapy, delivery, safety, control and production for their use.
- For plasmid DNA, via bacterial vectors disclosure of the plasmid backbone, transgene and selection gene or regulatory nucleotide sequences to generate RNA.
- For viral vectors, details of the virus backbone, transgene and regulatory sequences.
- For bacteria vector, details of plasmid origin, identification and isolation of nucleotide sequences and regulative functions with gene coding capacity.
- The details of therapeutic gene sequences of any modifications to wild-type sequences with codon optimization, site-specific mutations, deletions and rearrangements.
- The details of therapeutic sequence transcriptional elements to control the expression of a transgene in a temporal or tissue-specific manner for product.
- Use of DNA element selection and urgency of minimal use of antibiotic-resistance genes in the final GTMP.
- The purity and characterization of the genetic material with batch analysis and use.
- Any cross-contamination by recombination with endogenous sequences in the cell substrate during design, construction or production of geno-ceuticals
- Contamination of the final geno-ceutical GTMP with sequences present during manufacturing (e.g., read-through from production vectors).
- Data on the control and stability of the vector and the therapeutic sequences during development and in production should be provided. The degree of fidelity of the replication systems should ensure the integrity and homogeneity of the amplified nucleic acids.
- Complete details of history of the cell line, origin, identification, characteristics and potential contamination with other cells, bacteria, viruses or extraneous genetic sequences to ensure genetic stability during production.

- Full details of the origin, identity and biological characteristics of the packaging cell line or helper virus together with details of the presence or absence of endogenous viral particles or sequences, along with any lacuna in knowledge or risk assessment (2).
- During development, details of any changes to the vector design to improve product characteristics to comply with ICH guideline Q5E (see Table 14.1) (9).

14.4.2 Vectors for Gene Therapy

In the following discussion, vectors using GTMPs/ATMPs as substances are described for industry along the same lines as non-drug live 'orphan' biological substances recommended by FDA. However, the FDA and EC still have incomplete guidelines on the genetic origin of GTMP (geno-ceutical) substances and regulating GTMPs and ATMPs in side tissue cells. Moreover, attention needs to be paid to more specific transgene action inside cells to define geno-ceutical toxicity or adverse actions.

14.4.2.1 Manufacturing

Vectors should be produced from well-characterized bacterial or virus seeds and/or cell banks. Master and working seed/cell banks should be established and subjected to an appropriate quality control strategy. Appropriate control of the risk of contamination with adventitious agents is essential to ensure the microbiological safety of the product.

Production may involve the establishment of working virus seeds before inoculation of the production cell culture, or may involve the use of DNA plasmids to transfect the production cell culture in addition to or instead of infection with a virus. The number of steps between the working seed/cell lot and vector production should be almost equal to the steps used for production of the vector used in clinical studies.

Mention the rationale of using different substrates for production. This might include primary cells, diploid cells and/or continuous cell lines. The rationale for the use of genetically engineered cells should comply with norms for production, in accordance with the principles outlined in ICH guideline Q5D.

Mention the effective purification process used to reduce or eliminate impurities to acceptable levels. Mention the contamination of the final GTMP with manufacture-derived sequences, such as read-through from the production vector or contamination with helper sequences. Ideally, steps should be taken in production to minimize or eliminate these. In some cases, there may be minimal downstream processing of viral vectors. In such cases, justify the absence of purification steps to reduce unwanted product- and process-related impurities based on technical considerations, product quality and clinical safety and efficacy. The use of maximum purification steps is encouraged for all gene therapy vectors. Substances such as diluents or stabilizers or any other excipients added during preparation of the final vector or final product should be shown not to impair the efficacy and safety of the vector in the concentrations employed.

14.4.2.1.1 Requirement of Vector Manufacturing Process and Process Controls

A clear definition of the vector-origin drug substance should be provided. A flow diagram should be provided to illustrate the manufacturing route from the bacterial seed, virus seeds and/or cell banks or sources of nucleic acids up to the GTMP substance. The flow diagram should include all steps (i.e., unit operations) of the manufacture of the purified GTMP substance, including inoculation, fermentation/culture, harvesting, clarification, pooling, purification and concentration. It is expected that process parameters and control procedures are implemented to ensure an acceptable level of consistency of production conditions of the expected product, at least within the parameters of the clinically tested batches. Unintended variability—for example, in culture conditions or inoculation steps during production—may cause alteration to the gene product, reduce the yield of the gene product and/or result in quantitative and qualitative differences in the quality of the vector or the impurities. For the process description, information should be included on individual process steps—for example, scale, culture media, additives and major equipment. For each stage of the vector manufacturing process, all relevant information (such as DNA and virus concentrations, cell densities, cultivation times, holding times, process intermediates and temperatures as appropriate) should be provided. Critical steps and critical intermediates should be identified, and acceptance criteria should be set and justified.

For non-replication–competent viral vectors and conditionally replicating virus vectors, information should be provided on process parameters and controls and testing conducted to prevent infection/contamination of the packaging cell line by wild-type, helper or hybrid viruses, which might lead to the formation of replication-competent recombinant viruses during production. For non-replication–competent viral vectors, the absence of RCV should be demonstrated with an assay of suitable sensitivity. The manufacturing process must be set up to minimize the risk of microbiological contamination.

To ensure the control and consistency of the vector GTMP substance process and product at the end of harvesting, analytical and control parameters should be developed and established. These may include the following: number of passages, growth rates and viability, bio-burden and endotoxin, identity (desired transgene and vector), purity and yield. If testing is made more sensitive by initial partial processing (e.g., unprocessed bulk may be toxic in test cell cultures, whereas partially processed bulk may not be toxic), then this should be explained in the MAA. Sensitive molecular methods may be used as alternatives to test for the presence of specific extraneous viral sequences.

For viral vectors, titers and particle-to-infectivity ratios should be determined on harvests, and minimum acceptable titers should be established. Tests for RCVs may be necessary for certain replication-defective or conditionally replicating viral vectors. For products containing replication-deficient viruses, a test to detect replication-competent viruses in supernatant fluids of producing cells and in the viral fraction at appropriate stages of production is essential. A clear definition of a batch of vector drug substance should be provided, including details on batch size and scale of production. An explanation of the batch numbering system, including information regarding any pooling of harvests or intermediates, should be provided. If nucleic acid constructs are complexed with polycations, proteins or polymers or are linked to carriers, details of the production process, parameters and controls for all components of the final gene therapy vector should be provided.

14.4.2.2 Controlled Materials

14.4.2.2.1 Starting 1 Materials in Gene Delivery

All starting materials used for manufacture of the active vector substance should be listed with information on their source, quality and control of these materials. The bacterial/cell/virus seed or banks for starting materials should be mentioned, with the source and history of the first-time cells or bacterial or virus seeds used for generation of the respective bank with genetic stability of the parent material. All starting materials at working cell banks and viral seeds should be characterized and monitored. Evidence of freedom from contamination with adventitious agents is essential. For all starting materials, the absence of microbial/viral and fungal contaminants should be ensured through testing after expansion to the limit of in vitro cultivation used for production.

If materials of ruminant origin are used in preparation of the master and working seeds or cell banks, compliance with the relevant transmissible spongiform encephalopathy (TSE) note for guidance is required (10). Moreover, a separate guideline exists on the use of bovine serum or porcine trypsin used in the manufacture of human biological medicinal products (see Table 14.1) (11). Genetic stability of the starting materials should be demonstrated at the beginning and the end of the culturing process.

The following sections provide an indication of the tests expected to be conducted on different types of starting material tests required as product- and production process-specific:

14.4.2.2.1.1 Virus Seed Banks Control of virus seed banks should include identity (genetic and immunological), virus concentration and infectious titer, virus genome integrity, expression of the therapeutic sequences, biological activity of the therapeutic sequence or the derived product (protein or RNA), sterility (bacterial, and fungal), absence of *Mycoplasma* and *Spiroplasma* (in case insect cells are used during virus seed production), absence of adventitious/contaminating viruses and RCVs (where the product is replication deficient or replication conditional), intervial homogeneity and other relevant characteristics of the virus seed bank. The complete sequence of the therapeutic and the regulatory elements and, where feasible, the complete sequence of the virus in the seed bank should be confirmed as part of the characterization (see Table 14.1).

14.4.2.2.1.2 Eukaryotic Cell Banks Testing conducted on producer/packaging cell lines should include identity, purity, cell number, viability, strain characterization, genotyping/phenotyping and, if appropriate, verification of the plasmid/transgenic/helper sequence structure (e.g., restriction analysis or sequencing), genetic stability, copy number, identity and integrity of the introduced sequences.

Testing of the producer/packaging cell bank for the presence of adventitious viruses should be conducted according to the guidelines given in Table 14.1. Tests for contaminating and endogenous viruses, including wild-type forms of any viral vectors used, should be included if appropriate. The absence of bacterial and fungal contamination, as well as *Mycoplasma* and *Spiroplasma* (insect cells), should be determined.

For the packaging cell lines, detailed descriptions of their design, construction, production and the banking system used should be provided.

14.4.2.2.1.3 RNA or DNA Vectors and Plasmids Testing of RNA and DNA vectors, plasmids or artificial chromosome DNA should include tests for genetic identity and integrity, including confirmation of the therapeutic sequence and regulatory/controlling sequences, freedom from extraneous agents, sterility and endotoxin levels. The presence or absence of specific features such as CpG sequences should be confirmed by suitable methods.

14.4.2.2.1.4 Bacterial Cell Banks Bacterial cell banks should be tested for phenotypic and genomic identity. The presence or absence of inserted or deleted sequences necessary for the safe use of the GTMP should be confirmed. The immunological identity, including the genetically modified components, should be determined, for instance, by serotyping. Absence of contaminating bacteria, contaminating plasmids and contaminating bacteriophage particles that can infect the bacterial producer strain, fungal sterility, and intervial homogeneity of cell bank stocks should be assured. For transformed bacterial cell banks, testing should include the presence of plasmid or genome sequences containing the therapeutic sequence and associated regulatory/control elements, plasmid copy number and ratio of cells with/without plasmids. The principle is described in ICH guideline Q5D on derivation and characterization of cell substrates.

14.4.2.2.1.5 Complex Making Materials Complexing materials (such as nanoparticles or lipids) used during the manufacturing of the GTMP substance are considered as starting materials and have to be mentioned for their intended purpose. The quality and purity of the complexing materials is essential for the said quality of the GTMP; therefore, the appropriate characterization and specification of the complexing materials is considered vital in process controls. The level of information depends on the nature of the complexing material and resulting vector gene product. If multiple sources (e.g., animal, plant, synthetic sources) or suppliers for the complexing materials are used, information should be provided for each, along with additional characterization and comparison studies to demonstrate equivalence of batches (physico-chemical and purity profile and complexing performances) manufactured with each source or supplier.

14.4.2.2.2 Raw Materials

Source, characteristics and testing of all materials used during manufacture should be provided. Data should be provided to demonstrate that all materials used during production are of suitable quality and are consistent between batches and/or between suppliers, in case multiple sourcing is envisaged for some of them, as per the reference given on raw materials of biological origin for the production of cell-based and GTMPs (see Table 14.1). Information should be provided on the residual level of raw materials (or significant components of raw materials such as helper virus/packaging sequences or media) in the final GTMP, and an assessment of the significance of these residuals should be made.

For the helper viruses, detailed descriptions of their design, construction, production and the banking system used should be provided, with the same level of detail and amount of confirmatory data as is required for the starting materials addressed in Section 4.2.2.1.

All raw materials consisting of animal tissue or fluids or containing products of animal origin or materials that have come in contact during production with materials of human or animal origin should comply with the relevant TSE note for guidance and with viral safety and microbial safety requirements (see Table 14.1). Penicillin, all other β-lactam antibiotics and streptomycin should neither be used during production nor added to the final product, as they are known to provoke sensitivity in certain individuals. This would apply to other toxic reagents such as ethidium bromide.

14.4.2.3 Characterization of the Gene Delivery Vector or GTMP Substance

Characterization studies should be conducted throughout the development process, resulting in a comprehensive picture and knowledge of the GTMP, which takes the individual components (including starting materials, intermediates, GTMP substance and GTMP product) into full consideration. Characterization of the vector should include all components, in particular those present in the final product. Ensure that characterization data obtained throughout gene delivery trials is significant in the development and/or manufacturing process. Clear identification of the batches (development, pilot, full-scale details) used for characterization studies should be disclosed. Batches used for setting specifications should be based on manufacturing experience during clinical development, as mentioned later. An extensive characterization of the geno-ceuticals should be established in terms of genotypic and phenotypic identity, purity, biological potency/therapeutic sequence activity, infectivity/transduction efficiency and suitability for the intended use, unless otherwise justified. Characterization studies should use a range of orthogonal state-of-the-art techniques, including molecular, biological and immunological tests. The methods used should be described.

14.4.2.3.1 Structure and Other Characteristics of the Gene Delivery Vector

The data confirming the sequence of the therapeutic gene and genetic elements required for selectivity, regulation and control of the therapeutic sequence should be provided. Mapping data (e.g., via restriction endonucleases) should be provided to complement sequence data and transcription/translation elements and open reading frames analyzed. It should be demonstrated that there is no inclusion of known oncogenic/tumorigenic sequences. Tests should be included to show the integrity and homogeneity of the recombinant viral genome or plasmid and the genetic stability of the vector and therapeutic sequence. Phenotypic identity and analysis of the therapeutic sequences and selectivity/regulatory elements delivered by the vector should be included. Physicochemical characteristics such as refractive index, particle or molecular size average and distribution and aggregation levels should be determined in characterization studies.

For viral vectors, the tissue tropism, infectivity (in a variety of cell cultures), virulence, replication capacity, ratio of infectious to non-infectious particles and immunological characteristics (where appropriate) should be documented. Mean particle size and aggregates should be analyzed. For viral vectors, insertion sites should be determined where appropriate and the potential for insertion mutagenesis established and associated risks fully evaluated.

For plasmids, the transfection efficiency and copy number should be demonstrated in the relevant cell types, and the different plasmid forms should be identified and quantified. The ratio of circular to linear forms, the locations of replication origins and, if relevant to the design of the product, the presence or absence of CpG sequences should be demonstrated.

For a complexed nucleic acid vector, the characteristics of the vector, the complexing components and the resulting complexed nucleic acid sequence should be investigated. This includes the structure of the complex and the interaction between the vehicles and the negatively charged DNA. The properties of the complexing/delivery systems should be adequately characterized and include form, particle size distribution, surface charge, stability under a given condition or in a particular biological environment (such as the one expected for the transfection step), and distribution of nucleic acid within the complexing structure. Suitable tests should be included to establish, for example, that the complexed nucleic acid has the desired biochemical and biological characteristics required for its intended use.

14.4.2.3.2 Biological Activity

The intended action of regulating, repairing, replacing, adding or deleting a genetic sequence should be demonstrated. The in vitro biological activity of all transgenes and any other expressed sequences should be determined. The level of transgene expression, associated biological activity and factors associated with the proposed mechanism of action of the vector and delivery system, including maintenance of the therapeutic sequence in the target cell, should be analyzed. Any selectivity claimed for the host range and tropism of a viral vector or selectivity of delivery of a complexed nucleic acid should be demonstrated, as should selectivity of transgene expression where it is claimed.

14.4.2.3.3 Impurities

Potential impurities in the GTMPs and/or ATMPs will be influenced by the nature of the product and the choice of production or manufacturing process. These include host cell proteins, host cell DNA, helper viruses/sequences, packaging viruses or sequences, residues of biological materials introduced during productions such as bovine serum or albumin, antibiotics, leachable molecules from equipment, endotoxins, RCVs and any proteins co-expressed with the transgene. Additional impurities needing consideration may include hybrid viruses in the case of virus vector production, lipids and polysaccharides in the case of production systems which involve bacterial fermentations and RNA and chromosomal DNA in the case of plasmid purification.

Product-related impurities, such as vectors with deleted, rearranged, hybrid or mutated sequences, should be identified and their levels quantified. The possibilities for co-packaged extraneous DNA sequences being present in the vector should be explored. Reference should be made to potential degradation during the manufacturing process affecting key properties of the vector such as infectivity/

non-infectious forms, plasmid forms with reduced transduction efficacy or degradation of nucleic acid complexes through, for example, oxidation or depolymerization. In the case of vectors designed to be replication deficient or conditionally replicating, the absence of an RCV should be demonstrated and/or conditional replication demonstrated.

Process-related impurities include residues of starting materials (residual DNA and residual host cell protein from each cell bank), raw materials (culture reagents, purification reagents and equipment materials, helper viruses and helper virus nucleic acid used in production), adventitious agents and leachable molecules and extractable products from the process. In the case of complexed nucleic acids, by-products or impurities arising from the formation of the complex during production should be addressed with respect to their impact on the safety and performance of the complex when administered to patients.

The characterization data generated should serve as an input into the specification setting for the drug substance and drug product, along with data from batch analysis. In the case of drug substances that are combined with materials acting as carriers or supports, the characterization studies should be repeated for the substance in the combined state. The nature and strength of the combination involved should be explored in the studies.

14.4.2.4 Specifications for the Drug-Like Vector Substance in Gene Therapy

The criteria for acceptance or rejection of a production batch must be provided. Gene delivery specifications should be given and justified. All specification of parameters, methods and specifications or criteria for acceptance should be provided. The specifications for the vector or complementary drug substance should normally encompass tests for identity, purity, content, activity, sterility, endotoxin level and *Mycoplasma*. The analytical methods should be relevant and techniques validated.

The following sections indicate a set of general specifications. However, a detailed list of the tests required is essentially product and production process specific.

14.4.2.4.1 Identity and integrity

The genetic identity and integrity of the drug substance should be assured using tests that identify both the therapeutic sequence and the vector. Such tests might include DNA sequencing or restriction enzyme mapping and immunological assays.

The identity of the drug substance may also be confirmed through infection/transduction assays and detection of expression or activity of the therapeutic sequences (see the section on potency assays). This identity test is especially important for complexed nucleic acid sequences.

14.4.2.4.2 Content

The quantity of the GTMP substance should be established. For viral vectors, infectious titers should be quantified; the number of particles (infectious/non-infectious, empty/genome containing) should also be determined. The particle-to-infectivity ratio should be included to define the content of the GTMP substance. For plasmids and other forms of nucleic acids, the quantity or concentration of nucleic acid should be established.

14.4.2.4.3 Potency Assay

A suitable measure of the potency of the GTMPs should be established. At least one biological potency specification should be established, the attributes reflecting the physiological mode of action and/or the pharmacological effects of the GTMP. The potency assay should normally encompass an evaluation of the efficiency of gene transfer (infectivity, transduction, delivery) and the level of expression of the therapeutic sequence or its direct activity. Where possible, the potency assay should include a measure of the functional activity of the therapeutic sequence or the product of it. This functional test may be supplemented with immunochemical methods to determine the integrity and quantity of an expressed protein product if appropriate. For release testing, simpler surrogate assays (e.g., based on nucleic acid amplification) may be acceptable, provided a correlation to the more functional test or the clinical outcome has been established in bridging studies.

In vitro biological potency tests should be developed. If not feasible, biological potency tests in animal tissues maintained ex vivo or in whole animals can be considered. Transgenic animals or animals with transplanted human tissues or systems (e.g., a suitable xenograft model) may be suitable for this purpose. In order to reduce the use of animals in accordance with the 3R principles, a validated in vitro method is generally preferred over animal testing wherever possible.

Suitable ways for expressing the potency of GTMP vectors in reference to an appropriately qualified reference material should be established with a range and specifications whenever possible.

14.4.2.4.4 Product-Related Impurities

The presence of product-related impurities such as non-functional forms of the vector or the presence of co-packaged unwanted genetic sequences should be included in the specification and acceptance limits set to exclude or limit these impurities as appropriate and justified.

For viral vectors, empty particle number, aggregates and RCVs should be controlled. For plasmid DNA, limits for different forms of plasmid should be included. Other impurities may need to be considered. Impurity limits should be justified with respect to clinical safety.

14.4.2.4.5 Process-Related Impurities

Specifications should be set for materials used in vector production, unless process validation data have been provided to demonstrate that such residues are consistently reduced to acceptable levels. For the release specifications, tests should be developed and relevant (upper) limits set to monitor the residual levels of contaminants of cellular origin (e.g., host cell protein, including helper virus protein) or DNA from the bacterial or packaging cell line, as well as raw materials that may have been used during the production process such as benzonase or resins. Other process-related impurities may include nucleic acids derived from bacteria used for the production of plasmid DNA, extraneous nucleic acids in vector preparations, helper viruses or other impurities such as residual animal serum proteins (e.g., bovine serum albumin [BSA]) used in production. If tumorigenic/immortalized cell lines are used during production, the total residual DNA level should be strictly controlled and kept at a minimum unless otherwise justified. Impurity limits should be justified with respect to clinical safety and efficacy.

14.4.2.4.6 Extraneous Agents

Tests for extraneous agents should be included to ensure the safety of the vector. For replication-deficient or conditionally replicating viral vectors, a test for RCV should be included. In the case of vectors that are potentially hazardous to patients' health in their replication-competent forms, such as members of Retroviridae, the absence of replication competence should be demonstrated using a validated assay. In other justified cases, it may be acceptable to release vector lots with an upper limit for RCVs. In these cases, the justification for the limit should include qualification on the basis of non-clinical and/or clinical data for batches with similar levels.

14.4.2.4.7 Physicochemical Properties

Limits should be applied to measurement of pH and any other relative physicochemical properties such as opalescence and refractive index. Particle number, molecular size average and size distribution should be controlled, as appropriate.

14.4.2.4.8 Geno-pharmacopeial Tests

Depending on the nature of the GTMP substance, other pharmacopeial tests will apply for sterility testing and bio-burden, which should be done in accordance with requirements (see Table 14.1).

14.4.3 Gene Therapy Product Manufacturing

Most of the considerations made for GTMPs are similar to drugs. Recommendations applicable to ATMPs are the same as those described earlier as well (12). However, some specific requirements apply to the GTMPs as discussed next.

14.4.3.1 Description of the GTMP Product and Genoceutical Development

Definition of the GTMP's qualitative and quantitative formulation should be provided along with the generic trade name proposed. The description should take into account the origin, identification, physico-chemical and functional characterization studies and the expected function of all components in the final product.

14.4.3.2 Manufacturing of the GTMP Product and Process Controls

A clear description of the GTMP's mass-scale manufacturing process and the in-process controls should be provided. A flow diagram should be provided to illustrate the manufacturing route from the purified drug substance up to the final drug product in its primary packaging. The diagram should include all steps (i.e., unit operations), including formulation, filtration, filling and, where relevant, any further freeze-drying or freezing steps. For each stage of the GTMP manufacturing process, all relevant information in terms of holding times, temperatures or any parameter relevant for the final quality of the GTMP should be provided. Process intermediates should be defined. Process parameters and procedures should be defined to ensure consistency of production conditions. The quality controls and critical manufacturing steps should be identified and the control strategy justified. The manufacturing process must be set up to minimize the risk of microbiological contamination.

14.4.3.3 Excipients

Complexing materials for formulating the GTMP product are considered excipients and have to be qualified for their intended purpose. The quality and purity of the complexing materials or excipients are essential for the final quality of the GTMP; therefore, the appropriate characterization and specification of the complexing materials are considered vital. The level of information to be provided will depend on the nature of the complexing material and resulting final GTMP product (see Table 14.1) (13). When multiple sources (e.g., animal, plant, synthetic sources) or suppliers for the complexing material are used, fulfill the requirements as described in Section 4.2.2.1.

14.4.3.4 Characterization for the GTMP Product

Characterization of the GTMPs is not expected at this start stage (see Section 4.2.3 earlier). The GTMP can be presented with medical devices. The compatibility of the GTMP with the medical device will have to be demonstrated. However, specific requirements for ATMPs containing devices are more stringent.

14.4.3.5 GTMP/ATMP Product Specification

Quality control tests should be performed at the final product level, unless appropriate justification can be provided based on release testing at the GTMP substance level. Tests on attributes that are specific to the formulated product in its final container and quality attributes that may have been impacted by the formulation steps should be included in the release testing.

Unless otherwise justified, the release specifications for each batch of ATMPs are expected to embrace the following:

- The range of quality attributes listed under 'GTMP substance' earlier, including identity and potency. Tests for impurities and process-related impurities from the first step could be omitted based on relevant justification and validation data.
- Infectivity or transduction efficiency: in vitro infectivity or transduction efficiency of the GTMP in its final formulation should be included.
- Specification should be applied for appearance and physicochemical properties (e.g., pH and any other relative physicochemical properties such as opalescence, refractive index and osmolality, visible and sub-visible particles) specific to the GTMP product.
- Sterility, endotoxin, particulate matter and other genocopoeial tests such as extractable volume or residual moisture should be included as appropriate.

- Where appropriate, and subject to a risk-based approach, RCV acceptance criteria should be applied to ensure the safety of the GTMPs.
- Assays for critical excipients, such as albumin or complexing materials used in the formulation of either GTMPs or ATMPs should be included, particularly where these ensure the expected bioactivity and/or maintain the stability of the final formulated vector.
- Specifications should also be set for gene delivery vector materials used in the gene therapy formulation and filling unless process validation data have been provided to demonstrate that such residues are consistently reduced to acceptable levels.
- Where the GTMP contains a device, specific release testing, including functional release tests (e.g., for syringes), may be required.

14.4.4 Process Development and Process Validation for GTMP Substance and Gene Therapy Products

Changes in the manufacturing process, such as scale-up of culture and/or purification, often occur during development as product development progresses to full-scale commercial production. These changes are usually introduced before final validation of the process. This may have consequences for the quality of the product, including effects on its biochemical and biological properties, and thus implications for control testing.

Approaches to determine the impact of any process change will vary, depending on whether this is at the GTMP or gene delivery stage and with respect to the specific manufacturing process step concerned. It will also depend on the extent of the manufacturer's knowledge and experience with the process and development data gained. Appropriate studies should be conducted in order to demonstrate comparability of the pre- and post-change product. The criteria for determining comparability of GTMP medicinal products after manufacturing changes also should be justified (14).

For complexed nucleic acids, it is known that small changes to complexed products and the materials used can significantly influence their performance. In vivo studies may be necessary to demonstrate that any process changes do not affect the safety and efficacy profile of the product when results from physicochemical and in vitro testing indicate a change in the properties of the product.

At the end of the process development and when the manufacturing process for both GTMPs and ATMPs is deemed finalized, the validation of the entire manufacturing process should show consistency of the production process using a sufficient number of consecutive production runs as representative of the commercial-scale manufacturing process. The number of required batches depend on several factors: (1) the complexity of the process being validated, (2) the level of process variability and (3) the amount of experimental data and/or process knowledge available on the specific process. Deviations from the validation protocol and acceptance criteria should be investigated (15).

In particular, the ability of the process to remove or inactivate any helper, hybrid or RCV generated or used during manufacture or components of the production system that may support their formation should be demonstrated where appropriate. If scaled-down experiments are used, they should be fully described and justified, and such scale-down models should be demonstrated to be representative of the full-scale commercial manufacturing process. If the product is subject to hold times during the manufacturing process, these must also be validated. The validation section should include validation of shipping and transport and reconstitution of the GTMP.

14.4.5 Analytical Method, Validation and Reference Standards for GTMP Substances and ATMP Products

Details of all non-genocopeial tests used for batch release of GTMPs and ATMPs should be provided, including their analytical performances within their designated use. Individual tests may serve more than one purpose (e.g., identity and potency). All analytical methods used for release of geno-ceutical substance and geno-ceutical product batches should be fully validated according to ICH guidelines and suitable for their purpose. For assays related to impurities which may affect the safety of the product, such as tests for toxic impurities and tests for RCVs, it is essential to establish the suitability and the sensitivity of the tests. The limit of detection must be such that the test provides assurance of the safety of the vector product. Also, the appropriateness of the permissive cell types used in the assays for RCVs should be established. Each reference material used in control tests should be described in full and demonstrated to be suitable for its intended purpose. A reference batch of vectors of an assigned potency should be established and, where appropriate, used to standardize the assays. The stability profile and relevant storage conditions of those reference batches should be established.

If the tests proposed for the release of commercial batches are different from those used throughout clinical development, the differences should be discussed and justified, and comparison of the old and the new method should be performed to demonstrate equal performance of the methods.

14.4.6 Stability for GTMP Substances and ATMP Products

Stability protocols, stability data, justifications for the container-closure system used and proposed shelf-lives and storage conditions should be presented for the GTMP substance, GTMP product and any intermediate product stored during production (i.e., intermediates for which a holding time is scheduled on the production process scheme). The principles outlined in ICH stability guidelines should be followed (see Table 14.1) (16). Real-time stability studies should be undertaken, in particular for the GTMPs and ATMPs intended for marketing. However, it is acknowledged that accelerated stability studies (e.g., at elevated temperatures or under other stress conditions relevant for the product of interest) may provide complementary supporting evidence for the stability of the product and help to establish the stability profile. Forced degradation studies provide important information on degradation products and identify stability indicating tests.

In general, the shelf-life specifications should be derived from the release specifications, with additional emphasis on the stability-indicating features of tests used and tests and limits for degradation products. Vector integrity, biological potency (including transduction capacities) and strength are critical product attributes that should always be included in stability studies. In the case of products formulated with carrier or support materials, the stability of the complex formed with the drug substance should be studied. Where relevant, the in-use stability of the drug product (after reconstitution or after thawing) should be properly investigated, including its compatibility with any diluents used in reconstitution and, if appropriate, devices used for administration. The recommended time-in-use period should be justified. The impact of the transport conditions on the stability of GTMPs and ATMPs with a short-term shelf-life should be considered.

14.4.7 Adventitious Agent Safety Evaluation

The risk of contamination of the GTMP substance or product with adventitious agents must be minimized by the control of starting and raw materials and excipients, facility controls and production controls and procedures. It should be demonstrated that the production process consistently yields batches that are free from contaminating agents. Depending on the product, the potential contaminating agents to be considered may be of human, animal, arthropod and/or plant origin. The adventitious agent safety information should be presented under the respective non-viral and viral headings.

14.4.7.1 Non-Viral Adventitious Agents

Gene therapy vectors other than bacterial vectors are required to be microbiologically sterile. Since it may not be possible to apply direct sterilization methods such as heat or irradiation, the microbiological sterility of gene therapy vectors should be ensured by application of a combination of measures, including the following:

- Selection and control of starting material (including seed and cell banks), reagent and excipients and equipment.
- Exclusion of ingress of extraneous material during the production process.
- In-process tests and controls focusing on limiting bio-burden levels.
- The application of bio-burden reduction process steps and sterilization by filtration. The control of endotoxins and the presence of bacteria other than the strain required should also be addressed in this section.

14.4.7.2 Viral and Non-Conventional Adventitious Agents

The viral safety of each GTMP has to be ensured. Contamination with extraneous viruses and residues of viruses used during production, such as production and helper viruses, needs to be excluded as far as possible. Bacteriophages are relevant contaminating viruses for vectors that are produced on bacterial substrates. Specific guidelines should be ensured if biological material from animal species susceptible for TSE is used in the production process. Rigorous testing of seed and cell banks, intermediates and end products for the presence of adventitious virus needs to be conducted. Where appropriate, viral clearance studies should be undertaken to determine reduction factors for the relevant steps of the production processes. In addition, raw materials of biological origin should be thoroughly tested or manufactured by a process validated for the removal of adventitious and endogenous viruses.

Since the possibilities for applying virus clearance steps during production are limited for many types of GTMPs, the viral safety of these products should be ensured by applying a combination of measures, including the following:

- Selection and control of starting materials (including seed and cell banks), raw materials and equipment.
- Application of measures which exclude ingress by extraneous material during production.
- Exclusion of extraneous agent ingress during the production process.
- Application of vector purification process steps which, where feasible, provide elimination and inactivation capacities vis-a-vis relevant viruses.

14.5 NON-CLINICAL DEVELOPMENT

14.5.1 INTRODUCTION

14.5.1.1 General Principles

The aim of the non-clinical study program during the development of GTMPs is to provide sufficient information for a proper benefit–risk assessment for the use of such products in humans. This section provides considerations on this program in order to support the MAA for GTMPs.

Features of GTMPs which are specific to this class of medicines and which affect the requirements for the non-clinical development include the potential in vivo effects of the transgene or other recombinant nucleic acid sequences, the vector backbone (i.e., viral, bacterial or plasmid-derived sequences) and the excipients, including any carrier or support medical device employed.

The nature and extent of non-clinical development will be dependent on the nature of the GTMP and the availability of relevant models, the clinical use, the targeted clinical population, the intended route of administration and the treatment regimen. The non-clinical development could be designed on a risk-based approach. The non-clinical studies can be carried out as stand-alone or as combined studies. The selection of suitable control groups should be considered based on the established knowledge of the vector. For example, studies may need to be conducted using the vector with no transgene or using an empty vector or vector containing a non-function transgene as a control.

Generally, use of the same animal model in both toxicology investigations and pharmacokinetic studies is recommended, in particular when vector-related toxicity signals are observed. Consideration should be given to interim sacrifice groups if it is important to monitor any changes at the time of maximum inflammatory response (e.g., to an adenoviral vector) or when gene expression is maximal. When a GTMP is combined with a medical device, the medical device should comply with the applicable legislation. Depending on previous experience with delivery devices and/or excipients, non-clinical studies addressing their contribution to GTMP activity may be required. Pivotal first-time non-clinical safety studies should be carried out in conformity with the principles of 'Good Laboratory Practices (GLP) in relation to ATMPs' (see Table 14.1) (17).

14.5.1.2 Characterization

The applicant should carefully consider the quality development before progressing with non-clinical development. Consideration should be given to adequately define the GTMPs and ATMPs.

Products used in non-clinical studies should be sufficiently characterized to provide reassurance that the non-clinical studies have been conducted with material that is representative of the product to be administered to humans in clinical studies. The potential impact of any modifications to the manufacturing process and the test article during the development program on extrapolation of the animal findings to humans should be considered. Any modification of the nucleic acid sequence of the GTMP or any other sequence that might affect the characteristics of the final gene product may require additional safety evaluation. The scientific rationale for the chosen approach should be provided.

14.5.1.3 Methods of Analysis

Methods of analysis used in the non-clinical program should be technically validated with the test article in the appropriate matrix. Applicants should justify the selection of assays used for these studies and their specificity and sensitivity. The sensitivity limits of the chosen assay should be based on properly validated procedures.

When developing a method of analysis to be used in the non-clinical program, considerations should be given to the procurement of the cells/tissue and the quality and suitability of the sample preparation for the intended assay. For example, in the case of *n*ucleic *a*cid *a*mplification *t*esting (NAAT), the specificity of NAAT methods depends on the choice and design of the primers and probes, as well as on the reaction conditions and the method of detection; thus, the rationale for the selection of the primer and probe sequences should be carefully justified. Owing to its high sensitivity, NAAT assays are prone to cross-contamination and false-positive results unless proper precautions are taken. Details of assays used should also be discussed, and the negative and positive controls used should be indicated.

When performing NAAT-based assays to measure vector copy number for integrating vectors, the limits of detection and quantification should be expressed preferably as vector copy number/genome. For episomal vectors, the limits of detection and quantification should be expressed as copy number/µg host cell DNA analyzed. Advancing developments in in situ nucleic acid amplification and hybridization techniques may allow localization of vector DNA or transgenes within cells or tissues.

14.5.2 Animal Species and Model Selection

Non-clinical studies should be done with the most appropriate pharmacologically relevant in vitro and in vivo models available. The rationale for the non-clinical development and the criteria used to choose these models should be discussed and justified in the non-clinical overview. In case no appropriate animal models are available to address all aspects of non-clinical testing, based on a scientific justification, the applicant should either endeavor to develop such models or perform in vitro evaluations using systems appropriately reflecting the disease state.

The following aspects should be considered when selecting the experimental animal model:

- The ability of the intended vector to transfect/transduce/infect and to replicate in the chosen animal species/models. For GTMPs based on a replication-deficient viral vector, the animal model should be sensitive to the viral infection. For GTMP based on an RCV or microorganism, the ability to replicate needs to be taken into consideration when selecting the animal model. For oncolytic viruses which are classified as GTMPs, it may be important to include a tumor-bearing human xenograft in immune-deficient or immunocompromised animals or a syngeneic animal tumor model in order to assess the effects of viral replication in tumor cells in the non-clinical studies.
- The expression and tissue distribution of cellular receptors for a virus/virion/bacteria in the animal model that might affect the efficiency of the uptake by the host and the cellular and tissue sequestration of the vector. Depending on the type of gene therapy vector, tissue tropism may occur or be intended to occur via selective presence of the GTMP in tissues or organs, as well as selective infection of cells and tissues or selective expression of the therapeutic genes. When selecting the animal model for such vectors, the comparability of the tissue tropism in the selected animal model and humans should be discussed and justified. Specific guidance on tissue tropism is provided in the reflection paper on the development of recombinant adeno-associated viral vectors and the ICH considerations on oncolytic viruses (see Table 14.1) (18–20).
- The activity of regulatory elements and their control to drive tissue-specific expression and the expression level of the transgene.
- The biological response to the transgene product, including its target expression, distribution, binding and occupancy, functional consequences (including cell signaling) and also regulation of associated gene(s) if relevant.
- The immune status of the animal, its immune response and potential preexisting immunity. The immune status and preexisting immunity in humans should be taken into account when selecting the animal model. The persistence and clearance of the administered nucleic acid will largely depend on immune surveillance; therefore, the immune status of the animal model should mimic the patient's situation as closely as possible. The animals' immune reaction to the parental virus or bacteria used to derive the GTMP should be taken into consideration, if applicable, and any potential impact on study outcomes or interpretation should be assessed. Effects of preexisting immunity against the

vector vehicle and/or vector gene products in the patient may be mimicked by pretreatment of the animals with the vector.

- Presence of animal genes or gene products homologous to the therapeutic gene or transgene product. For example, a vector expressing a human cytokine would best be tested in an animal species in which that cytokine binds to the corresponding cytokine receptor with affinity comparable to that seen for human receptors and initiates a pharmacologic response comparable to that expected in humans.
- Transgenic animals are used to model various human diseases. Nevertheless, the choice of transgenic animal model should be properly discussed.
- Metabolism and other geno-pharmacokinetic aspects, if needed. Use of large or diseased animal models may be considered in order to mimic particular clinical conditions or biodistribution of the GTMP depending on the nature of the product, its route of administration and, optionally, the delivery system employed (e.g., intracerebral administration).
- Consideration should be given to biological characteristics of the components of the product in the species being used in relation to the dose administered together with the volume that can be safely administered to the test animals.
- The active and/or passive distribution of the virus or vector in the model organism and the possibility of recombination of the GTMP (or parts of the GTMP) with endogenous viruses of the host.

In case a single animal model might not suffice to address relevant aspects, various different animal models should be employed in these studies. The chosen animal models may include wild-type, immunocompromised, knockout, knockin, humanized or transgenic animals. The use of experimental disease models or homologous models can be considered. Small rodent animals, including transgenic, knockout, and natural disease models, may represent relevant models, but limitations due to small size and brief life span should be considered. The number of animals used per dose level tested has a direct bearing on the ability to detect toxicity. A small sample size may lead to failure to observe toxic events due to low frequency, regardless of severity. The limitations that are imposed by sample size, as often is the case for non-human primate studies, may be in part compensated for by increasing the frequency and duration of monitoring. Both genders should generally be used or justification given for specific omissions. To improve safety assessment, special consideration should be given to the size of the control groups, especially when historical data are lacking or limited for the chosen animal model or species.

14.5.3 Genotoxicity

14.5.3.1 Primary Genodynamic Proof-of-Concept Studies

These studies should generate non-clinical evidence supporting the potential clinical effect, or at least provide information on the related biological effect and molecular mechanism of vector action. This can be shown by in vivo studies and/or in vitro studies, especially when relevant in vivo disease models are not available. In vitro and in vivo studies performed to unravel the mechanism of action relating to the proposed therapeutic use (i.e., genodynamic 'proof of concept' studies) should be performed using relevant animal species and models suitable to show that the nucleic acid sequence reaches its intended target (target organ or cells) and provides its intended function (level of expression and functional activity). It should be taken into consideration that counteractive mechanisms may exist in animals that could impair the function of the GTMP. The use of homologous animal models to explore potential biological effects is encouraged if useful. Specific control of expression and production of the expected transgene product in the appropriate target organ should be demonstrated. If synthesis of an aberrant or unintended gene product from the GTMP cannot be excluded by quality data, the presence, and if relevant, the biological consequences of the aberrant gene product formation should be investigated.

The duration of the transgene expression and the therapeutic effect associated with the nucleic acid sequence and the rationale for the proposed dosing regimen in the clinical studies should be described. When the GTMP is intended to have a selective or target-restricted function, studies to confirm the specificity of this function in target cells and tissues should be performed.

In order to demonstrate the therapeutic effect and evaluate the level of gene expression and functional activity, it is recommended to select and test a relevant choice of markers for the disease and safety. Moreover, it is expected to determine the best effective dose without toxic effects of the product which exerts the desired pharmacological activity in the most suitable animal model.

During insertion into the host chromatin, expression cassettes of integrating vectors (e.g., gamma retrovirus, lentivirus) will be present within a native chromatin environment and thus be subject to host epigenetic regulatory machinery (3). It has been shown, for example, that epigenetic modifications such as DNA methylation and histone modifications can negatively affect the transgene expression profile by reorganizing the local chromatin environment that ultimately leads to a loss of therapeutic gene expression, either via a complete gene silencing or position effect variegation. When designing such vectors, applicants should take into account that epigenetics could interfere with the efficacy and safety of the final GTMP (21). Therefore, applicants are encouraged, where relevant, to investigate these issues further by performing ex vivo analysis of genomic distribution of integrating vectors, which will provide crucial information about 'host-on-vector' influences based on the target cell genetic and epigenetic state during early development.

14.5.3.2 Safety Genotoxicology

Safety genotoxicology studies may be required in order to investigate the potential undesirable genotoxic or dynamic effects of the GTMP (both the vector and the transgene) on vital physiological functions (central nervous system, cardiovascular system, respiratory system) and any other organ system based on the biodistribution of the GTMP product in relation to exposure in the therapeutic range. Appropriate safety therapeutic genoceutical studies should be conducted or its absence justified and agreed to by the appropriate authorities (22). This will be on a case-by-case basis and dependent upon the intended route of administration to patients, the existing knowledge of the vector class and distribution and the mechanism of action of the transgene product. A risk-based approach can be applied. Safety genoceutical studies are generally performed by single-dose administration; therefore, safety genopharma study endpoints should, where possible, be combined with toxicity and biodistribution studies (e.g., to investigate persistence).

However, when genotoxic effects occur only late after treatment, or when results from repeat-dose non-clinical studies or results from use in humans give rise to concerns about safety genotoxic effects, the duration of the safety pharmacology studies should be adjusted accordingly.

14.5.4 Genotoxic Kinetics

The standard absorption, distribution, metabolism and excretion studies for conventional medicinal products may not be relevant for GTMPs. Genotoxic kinetic studies should focus on the distribution, persistence, clearance and mobilization of the GTMP and should address the risk of germline transmission. Genotoxic kinetic studies should, where possible, be combined with non-clinical safety studies (23).

Genotoxic kinetic studies are based on the detection of the administered nucleic acid (vector and/or transgene) and should include all relevant organs and tissues, whether target or not. The pharmacokinetic behavior of the expressed gene product should also be investigated with regard to duration and site of expression and/or release.

Investigations of shedding should be performed in accordance with the European Medicines Agency 'ICH considerations on general principles to address virus and vector shedding' for environmental risk assessment in MAA (24).

For genotoxic kinetic studies, only validated methods such as NAAT assays should be used to investigate tissue distribution and persistence of the GTMP. Applicants should justify the selection of assays and their specificity and sensitivity.

14.5.4.1 Biodistribution Studies

14.5.4.1.1 Biodistribution, Persistence and Clearance of Administered GTMP

The dosing used for biodistribution studies should mimic clinical use, with appropriate margins (e.g., 10-fold the clinical dose) adjusted to the characteristics of the animal model used. The route of administration and the treatment regimen (frequency and duration) should be representative for the clinical use. In addition, evaluation of biodistribution of the GTMP after a single administration may add information on the clearance of the administered GTMP. Under certain circumstances, the route of administration that gives the maximum systemic exposure of the GTMP may be included in the biodistribution studies as a worst-case scenario.

The sampling time points and frequency should be chosen to allow determination of the maximum level of administered GTMP present at target and non-target sites and GTMP clearance over time. The observation period of the study should continue until there is no signal detection or until a long-term signal plateau phase is reached. All relevant organs and tissues should be harvested and investigated for presence and clearance of the administered GTMP. If the administered nucleic acid is detected in unintended tissues or organs using a NAAT-based assay, expression of the gene product, as well as its duration and level of expression, should be determined on a case-by-case basis using reverse transcriptase–polymerase chain reaction (RT-PCR) immunological assays and/or assays to detect functional proteins.

If the administered vector is replication competent, the detection of viral sequences in non-target sites by NAAT techniques should be followed by appropriate quantitative infectivity assays in order to evaluate the infectious potential of the detected nucleic acid. The infectivity assay should be validated, and justifications for the specificity and sensitivity of the assay should be provided. Biodistribution studies should be designed to cover a second viraemia as a result of replication of the vector/virus in vivo. If the animal model used does not support in vivo replication of the vector/virus, replication could be mimicked by repeated administration of the GTMP. Any specific characteristic of the GTMP with potential influence on biodistribution, such as latency/reactivation or vector genome mobilization, has to be taken into consideration for the design of biodistribution studies. Moreover, existing biodistribution data from the same vector but with a different transgene can be taken into account when determining the need for and extent of biodistribution studies.

14.5.4.1.2 Intended Genomic Integration

If the whole vector (e.g., retro/lentiviruses) or part of it (e.g., chimeric vectors with retroviral/lentiviral portions) is intended for integration in the host genome, this feature of the vector should be studied by integration studies (*ex vivo* tissue culture or in vivo). Integration studies should focus at least on the following issues unless otherwise justified:

- Tissues/organs where the integration takes place. Not only the intended targets, but an analysis in all tissues where biodistribution has been observed should be considered.
- Copy number and localization of the integrated vector copies in the host genome. Information should be provided regarding the frequency and localization of potential off-target integration events.
- Structural integrity of the integrated vector (in particular the transgene expression cassette of interest) to detect rearrangements/recombination events.
- Genomic stability of the integrated vector over time and persistency of the average vector copy number in the cells.
- On-target/off-target genomic integration and the likelihood of off-target integration in case targeted integration is anticipated.

Nucleic acids with integrating properties (e.g., as in the case of mobile elements or when a site-specific recombinase is used) should be treated as integrative vectors. Suitable methods for determining vector presence and copy number of vector DNA in the genome may include NAT and sequencing assays. The basis for any integration assay used, including its potential deficiencies, should be described, as well as the limits of sensitivity and the negative/positive controls used. In addition to investigating the potential for integration of the nucleic acid into the host cell genome, information on the potential for oncogenesis may also be obtained from in vitro studies using appropriate cell lines and/or primary target cells, if feasible, to investigate changes in cell morphology, function and behavior due to the integration events. When dealing with non-integrating vectors and if there are signs of long-term expression, applicants should investigate if unintended integration is occurring. For some aspects of non-clinical testing of GTMPs, a risk-based approach may be used. The approach taken to address genomic integration needs to be justified.

14.5.4.1.3 Risk of Germline Transmission

Administration of certain GTMPs to patients or subjects raises the possibility of vertical germline transmission of vector DNA, which needs to be investigated, unless otherwise justified (e.g., if the clinical indication and/or patient population indicate that such studies are not warranted). The risk for germline transmission should be addressed primarily at the biodistribution level (signal in gonads, signal in gametes, semen fractionation studies and integration analysis) according to the guideline on non-clinical testing for inadvertent germline transmission of gene transfer vectors.

14.5.4.2 Shedding

Shedding is defined as the dissemination of vector through secretions and/or excreta and should be addressed in animal models. While shedding should not be confused with biodistribution (i.e., spread within the body from the site of administration), it is advised to integrate shedding studies into the design of biodistribution studies or other non-clinical studies when feasible. The aim of shedding studies is to determine the secretion/excretion profile of the virus/vector. Information collected from non-clinical shedding studies can then be used to estimate the likelihood and extent of shedding in humans and to guide the design of clinical shedding studies. If the shedding pattern is known, there is no need for additional non-clinical evaluation. This information would be sufficient to guide shedding studies in humans.

14.5.4.3 Other Genotoxic Kinetic Studies

The genotoxic kinetic behavior of any device or structural components of a GTMP should be investigated. For example, the distribution and clearance of material used to deliver non-viral or viral vectors (e.g., cationic lipid complexing material, materials for controlled vector release) should be studied. The impact of these components on temporal and spatial distribution of the vector should be analyzed if applicable.

14.5.5 Toxicology

Genotoxicity should be assessed for the whole GTMP (virus/vector particle/delivery system, nucleic acid sequences, etc.) and for the transgene products in order to determine unwanted consequences of the distribution and persistence of the vector, its infection/transduction/transfection, the expression and biological activity of the therapeutic gene(s) and vector genes, if applicable, as well as immunogenicity or unwanted genotoxic effects such as apoptosis, necrosis, cell killing and proliferation (24). The extent of non-clinical safety assessment and the design of the safety studies should not only be based on the type of product but should also depend on the tissue tropism/biodistribution and persistence of the GTMP. The possibility of reassortment and/or recombination with wild-type pathogens should be taken into consideration.

For toxicology studies, appropriate GTMP/ATMP dose levels, route and methods of gene delivery should be chosen to represent clinical use with appropriate safety margins. The applicant should justify the choice of endpoints and biomarkers predictive of toxicity in the animal model used.

Depending on the nature of the GTMP, it should be considered to include additional groups that are treated with the route of administration that is considered as the worst-case scenario (e.g., intravenous, representing the effect of widespread dissemination of the GTMP). Applying a risk-based approach, the applicant should consider including endpoints addressing the safety profile of potential final medicinal product impurities (e.g., toxicological consequences of any unforeseen aberrant gene products and of vector-encoded proteins). It is important to employ a safety margin in the animal.

14.5.5.1 Genotoxicity Study Design

For GTMPs intended for single administration, single-dose toxicology studies with an appropriately extended post-dose observation period should be performed. Such studies should include endpoints covered by the 'ICH guideline on repeated dose toxicity' such as necropsy, histopathology, clinical chemistry and hematology and the duration and reversibility of toxicity and should focus on endpoints relevant to the characteristics of the GTMP involved. Inclusion of interim groups to be evaluated at peak levels of biodistribution should be considered.

Single-dose toxicity studies for GTMPs should not be designed as acute toxicity studies with an endpoint of lethality.

The rationale for dose selection and choice of animal model should be justified, as expected for conventional repeat-dose toxicity. It is recommended to include in the studies a satellite control group to improve the historical data set regarding the species used, if needed. Repeated-dose toxicity studies should be provided when multiple dosing of human subjects is intended. The mode and schedule of administration should appropriately reflect the clinical dosing. For those cases where single dosing may result in prolonged function of the nucleic acid sequence and/or its product in humans but not in the animal model, or in case replication kinetics of replicating vectors in animals are not reflecting the situation in humans, repeated-dose toxicity studies should be considered to mimic the human situation.

The duration of the single-dose and repeated-dose studies may be longer than standard toxicity studies for other biopharmaceuticals, depending on the persistence of the GTMP, level and site of expression and the anticipated potential risks. A justification for the duration of the studies should be provided, as well as the duration of the recovery phase investigations, which should rely on the persistence of the vector and the transgene expression. The use of one relevant species for the single- and repeat-dose toxicity studies may be sufficient unless specific safety concerns require the use of a second animal species.

14.5.5.2 Genotoxicity Objectives

Genotoxicity studies might be required depending on the nature of the GTMP. The objectives of such studies can be addressed by a three-step approach as follows:

i) To investigate occurrences of genomic modification and detect any subsequent abnormal cell behavior;

ii) To evaluate toxicity issues due to insertion mutagenesis and investigate the mechanism driving these adverse toxicity effects. Toxicity issues due to off-target modifications when an on-target approach is intended should also be evaluated;
iii) To identify/characterize genomic integration sites and evaluate possible cross-talk between the transgenic and neighboring sequences.

14.5.5.2.1 Insertional Mutagenesis

Genotoxicity issues, including insertion mutagenesis and consequent tumorigenicity, should be evaluated carefully in relevant in vitro and in vivo models. If a positive finding occurs, additional testing will be needed to ensure the safety of the product. In these studies, standard genotoxicity assays are generally not appropriate but may be required to address a concern about a specific impurity or a component of the delivery system (e.g., complexing material). In particular, the use of some type of genotoxicity testing as outlined may be necessary to rule out any possible genotoxic effect that might be attributed to elements present in the formulated final drug product.

Insertion mutagenesis by genomic integration of vector DNA can lead to several scenarios, including altered expression of host genes (activation/inhibition), their inactivation (destruction of the open reading frame), activation/repression of neighboring silent/active genes and generation of a new entity encoding an active fusion protein. Insertion mutagenesis may have different outcomes. It may not affect cell growth, or it may induce a growth advantage or disadvantage. Insertion mutagenesis could be addressed in in vitro and/or in vivo studies, which should be designed to investigate any adverse effects induced by this genetic modification. Performing genotoxicity studies in established cell lines, primary cells or animal models should be considered to be able to estimate the safety profile of any GTMP.

14.5.5.2.2 Gene Delivery Vector–Specific Considerations

The potential for integration of the transgene expression cassette into the host genome should be investigated and discussed, both where it is intended and inherent to the method of expression (e.g., when retroviral/lentiviral vectors are used) and in cases where integration is not intended (e.g., when adenoviral, adeno-associated viral or plasmid vectors are used). Requirement for genotoxicity studies of GTMPs with host-DNA integrative capacity will depend on the way the final product will be delivered (local versus systemic), to which tissue/organ the GTMP will be targeted and the biological status of the cells to be targeted.

For GTMPs containing an active pharmaceutical ingredient that is not intended for integration, data from in vivo or in vitro studies that detect integration may still be required to rule out any possible safety concern. When expression of a therapeutic gene is lasting over a prolonged period of time, the persistence of the GTMP and likely the integration of the DNA vector into the genome should be carefully investigated. If integration is being confirmed, copy number determination, integration site identification and any subsequent adverse biological effects and change in cell behavior monitoring should be performed. Depending on the nature of the vector used, extended in vitro and in vivo assays addressing insertion oncogenesis may be warranted before initial administration in humans.

Bacteriophages and genetically modified microorganisms (e.g., *Lactobacillus*, *Salmonella*) can be considered out of the scope of genotoxicity studies because of the unlikelihood of safety issues raised by DNA transfer and integration into the host cell genome. The inability to predict the genotoxic risk of a GTMP simply on the basis of the choice of vector and the total integration load in the cells arises from the lack of comprehensive understanding of all factors that determine whether a cell bearing a genotoxic insertion remains established in vivo and whether its outgrowth eventually progresses to malignancy. The potential for vector integration into the human genome and the risks associated with it should always be taken into account.

14.5.5.3 Tumorigenicity

Standard lifetime rodent carcinogenicity studies are usually not required in the non-clinical development. However, depending on the type of product, the tumorigenic and oncogenic potential should be investigated in relevant in vivo/in vitro models for neoplasm signals, oncogene activation or cell proliferation index. The decision whether the tumorigenic or oncogenic potential of a GTMP needs to be investigated should be guided by the weight of evidence approach of carcinogenicity in 'ICH guideline S6' which includes, for example, the following outcomes:

i) Knowledge of intended gene target and gene expression pathway (e.g., issues with growth factor transgene product);
ii) Target- and pathway-related mechanistic/pharmacologic and known secondary pharmacologic characteristics relevant for the outcome of tumorigenicity studies and the prediction of potential human oncogenes;
iii) Potential genetic insertion mutagenesis study results;
iv) Histopathologic evaluation of repeated-dose toxicology studies such as histopathologic findings of particular interest, including cellular hypertrophy, diffuse and/or focal cellular hyperplasia, persistent tissue injury and/or chronic inflammation, preneoplastic changes and tumors;
v) Evidence of hormonal perturbation;
vi) Immune suppression: a causative factor for tumorigenesis in humans;
vii) Special studies and endpoints: data from special staining techniques, new biomarkers, emerging technologies and alternative test systems can be submitted with the scientific rationale to help explain or predict animal and/or human tumorigenic pathways and mechanisms when they would contribute meaningfully.

14.5.5.4 Immunogenicity and Immunotoxicity Toxicity Studies

Delivery of GTMPs can result in immune responses of the innate (systemic cytokine elevations, multiorgan inflammation) and adaptive immune system (antibodies against the vector and transgene product, cytotoxic lymphocytes raised against transfected/transduced/infected cells cytokine-secreting T lymphocytes specific for the transgene product). Many parameters can significantly influence the innate and adaptive responses towards various GTMPs such as host-factors (prior exposure to virus and/or transgene product, status of the immune system), gene transfer protocols (type of the delivery system, route of transgene delivery and target tissue), transgene delivery vehicle (type of viral vector, serotype, vector dose and type of transgene promoter, presence of selection markers or suicide genes that could have an immunogenic potential) and the transgene product (25). These aspects should be considered by the applicant during the non-clinical development. Special care should be addressed to complement activation and its consequences. Risk of cross-reactive or bystander autoimmune responses should also be considered. If repeat-dose administration can lead to complement activation, markers of complement activation should be investigated in animal and human sera.

14.5.5.5 Reproductive and Developmental Toxicity

The potential for reproductive and developmental toxicity needs to be addressed depending on the product type, mechanism of action, distribution and shedding profile and patient population. General principles to detect toxicity to reproduction are provided with ICH guidelines S5-R2 (26). If the risk for germline transmission cannot be unequivocally determined according to principles as described in the 'Guideline on non-clinical testing for inadvertent germline transmission of gene transfer vectors', then breeding studies should be performed in order to directly address whether the administered nucleic acid is being transmitted to the offspring. In addition, the time course of spermatogenesis and oocyte maturation, respectively, will have to be carefully considered when performing breeding studies. Embryo-fetal and perinatal toxicity studies and germline transmission studies should be provided, unless otherwise duly justified on the basis of the type of product concerned.

Similarly, embryo-fetal and perinatal toxicity studies may be required if women of child-bearing potential are to be exposed to GTMPs, depending on the clinical use and clinical population in order to investigate the effect on the fetus such as placental transfer of cytokines produced locally.

In any case, flexibility needs to be applied to employ a scientifically valid testing strategy aiming clinically translatable results, in line with the 3R principles. While recognizing that for certain product types routine non-clinical studies on reproductive toxicity lack predictivity, it is important for human risk assessment to address any limitations, uncertainties and data gaps of the testing program.

14.5.5.6 Local Tolerance

Local tolerance studies may be relevant for some GTMPs, depending on their type, route and protocol of administration (e.g., intraocular, intramuscular, intravenous, intratumoral). If the proposed clinical formulation and route of administration have been examined in other animal studies, then separate local tolerance studies are not necessary. If needed, they can be addressed as part of the general toxicity study and follow the 'Guideline on non-clinical tolerance testing of medicinal products'.

14.5.6 Geno-ceutical and Medical Product Interactions

As for any other medicinal products, the effects of co-medication should be investigated on a case-by-case basis if they could affect transfection/transduction/infection, tropism and efficacy of the vector, therapeutic gene expression, biological activity of the expressed proteins and tissue distribution of the vector. For instance, clearance of the vector or virus may be altered under an immunosuppressive co-treatment, and therefore this point has to be addressed. For example, this point would have to be addressed if an immunosuppressive co-treatment was expected to alter clearance of the vector/virus or if a GTMP that causes inflammation or cytokine release in the liver could affect the liver metabolism of co-administered pharmaceuticals.

14.6. CLINICAL DEVELOPMENT

14.6.1 General Considerations

In general, for GTMPs, product clinical development needs current guidelines relating to specific therapeutic areas. Any deviation from existing guidelines needs to be justified. For new therapeutic indications and conditions where limited guidance exists, consultation of national regulatory authorities and/or scientific advice on the clinical development plan, including the confirmatory studies, is recommended.

In view of the complexity of gene therapy, the potential benefits and risks of a GTMP approach versus existing conventional treatments, including consideration of the medical need, should be discussed in the clinical overview (e.g., GTMP factor IX vs. plasma-derived or recombinant factor IX). Ideally, full compliance with current guidelines is not possible. In such cases, proper justification with feasible, alternative approaches is expected to obtain comparable information. All studies should be adequately planned to allow assessment of the feasibility and risks of the gene therapy approach. In cases where randomized controlled clinical trials are not feasible, alternatives (e.g., well-documented natural history data or using the patients as their own control) might be acceptable if appropriately justified, and the caveats for using these alternatives should be discussed. The ICH guideline E10 and FDA guidelines on the choice of control groups in clinical trials should be consulted (27). The absence of control groups in the clinical design should be justified based on the objectives of the study, the disease and the GTMP under investigation. For certain conditions targeted for treatment with a GTMP, follow the 'Guideline on clinical trials in small populations' (28). However, it should be noted that the database on the recruited patients should be as complete as possible. Clinical scientists are advised to develop and use technical validation methods for patient monitoring as early as possible during clinical development. If surrogate parameters are used to monitor clinical efficacy (e.g., replaced level of secreted protein), they have to be proven clinically meaningful.

Long-term monitoring of patients treated with a GTMP is also the legal requirement of long-term efficacy and safety follow-up according to regulation (EC) No. 1394/2007 and FDA regulations (see Table 14.1). Those long-term studies should be appropriately designed (e.g., sampling plan, sample treatment, analytical methods, endpoints) in order to maximize information output, especially when invasive methods are used. If GTMP is intended to provide lifelong persistence of gene therapy and genetic therapy effects, see the 'Guideline on follow up of patients administered with GTMPs' (4). General rules may be followed as discussed in the following sections.

14.6.1.1 Patient Screening/Eligibility

The immune status of the patient (i.e., immunocompromised or immunocompetent), as well as preexisting immunity against the vector, should be determined before treatment.

14.6.1.2 Vulnerable Populations

Vulnerable populations, such as children and the elderly, should be considered when developing a GTMP. The target population might be vulnerable, such as pregnant women, children, the elderly and the immunosuppressed. For example, the immunogenicity of a viral vector may vary between children and adults, depending on preexisting exposure to the virus. As GTMP development is indication and product specific, no specific guidance can be given regarding the extent of data to be generated.

When the medicinal products are likely to be of significant clinical value in such populations and where appropriate animal models exist, robust evidence from the non-clinical development program should be available to support the safe use in the target population. The clinical development will have to take into account the epidemiology of the disease and specificities of the populations in the claimed indication.

In case a GTMP is specifically indicated for use in pregnant women (i.e., applied during pregnancy), careful antenatal monitoring of mother and fetus should be conducted. In addition, postpartum long-term follow-up of the child and the mother should be performed.

For children, long-term effects of administration of the GTMP should be specifically considered and monitored adequately, as defined in Regulation (EC) 1901/2006 (Pediatric Regulation) and relevant pediatric guidelines. For the duration of long-term follow-up of pediatric patients treated with a GTMP, read Section 14.6.8.

14.6.2 Genotoxic Kinetic Studies

Classical pharmacokinetic studies based on absorption, distribution, metabolism and excretion (ADME) studies are usually not required for GTMPs. However, kinetics studies need to be carried out on a case-by-case basis, depending on the specific GTMPs (e.g., if the gene product is a protein excreted in the blood circulation) (29).

However, it is expected that the following studies will be carried out:

i) Usually, shedding studies are required to address the excretion of the GTMPs. Investigations of shedding and risk of transmission to third parties should be provided with the environmental risk assessment, unless otherwise justified, in the application on the basis of the type of product concerned;
ii) When possible, dissemination in the body, including investigations on persistence, clearance and mobilization of the gene therapy vector, should be investigated. Biodistribution studies shall additionally address the risk of germline transmission;
iii) Finally, kinetic studies of the medicinal product and the transgene product (e.g., expressed proteins) should be carried out.

For oncolytic viruses, specific guidance is provided in ICH 'Considerations on oncolytic viruses' (19).

14.6.2.1 Shedding Studies

Shedding studies to address the excretion of the GTMP should be performed. When shedding is observed, the potential for transmission to third parties needs to be investigated, if relevant (e.g., with RCVs/oncolytic viruses), or a justification for not doing this should be provided. The ICH 'Considerations and general principles to address virus and vector shedding' and the 'Guideline on environmental risk assessment' provide comprehensive recommendations for the design of shedding studies, as well as the interpretation of clinical data in assessing the need for virus/vector transmission studies (30). Those data also contribute to appropriate planning of the long-term follow-up program.

Apart from contraceptive measures requested for clinical trials (CTFG 'Recommendations related to contraception and pregnancy testing in clinical trials'), when there is a risk of shedding through the seminal fluid, at least two means of contraception—including barrier contraception—should be recommended beyond one cycle of spermatogenesis after the last positive sperm sample (30).

14.6.2.2 Biodistribution Studies

The cell tropism, the route of administration, the target organ/cells, the vector type, the kinetics of viremia and the indication, as well as the clinical feasibility and ethical acceptability, should be taken into consideration when designing dissemination studies (e.g., choosing the target and non-target organs, cells and body fluids). Also special attention should be paid when a GTMP will be applied under conditions in which impaired blood–brain barrier integrity can be expected.

Invasive techniques (e.g., biopsies, fluid collection) may not always be feasible and ethically appropriate. Thus, the use of other, less invasive techniques (e.g., imaging techniques) might prove useful in some cases to study GTMP dissemination whenever possible. Special attention should be paid to dissemination when using a replication-competent GTMP. In such cases, patients should be monitored for clinical signs of productive infection with the RCV or for signs of unwanted dissemination.

14.6.2.3 Genokinetic Studies of the Transgene Product (e.g., Expressed Proteins or Genomic Signatures) as Orphan Drug

Different kinetic behaviors of transgene products or GTMPs/ATMPs orphan drugs are different from conventional pharmacokinetic studies. Genokinetic studies may include a minimum determination of plasma concentration and half-life for the therapeutic GTMP gene product (i.e., therapeutic protein); in some cases, there might be a need to assess this also for other vector genes expressed in vivo as shown in non-clinical studies. A correlation between the levels and duration of expression and clinical efficacy and safety should be investigated. For gene expression products such as enzymes or proteins, differences in their kinetics and elimination should be taken into consideration depending on genetic polymorphism.

For the treatment of genetic diseases by gene correction/addition strategies, the therapeutic effects of the product on different causative gene mutations should be taken into consideration and investigated as justified. The potential interference of residual endogenous proteins with the therapeutic product should be addressed. For example, the presence of endogenous proteins coded by genes with hypomorphic or dominant negative mutations may interfere with the half-life and function of the protein product expressed from the delivered gene, and thus respective effects should be carefully considered.

14.6.3 Gene Dynamic Studies

Gene dynamic (GD) studies are performed to study the function and/or expression of the therapeutic nucleic acid sequence (orphan drugs). In most cases of GTMP, GD studies address the expression and function of the gene expression product (e.g., as a protein or enzyme, including conversion of pro-proteins by expressed enzymes or induction of immune response), while in other cases the effect of the vector itself is addressed (e.g., recombinant oncolytic virus). The selected GD markers should be relevant to demonstrate therapeutic efficacy of the product, and in cases where the GD effects are proposed as surrogate efficacy endpoints, this needs to be justified. The proposed GD marker should be linked to clinical benefit.

14.6.4 Dose Selection and Gene Delivery Schedule

In general, the dose response effect should be evaluated; reference is made to ICH 'Guideline E4 dose response information to support gene drug registration' (31). The selection of the dose should be based on the findings obtained in the quality assessment and the non-clinical development of the product, and it should be linked with the potency of product. When a classical dose finding is not possible, a minimal effective dose and a maximum tolerable dose may provide useful information on the relationship between exposure and effect. The proposed dose has to be justified by scientific data.

14.6.5 Immunogenicity of GTMPs/ATMPs

Prior infection or vaccination with related viruses may affect the safety and efficacy of the GTMP (e.g., adenoviruses, poxviruses [smallpox vaccine]); thus, the preexisting immunity to the vector itself should be determined prior to initiation of the therapy if a vector is chosen for which preexisting immunity can be assumed. These data might also determine the need for immune suppression. An immune response to the transgene product might eventually compromise the efficacy of the product and might have an impact on safety. Thus, evaluation of the immune response to the transgene product (i.e., determination of antibodies against the expressed protein) should also be part of the clinical development. In case repeated administration of the GTMP is foreseen, early considerations of the most appropriated vector (sero) type should be conducted, as well as the need for immune suppression of the patients. A comprehensive evaluation of the immune response to the vector and the transgene product has to be performed. This might include the evaluation of the cellular and humoral immunity to the vector as well as to the transgene product (e.g., titer and avidity of antibodies and information on whether the antibodies are neutralizing or not). The results should be documented in relation to the timing of the treatments, and correlation of the immunogenicity results with concurrent safety and efficacy should be provided.

14.6.6 Efficacy of Gene Delivery

Existing guidelines for the specific therapeutic area (e.g., cancer, rare diseases) should be followed with regard to study design (e.g., choice of endpoints, choice of comparator, inclusion/exclusion criteria). Any major deviations from these guidelines should be justified. Ideally, randomized controlled and blinded confirmatory studies should be conducted. However, this may not always be possible, and other controls (i.e., historical controls, patient's own control) could be acceptable. The ICH 'Guideline on clinical trials in small populations' provides guidance on the choice of control groups (28, 32). The applicant has to justify the approach scientifically. The efficacy studies should be designed to demonstrate efficacy in the target population, to support the proposed posology and to evaluate the duration of the therapeutic effect of the GTMP.

Clinically meaningful endpoints, which include previously validated or generally accepted surrogate endpoints (e.g., threshold of FIX or FVIII in case of hemophilia), are generally required to demonstrate efficacy. In certain situations the use of other endpoints is possible, provided that there is a correlation between this endpoint and the clinical meaningfully outcome. However, a clinically meaningful endpoint has to be investigated in the long-term follow-up (see ICH 'Guideline on follow-up of patients administered with gene therapy medicinal products' (33). Another important factor is the timing of the efficacy assessment; therefore, the schedule of clinical evaluation should be planned accordingly. If the intended outcome of the treatment needs long-term persistence and functionality of the transgene expression product (e.g., genetic diseases), it should be reflected with an adequate duration of follow-up. The design and duration of follow-up have to be specified also, considering potential loss of efficacy and might be completed post-marketing if justified.

14.6.7 Clinical Safety of GTMPs/ATMPs Delivery

A safety database should be set up, including any adverse events which are linked to the transgene product and/or to the vector or the transduction mechanism. Risks of the administration procedure—for example, invasive procedures to administer the GTMP (e.g., multiple injection, intracerebral application), the use of general or regional anesthesia or the use of immunosuppressive and chemotherapeutic therapy—should be addressed. Special consideration should be taken in the design of the clinical study and risk evaluation when medical devices are used for the delivery or implant of a GTMP. The medical device effect should be evaluated in the intended use of the GTMP. The use of the medical device with the GTMP should be adequately explained in the product information (34). In case of an anticipated risk, including events with a late onset (e.g., tumorigenicity), measures to detect the signal and to mitigate this risk should be implemented.

14.6.8 Adverse Effects of Gene Delivery in Gene Therapy by Orphan Drugs

Particular attention should be paid to:

- *Infusion-related reactions and cytokine release*: Short-term tolerability after administration of the GTMP, such as infusion-related reactions including cytokine release to the vector itself or any compound of the product, should be considered.
- *Infection and inflammatory responses*: Reassortment and/or recombination with wild-type pathogens, appearance of replication competent viruses or the change of tropism might lead to infection or an inflammatory response. Patients should be monitored carefully for signs and symptoms of infection.
- *Immune-mediated adverse effects*: Immune response to the vector itself, as well as to the transgene product, might lead in some cases to clinical consequences. Applying an exogenous transgene product might result in a break of tolerance to the endogenous protein counterpart if present.
- *Overexpression*: Overexpression of the transgene (e.g., coagulation factor VIII) might lead to severe clinical consequences. The level of transgene expression has to be monitored, and if relevant, the patient has to be monitored for clinical consequences.
- *Malignancy*: Several factors might contribute to tumor development in patients treated with a GTMP. These factors include product-related factors (e.g., insertional mutagenesis, altered expression of host genes), the transgene product itself (e.g., growth factors) or factors linked to the treatment procedure such as immunosuppressant therapy or chemotherapy (34). If malignancy occurs after treatment, a potential link with the GTMP should be investigated, taking into consideration both molecular and biological characteristics of the GTMP.
- *Any unintended transduction of tissues*: By its nature, the vector might have a specific tissue/cell tropism. However, unintended transduction of non-target tissues might occur. Information on the tissue specificity of the virus from which the vector is derived, focusing on the specific target according to the vector type, as well as the biodistribution obtained with the actual GTMP, and the experience with similar GTMP products should be provided. In case non-target specific tropism occurs, appropriate monitoring for the clinical consequences of such non-target tissue transduction should be in place.
- *Storage and retention samples*: In the conduct of clinical trials, samples of patients' sera and peripheral blood mononuclear cells (PBMCs) taken prior to treatment and at dedicated time points after treatment should be stored in order to allow for investigation of the potential for human infection with any adventitious agent transmitted by the GTMP. The duration of storage depends on patient population/disease, GTMP being administered and the integrity of the stored materials. Consent forms should be prepared and sample storage should be carried out according current rules and guidelines on biobanking.

14.6.9 Gene Therapy Geno-Vigilance and Risk Management Plan

For GTMPs gene therapy vigilance rules may be immediate or periodic reporting as per 'Guideline on good gene toxicity vigilance practices (GVP) on safety and efficacy follow-up and risk management of Advanced Therapy Medicinal Products' (33). Lack of efficacy should be followed in the long-term follow-up of patients treated with GTMPs during the clinical development—for example, insufficient expression of the transgene, preexisting immunity against the transgene product, any declining effect of the gene therapy over time such as transgene expression from the vector or a reduction of the number of vector-harboring cells.

Major points of discord in FDA guidelines are confusing with regard to if gene GTMPs are drugs or not. The reasons are:

i) Vectors from different virus classes (gamma retrovirus vs. adenovirus) and avian viruses show different drug-like actions expressing the same trans genes and so are not drugs (4).
ii) Transgenes encoding different enzymes for treatment of rare diseases do not have the same molecular structure and so are not drugs (5).
iii) The same viral vectors express the same transgenes to make the same final product to show a therapeutic effect or transduct the same cell type or regulatory elements, so they fall in 'sameness' orphan designation (6). In special circumstances, for the first time the FDA permitted GTMPs for neurodegeneration and COVID-19 treatments with clear guidelines to industries (35, 36, 37, 38, 39).

The Indian Council of Medical Research with the Department of Biotechnology released national guidelines for gene therapy product development and clinical trials (37). Many nations are also in the pipeline and following suit with their own regulations.

ACKNOWLEDGEMENTS

The literature-based survey is acknowledged with citations from the FDA and European guidelines for GTMPs to manufacturers. Authors acknowledge the support of Professor Aria A Tzika, Department of Surgery, Brigham Institute of Trauma and Burn, Massachusetts General Hospital, Harvard University, Boston to do edit manuscript.

REFERENCES

0. FDA Guideline 2021: 21 Code Federal regulations part 316-Orphan drugs: Designating an orphan product: Drugs and Biological Products: In section of Developing Products for Rare Diseases & Conditions. FDA 2021. http://www.accessdata.fda.gov/scripts/cpdlisting/oopd/
1. EU Guideline on the risk based approach according to annex I, part IV of Directive 2001/83/EC applied to Advanced therapy medicinal products (EMA/CAT/686637/2011).
2. EU Guideline on scientific requirements for the environmental risk assessment of gene therapy medicinal products (EMEA/CHMP/GTWP/125491/2006).

3. FDA guideline 2020: Retroviral vector based human gene therapy products for replication competent retrovirus during product manufacture and patient follow up. (CMC 2020).
4. FDA guideline 2020: Long term followup after administration of human gene therapy products.21CFR316.3(b)14.
5. FDA guideline 2020: Human gene therapy for rare diseases, retinal disorders, and hemophelia.
6. FDA guideline 2020: Interpreting sameness of gene therapy products under the orphan drug regulations (ODA) 21CFR316.3(b)12.
7. Guideline on quality, non-clinical and clinical aspects of medicinal products containing genetically modified cells (CHMP/GTWP/671639/2008).
8. EMA Note for guidance on minimising the risk of transmitting animal spongiform encephalopathy agents via human and veterinary medicinal products (EMA/410/01 rev.3).
9. EMA Guideline on the use of porcine trypsin used in the manufacture of human biological medicinal products (EMA/CHMP/BWP/814397/2011).
10. EMEA Guideline on Excipients in the Dossier for Application for Marketing Authorization of a Medicinal Product (EMEA/CHMP/QWP/396951/2006).
11. EMEA Reflection paper on quality, non-clinical and clinical issues related to the development of recombinant adeno-associated viral vectors (EMEA/CHMP/GTWP/587488/2007 Rev.1).
12. EMA Reflection paper on design modifications of gene therapy medicinal products during development (EMA/CAT/GTWP/44236/2009).
13. ICH considerations on oncolytic viruses (EMEA/CHMP/ICH/607698/08).
14. ICH considerations on general principles to address virus and vector shedding (CHMP/ICH/449035/09).
15. ICH guideline Q5A(R1) on Quality of biotechnological products: viral safety evaluation of biotechnology products derived from cell lines of human or animal origin (CPMP/ICH/295/95).
16. ICH guideline Q5C on stability testing of biotechnological/biological products (CPMP/ICH/138/95).
17. ICH guideline Q5D on derivation and characterization of cell substrates used for production of biotechnological/biological products (CPMP/ICH/294/95).
18. ICH guideline Q5E on Comparability of biotechnological/biological products (CPMP/ICH/5721/03).
19. ICH guideline Q6B on Specifications: test procedures and acceptance criteria for biotechnological/biological products (CPMP/ICH/365/96).
20. ICH guideline Q11 on development and manufacture of drug substances (chemical entities and biotechnological/ biological entities) (EMA/CHMP/ICH/425213/2011).
21. ICH guideline non-clinical testing for inadvertent germline transmission of gene transfer vectors (EMEA/273974/2005).
22. EMEA 2006: Guideline on the non-clinical studies required before first clinical use of Gene Therapy medicinal products (EMEA/CHMP/GTWP/125459/2006).
23. EMEA Guideline 2007: on strategies to identify and mitigate risks for first-in-human clinical trials within investigational medicinal products (EMEA/CHMP/SWP/28367/07).
24. ICH guideline 2009: M3 (R2) on non-clinical safety studies for the conduct of human clinical trials and marketing authorisation for pharmaceuticals (EMEA/CHMP/ICH/449035/2009).
25. ICH guideline S2 (R1) 2009: on genotoxicity testing and data interpretation for pharmaceuticals intended for human use (EMA/CHMP/ICH/126642/2008).

26. ICH guideline S5 (R2) 1995: on the detection of toxicity to reproduction from medical products and toxicity to male fertility (CPMP/ICH/386/95).
27. ICH guideline S6 (R1) 1998: on Preclinical safety evaluation of biotechnology-derived pharmaceuticals (CHMP/ICH/731268/1998).
28. ICH guideline S7A 2000: on Safety pharmacology studies for human pharmaceuticals (CPMP/ICH/539/00).
29. ICH guideline S8, 2004: Immunogenicity studies for human pharmaceuticals (CHMP/167235/2004).
30. EMEA Guideline 2007: on follow-up of patients administered with gene therapy medicinal products (EMEA/CHMP/GTWP/60436/2007).
31. CHMP Guideline 2005: on clinical trials in small populations (CHMP/EWP/83561/2005).
32. CPMP Guideline 1999: on repeated dose toxicity (CPMP/SWP/1042/99 Rev1 Correction).
33. EMA Reflection paper 2012: on management of clinical risks deriving from insertional mutagenesis (EMA/CAT/190186/2012).
34. ICH guideline E4 1995: on Dose response information to support drug registration (CPMP/ICH/378/95).
35. ICH guideline E10 1996: on choice of control groups in clinical trials (CPMP/ICH/364/96).
36. EMEA Guideline 2008: on safety and efficacy follow-up risk management of advanced therapy medicinal products (EMEA/149995/2008).
37. FDA Guidance 2020: document on human gene therapy for neurodegenerative diseases. Center for biologics evaluation and research (FDA-2020-D-2101).
38. FDA Guidance 2020: document on manufacturing considerations for licensed and investigational cellular and gene therapy products during covid-19 public health emergency (FDA-2020-D-1137) report.
39. ICMR_DBT 2019: National Guidelines for gene therapy product development and clinical trials (2019) https://main.icmr.nic.in/salient_features_gene_therapy.pdf https://icmr.nic.in/sites/default/files/guideleines/guidelines_GTP.pdf

15 iMRI for Clinical Gene Therapy

Disha Patel, Khushboo Faldu and Jigna Shah

CONTENTS

15.1 INTRODUCTION

Intraoperative magnetic resonance imaging (ioMRI) was first developed in the 1980s (1). Since then, ioMRI technology has contributed to significant advancement sin real-time imaging during surgeries. ioMRI is a safe, accurate, and minimally invasive alternative to conventional surgeries (2). The deployment costs of intraoperative units in surgical suites are high when compared to costs recovered and thus have limited the technological expansion. Some researchers have economically favored the interventional hybrid unit (iMRI) in the radiology suite (3–4). The hybrid surgical/magnetic resonance imaging (MRI) environment necessitates compliance with both surgical and MRI procedures as well as protocols, like surgical protocols for infection prevention and control and MRI protocols for adherence to magnet safety. This requires a multidisciplinary endeavor and flawless collaboration (5–6).

Gene therapy is an exciting medical field that has renewed the enthusiasm of researchers to discover the ultimate treatment modality that provides a permanent cure via genetic modification of the cells by repairing or reconstructing defective disease-causing genes. Gene therapy possesses the potential to cure complex pathophysiologies presented by diseases like neurodegenerative conditions (Parkinson's disease, Alzheimer's disease), neuronal disorders (epilepsy), and cardiac diseases (congestive cardiac failure [CCF], coronary artery blockage, and myocardial infarction [MI]) (7). The biodistribution and pharmacokinetic profile of genetic therapeutics are banked on in vitro cell line studies and laboratory analysis of tissue biopsy and autopsy, which necessitates the development of methods that can perform guided delivery and monitor gene therapy non-invasively. Gene therapy, being organ-specific,

DOI: 10.1201/9781003186069-15

requires localized administration for optimal results, which can be easily achieved with the use of iMRI technology (8).

Diverse imaging techniques like ultrasound, MRI, optical imaging, and nuclear medicine have been investigated for gene therapy monitoring (9). MRI offers substantial advantageous information of organ function and system morphology by providing high-contrast and high-resolution image output from multiple planes with minimal ionization risk. Modalities are being developed for the applicability of iMRI in monitoring gene administration, enhancing transfection and transduction of the gene, and tracking gene expression (10).

15.2 MAGNETIC RESONANCE IMAGING AND MAGNETIC RESONANCE SPECTROSCOPY IN GENE THERAPY

MRI provides a sensitive imaging method. It can detect micromolar (10 to 100 μm) concentrations of paramagnetic contrast dyes, resulting in higher spatial resolution with the help of powerful signal amplifiers. Biochemical amplification targeting magnetic resonance contrast agents has been extensively researched in gene therapy, as the reporter probes (i.e., metal ions) tend to accumulate inside the cells, causing magnetic resonance signal changes, but these changes can only be captured if the ions accumulate in higher concentrations in the cells (11).

Transferrin receptor (Tf-R) has continuously been studied as a receptor responsible for the transport and accumulation of contrast dyes inside the cells. These contrast agents involve human holotransferrin covalently bound to low-molecular-weight dextran that forms a cross-link with iron oxide (Tf-CLIO) (12) or blanket the nanoparticles of monocrystalline iron oxide (Tf-MION) (13–14). Transferrin is a glycoprotein responsible for ferric ion delivery from blood to various tissues. It facilitates endocytosis of the contrast agent into the cell, causing accumulation of the paramagnetic ferric ions that affect the T2 relaxation rate. Studies have reported that rat gliosarcoma overexpresses transferrin receptor, and Tf-MION leads to increased accumulation of ferric ions in the tumor implanted in mice cells, providing better contrast in MRI analysis. Tf-R engineering research is being conducted to study the effect of co-expression of therapeutic genes, Tf-R overexpression, and increased ferric ion concentration on cell physiology and functioning (12).

Transgene expression imaging has been studied with the use of contrast agents. Enzyme hydrolysis of these agents brings about changes in their magnetic properties. EgadMe is related structurally to gadoteridol [Gd(HP-DO3A)]. EgadMe possesses a chemically modified carbohydrate 'cap' bonded through a β-galactosidase-cleavable linker. This blocks gadolinium ion's water access, and thus signal enhancement does not materialize. Enzymatic hydrolysis separates the carbohydrate moiety, and gadolinium ion's water access is established, and thus signal enhancement by the contrast agent takes place (15). When Xenopus embryos were injected with EgadMe, regions that expressed β-galactosidase were seen as high-intensity regions in the MRI scan (15). This demonstrated that detection of gene expression in living animal systems is possible with the use of MRI, and refinement in contrast agent delivery should be developed.

Gene expression can be measured with the use of magnetic resonance spectroscopy (MRS), as it can distinguish magnetic resonance signals from distinct chemical entities. 19F MRS was utilized to observe the yeast cytosine deaminase (yCD) enzyme–catalyzed transformation of 5-fluorocytosine (5-FC), a prodrug to 5-fluorouracil (5-FU), an active chemotherapeutic moiety in a colorectal tumor xenograft rat model (16). This study highlighted that the MRS technique can be used in the non-invasive monitoring of transgene expression in tumors.

15.3 MRI-MONITORED GENE DELIVERY

Effectual gene delivery to the target organ is a crucial step in efficacious gene therapy. It is important to observe the biodistribution of administered genes and to observe the localization of the administered genes in the target location. A study monitored gene delivery to swine artery walls with the use of MRI (17). A lentiviral vector was utilized to carry a green fluorescent protein (GFP) gene with gadolinium (Gd), a T1 MRI contrast agent. The GFP-Gd mix was locally administered via a catheter, and the process was monitored by iMRI. Transfer of GFP-Gd in the artery wall was depicted by an enhanced bright ring in the cross-sectional MRI images, and the subsequent histological staining provided evidence of the presence of GFP-positive cells in that region (8).

MRI was utilized to study the systemic distribution of gadolinium (Gd)–trypan blue mix in the canine prostate gland (18–19). An MR-compatible biopsy needle was percutaneously positioned for injecting the Gd–trypan blue mix into the prostate gland. The study accurately correlated MRI and the histological result of the intraprostate biodistribution of the Gd–trypan blue mix (20).

Intraluminal MRI provides high-resolution images of the luminal walls and has been utilized in the cardiovascular system, hepatobiliary system (21), and esophagus (22). It can be developed to facilitate MRI-guided gene therapy delivery and to monitor transgene activity in the body (23).

15.4 ENHANCEMENT OF GENE EXPRESSION BY MRI

The low capability for successful transfection and transduction of the genes or vectors into the target limits the efficacy of gene therapy. In vivo vasculature gene transfection/transduction is approximately ~1% for non-viral vectors and <5% for viral vectors (24–25). Genetic transfer and expression can be enhanced by the usage of a combination of MR techniques with radiofrequency (RF) and focused ultrasound (26).

RF creates local heat that enhances gene transfection and transduction. Controlled heating enhances in vitro gene transfection by increasing cell metabolism, heat shock protein activity, or plasma membrane permeability (27–29). Feasibility for in vitro and in vivo studies to utilize MRI and RF combination systems was studied in a condition known as in-stent neointimal hyperplasia (30). The MR/RF system augmented vascular gene expression (31) by improving transfection of vascular endothelial growth factor (VEGF) gene therapy. The system utilized a loopless MR antenna that delivered RF heat intravascularly with the use of a heat delivery vehicle, which enabled MR thermal mapping of the target vessels for RF heat distribution and monitoring (32–33).

Low-frequency ultrasound facilitates the passage of genes and vectors through the cell membranes and thus improves transfection/transduction and expression of the transgenes. Low-frequency ultrasound can increase cell membrane porosity and decrease the unstirred layer's thickness on the cell surface (34–36). The use of low-frequency ultrasound is limited to superficial organs, as it cannot provide high-resolution images of deep structures or vessel walls for gene targeting. MRI is utilized to guide focused ultrasound energy at a target organ or tissue for improving gene expression via promoting the activity of heat shock protein (hsp) (8, 37). This technique is known as MRI-guided focused ultrasound (MRI-FUS). MRI-FUS mediated human heat shock protein 70 (hsp70) induction in a rat leg enhanced hsp70 messenger RNA (mRNA) expression at the MRI-FUS treated region (8, 29). Modified C6 glioma cells carried a fused gene code under control of the hsp70 promoter. The coding contained two genes: GFP and thymidine kinase (TK). Heat shocks at constant temperature were delivered using MRI-FUS for 3 minutes that elevated the temperatures of in vivo tumors. Increased TK-GFP expression was observed after 24 hours

TABLE 15.1
Application of Magnetic Resonance Imaging and Magnetic Resonance Spectroscopy in Gene Therapy

Method	Monitored Gene Therapy Stage	Reporter/ Marker Gene	Contrast Agent	Targeted Cell Line/Organism	Reference
MRI	Engineered human transferrin receptor (ETR) transgene expression	ETR	Tf-MION	Rat 9L gliosarcoma cells	(11, 13–14)
	Engineered human transferrin receptor (ETR) transgene expression	ETR	Tf-CLIO	Gli36∂EGFR human glioma cells	(11–12)
	Enzymatic activation of EgadMe by injecting β-gal mRNA in embryo	β-gal	EgadMe	Xenopus embryo	(11, 15)
MRS	Adenovirus-mediated arginine kinase (AK) gene transfer	Arginine kinase	Phosphoarginine	Skeletal muscle of neonatal mice	(11, 39)
	Adenovirus-mediated creatine kinase (CK) gene expression	Creatine kinase	Phosphocreatinine	Mice hepatocytes	(11, 40)
	Retrovirus-mediated cytosine deaminase gene expression	Cytosine deaminsase	[^{19}F]fluorocytosine	Colon cancer in rats	(11, 16)

of heat shock delivery (8, 37). Focused ultrasound can be utilized for opening the blood–brain barrier (BBB). Researchers have reported its opening with the use of ultrasound contrast agents. BBB opening during sonication can lead to changes in the signal intensity, which can be detected with the use of MRI (38). A polymer/liposome-based ultrasound contrast agent can be used to carry therapeutic genes across the BBB with the use of MRI-FUS. This can allow the higher passage of transgenes into the brain for enhanced brain targeting (35).

15.5 GENE EXPRESSION TRACKING BY MRI

Gene expression of delivered therapeutic genes should be tracked to discover the level of gene expression, as well as the duration for which the genes are functional at the targets. Direct visualization of genes and vectors cannot be achieved by any clinical imaging modality. MRI can detect gene expression of downstream metabolites (proteins and enzymes) and thus helps track gene expression (41).

Initially, MRI gene expression tracking was based on imaging of MR substrate-attractable receptors/enzymes, which were expressed when transgenes transduced the target. MR signals were generated due to the increased concentration of paramagnetic substrates at the target sites, as MR substrate-attractable receptors/enzymes had an increased affinity for binding or metabolizing the paramagnetic substrates (42). Tf-bound super-magnetic contrast dyes can be used for tumor cell imaging due to increased expression of human transferrin receptor (TfR) genes in these cells (14). Tyrosinase is an enzyme involved in melanogenesis. It has a higher affinity for binding to metal ions like ferric ions that leads to signal hyperintensity on T1-weighted images (43). This capability of tyrosinase is used for catalyzing the conversion of contrast agents to higher relaxivity in tyrosinase-induced MRI (41).

The development of smart contrast agents for gene expression tracking by MRI was enabled by nanotechnology. Smart contrast agents are biochemical pathway-specific and are ligated to magnetic resonance–detectable contrast agent molecules or nanoparticles. The transgene expression leads to activation of downstream receptors and enzymes, causing accumulation of smart contrast dyes on these receptors through receptor-ligand interactions (44). Novel gadolinium-bisamides have been designed and synthesized as enzyme-catalyzed MR contrast dyes for increasing longitudinal (R1) relaxivity (45).

As previously discussed gene-expressed receptors and enzymes are used as reporters or markers for image generation in MRI. Thus, developing real-time gene tracking with the use of MRI will require the development of novel dual gene carriers that can be utilized to transmit and express two genes: a reporter/marker gene and a therapeutic gene at the target site (46).

15.6 GENE THERAPY FOLLOW-UP BY MRI

MRI possesses the capability for anatomic imaging for organ morphology observation and functional imaging of organ perfusion, as well as metabolic and mechanical function assessment. The gene therapy follow-up can use MRI to evaluate post-reatment organ/system recovery (47–49). Evaluation of cardiac ischemia/infarction tissue recovery after gene therapy can be done by multiple magnetic resonance techniques like perfusion MRI, cardiac MR tagging for myocardial deformation analysis, and cardiac MR spectroscopy to assess cardiac energy metabolism. Gene therapy outcomes of the vascular system include the limited occurrence of restenosis after stenting and balloon angioplasty, preventing vein graft stenosis, preventing thrombus formation, and enhanced therapeutic angiogenesis for cardiac and limb ischemia (50). Catheter angiography is the gold-standard technique for follow-up of vascular gene therapy but is invasive. Non-invasive techniques like MRI angiography and perfusion MRI can also be beneficial for the assessment of the extent of the success of vascular gene therapy (50).

15.7 CONCLUSION

Genetic therapeutics is an encouraging approach used to address numerous diseases with a permanent cure. Molecular imaging technology in association with gene therapy will witness a research boom with the evolution of gene therapy. Genetic engineering will help with the development of robust viral and non-viral vectors, and the development of bicistronic vectors will enable targeting two target proteins from a single mRNA. Continued refinements in molecular probe chemistry will generate the next generation of probes that have enhanced specificity and sensitivity profiles. Intraluminal MRI allows precise biodistribution monitoring of the delivered transgenes. Gene expression enhancement by RF and focused ultrasound can utilize the MR thermomapping technique. Nanotechnology has boosted target-specific molecular MR imaging as a non-invasive in vivo evaluation technique for gene therapy. Pre- and post-gene therapy functional MRI scans can help assess gene therapy success. The ultimate goal is to develop molecular imaging technologies that can provide early data on gene delivery and expression to facilitate the evaluation of successful gene therapy in patients.

REFERENCES

1. Mislow JMK, Golby AJ, Black PM. Origins of Intraoperative MRI. Vol. 20, Neurosurgery Clinics of North America. Elsevier; 2009. p. 137–146.
2. Azmi H, Gibbons M, DeVito MC, Schlesinger M, Kreitner J, Freguletti T, et al. The interventional magnetic resonance imaging suite: Experience in the design, development, and implementation in a pre-existing radiology space and review of concepts. *Surg Neurol Int.* 2019;10(101):101.
3. Larson PS, Starr PA, Bates G, Tansey L, Richardson RM, Martin AJ. An optimized system for interventional magnetic resonance imaging-guided stereotactic surgery: Preliminary evaluation of targeting accuracy. *Oper Neurosurg* [Internet]. 2012 [cited 2021 Jul 6];70(1):95–103. Available from: /pmc/articles/PMC3249469/.
4. Scheer JK, Hamelin T, Chang L, Lemkuil B, Carter BS, Chen CC. Real-time magnetic resonance imaging-guided biopsy using smartframe® stereotaxis in the setting of a conventional diagnostic magnetic resonance imaging suite. *Oper Neurosurg* [Internet]. 2017 Jun 1 [cited 2021 Jul 6];13(3):329–337. Available from: https://academic.oup.com/ons/article/13/3/329/2966509.
5. Kettenbach J, Kacher DF, Kanan AR, Rostenberg B, Fairhurst J, Stadler A, et al. Intraoperative and interventional MRI: Recommendations for a safe environment

[Internet]. Vol. 15, Minimally Invasive Therapy and Allied Technologies. Taylor & Francis; 2006 [cited 2021 Jul 6]. p. 53–64. Available from: https://www.tandfonline.com/doi/abs/10.1080/13645700600640774.

6. Kettenbach J, Kacher DF, Koskinen SK, Silverman SG, Nabavi A, Gering D, et al. Interventional and intraoperative magnetic resonance imaging. *Annu Rev Biomed Eng* [Internet]. 2000 Nov 28 [cited 2021 Jul 6];2(2000):661–690. Available from: www.annualreviews.org.
7. Gene therapy : The future is now. 2020;(April):2020. Steve Silberberg, OD. *Optometry Times Journal*, April digital edition 2020, Volume 12, Issue 4.
8. Yang X, Atalar E. MRI-guided gene therapy. *FEBS Lett.* 2006;580(12):2958–2961.
9. Weissleder R, Mahmood U. Molecular imaging [Internet]. Vol. 219, Radiology. Radiological Society of North America Inc.; 2001 [cited 2021 Jul 6]. p. 316–333. Available from: https://pubs.rsna.org/doi/abs/10.1148/radiology.219.2.r01ma19316.
10. Yang X. Imaging of vascular gene therapy [Internet]. Vol. 228, Radiology. Radiological Society of North America; 2003 [cited 2021 Jul 6]. p. 36–49. Available from: https://pubs.rsna.org/doi/abs/10.1148/radiol.2281020307.
11. Min JJ, Gambhir SS. Gene therapy progress and prospects: Noninvasive imaging of gene therapy in living subjects [Internet]. Vol. 11, Gene Therapy. Nature Publishing Group; 2004 [cited 2021 Jul 6]. p. 115–125. Available from: www.nature.com/gt.
12. Ichikawa T, Högemann D, Saeki Y, Tyminski E, Terada K, Weissleder R, et al. MRI of transgene expression: Correlation to therapeutic gene expression. Neoplasia. 2002 Jan 1;4(6):523–530.
13. Weissleder R, Moore A, Mahmood U, Bhorade R, Benveniste H, Chiocca EA, et al. In vivo magnetic resonance imaging of transgene expression. Nat Med [Internet]. 2000 Mar [cited 2021 Jul 6];6(3):351–354. Available from: https://www.nature.com/articles/nm0300_351.
14. Moore A, Josephson L, Bhorade RM, Basilion JP, Weissleder R. Human transferrin receptor gene as a marker gene for MR imaging. *Radiology* [Internet]. 2001 Oct 1 [cited 2021 Jul 6];221(1):244–250. Available from: https://pubs.rsna.org/doi/abs/10.1148/radiol.2211001784.
15. Louie AY, Hüber MM, Ahrens ET, Rothbächer U, Moats R, Jacobs RE, et al. In vivo visualization of gene expression using magnetic resonance imaging. *Nat Biotechnol* [Internet]. 2000 [cited 2021 Jul 6];18(3):321–325. Available from: https://www.nature.com/articles/nbt0300_321.
16. Stegman LD, Rehemtulla A, Hamstra DA, Rice DJ, Jonas SJ, Stout KL, et al. Diffusion MRI detects early events in the response of a glioma model to the yeast cytosine deaminase gene therapy strategy. *Gene Ther* [Internet]. 2000 Jun 14 [cited 2021 Jul 6];7(12):1005–1010. Available from: www.nature.com/gt.
17. Yang X, Atalar E, Li D, Serfaty JM, Wang D, Kumar A, et al. Magnetic resonance imaging permits in vivo monitoring of catheter-based vascular gene delivery. *Circulation* [Internet]. 2001 Oct 2 [cited 2021 Jul 6];104(14):1588–1590. Available from: http://www.circulationaha.org.
18. Susil RC, Krieger A, Derbyshire JA, Tanacs A, Whitcomb LL, Fichtinger G, et al. System for MR image-guided prostate interventions: Canine study. *Radiology* [Internet]. 2003 Sep 1 [cited 2021 Jul 6];228(3):886–894. Available from: https://pubs.rsna.org/doi/abs/10.1148/radiol.2283020911.
19. Chowning SL, Susil RC, Krieger A, Fichtinger G, Whitcomb LL, Atalar E. A preliminary analysis and model of prostate injection distributions. *Prostate* [Internet]. 2006 Mar 1 [cited 2021 Jul 6];66(4):344–357. Available from: https://onlinelibrary.wiley.com/doi/full/10.1002/pros.20298.
20. Concilio SC, Russell SJ, Peng KW. A brief review of reporter gene imaging in oncolytic virotherapy and gene therapy. Vol. 21, Molecular Therapy—Oncolytics. Cell Press; 2021. p. 98–109.

21. Arepally A, Georgiades C, Hofmann LV., Choti M, Thuluvath P, Bluemke DA. Hilar cholangiocarcinoma: Staging with intrabiliary MRI [Internet]. Vol. 183, American Journal of Roentgenology. American Roentgen Ray Society; 2004 [cited 2021 Jul 6]. p. 1071–1074. Available from: www.ajronline.org.
22. Shunk KA, Lima JAC, Heldman AW, Atalar E. *Transesophageal Magnetic Resonance Imaging* 41:722–726 (1999), Wiley-Liss, Inc.
23. Liu Y, Li S, Wu Y, Wu F, Chang Y, Li H, et al. The added value of vessel wall MRI in the detection of intraluminal thrombus in patients suspected of craniocervical artery dissection. *Aging Dis* [Internet]. [cited 2021 Jul 6]. Available from: http://www.aginganddisease.org/EN/abstract/abstract148101.shtml.
24. Ylä-Herttuala S, Martin JF. Cardiovascular gene therapy [Internet]. Vol. 355, Lancet. Elsevier B.V.; 2000 [cited 2021 Jul 6]. p. 213–222. Available from: http://www.thelancet.com/article/S014067369904180X/fulltext.
25. Mazzolai L, Alatri A, Rivière AB, De Carlo M, Heiss C, Espinola-Klein C, et al. Progress in aorta and peripheral cardiovascular disease research. *Cardiovasc Res* [Internet]. 2021 Apr 23 [cited 2021 Jul 6]. Available from: https://academic.oup.com/cardiovascres/advance-article/doi/10.1093/cvr/cvab144/6248085.
26. Arrigoni F, Spiliopoulos S, de Cataldo C, Reppas L, Palumbo P, Mazioti A, et al. A bicentric propensity score matched study comparing percutaneous computed tomography—guided radiofrequency ablation to magnetic resonance—guided focused ultrasound for the treatment of osteoid osteoma. *J Vasc Interv Radiol*. 2021 Jul 1;32(7):1044–1051.
27. Doukas AG, Flotte TJ. Physical characteristics and biological effects of laser-induced stress waves [Internet]. Vol. 22, Ultrasound in Medicine and Biology. Pergamon Press Ltd; 1996 [cited 2021 Jul 6]. p. 151–164. Available from: http://www.umbjournal.org/article/0301562995020268/fulltext.
28. View of Maximizing Local Access to Therapeutic Deliveries in Glioblastoma. Part IV: Image-guided, remote-controlled opening of the blood—brain barrier for systemic brain tumor therapy | Exon publications [Internet]. [cited 2021 Jul 6]. Available from: https://exonpublications.com/index.php/exon/article/view/142/273.
29. Voellmy R, Zürcher O, Zürcher M, de Viragh PA, Hall AK, Roberts SM. Targeted heat activation of HSP promoters in the skin of mammalian animals and humans. *Cell Stress Chaperones* [Internet]. 2018 Jul 1 [cited 2021 Jul 6];23(4):455–466. Available from: /pmc/articles/PMC6045553/.
30. Gao F, Qiu B, Kar S, Zhan X, Hofmann LV., Yang X. Intravascular magnetic resonance/radiofrequency may enhance gene therapy for prevention of in-stent neointimal hyperplasia. *Acad Radiol* [Internet]. 2006 Apr [cited 2021 Jul 6];13(4):526–530. Available from: /pmc/articles/PMC1413577/.
31. Du X, Qiu B, Zhan X, Kolmakova A, Gao F, Hofmann LV., et al. Radiofrequency-enhanced vascular gene transduction and expression for intravascular MR imaging-guided therapy: Feasibility study in pigs. *Radiology* [Internet]. 2005 Sep 1 [cited 2021 Jul 6];236(3): 939–944. Available from: https://pubs.rsna.org/doi/abs/10.1148/radiol.2363041021.
32. Qiu B, El-Sharkawy AM, Paliwal V, Karmarkar P, Gao F, Atalar E, et al. Simultaneous radiofrequency (RF) heating and magnetic resonance (MR) thermal mapping using an intravascular MR imaging/RF heating system. *Magn Reson Med* [Internet]. 2005 Jul 1 [cited 2021 Jul 6];54(1):226–230. Available from: www.interscience.wiley.com.
33. Qiu B, Yeung CJ, Du X, Atalar E, Yang X. Development of an intravascular heating source using an MR imaging guidewire. *J Magn Reson Imaging* [Internet]. 2002 Dec 1 [cited 2021 Jul 6];16(6):716–720. Available from: www.interscience.wiley.com.
34. Unger EC, McCreery TP, Sweitzer RH. Ultrasound enhances gene expression of liposomal transfection. *Invest Radiol*. 1997 Dec;32(12):723–727.
35. Stavarache MA, Chazen JL, Kaplitt MG. Innovative applications of MR-guided focused ultrasound for neurological disorders. *World Neurosurg*. 2021 Jan 1;145:581–589.

36. Lawrie A, Brisken AF, Francis SE, Tayler DI, Chamberlain J, Crossman DC, et al. Ultrasound enhances reporter gene expression after transfection of vascular cells in vitro [Internet]. 1999 [cited 2021 Jul 6]. Available from: http://www.circulationaha.org.
37. Guilhon E, Quesson B, Moraud-Gaudry F, de Verneuil H, Canioni P, Salomir R, et al. Image-guided control of transgene expression based on local hyperthermia. *Mol Imaging* [Internet]. 2003 Jan 1 [cited 2021 Jul 6];2(1):153535002003021. Available from: https://journals.sagepub.com/doi/full/10.1162/15353500200302151.
38. Hynynen K, McDannold N, Vykhodtseva N, Jolesz FA. Noninvasive MR imaging-guided focal opening of the blood-brain barrier in rabbits. *Radiology* [Internet]. 2001 Sep 1 [cited 2021 Jul 6];220(3):640–646. Available from: https://pubs.rsna.org/doi/abs/10.1148/radiol.2202001804.
39. Walter G, Barton ER, Sweeney HL. Noninvasive measurement of gene expression in skeletal muscle. *Proc Natl Acad Sci* [Internet]. 2000 May 9 [cited 2021 Jul 6];97(10):5151–5155. Available from: https://www.pnas.org/content/97/10/5151.
40. Auricchio A, Zhou R, Wilson JM, Glickson JD. In vivo detection of gene expression in liver by 31P nuclear magnetic resonance spectroscopy employing creatine kinase as a marker gene. *Proc Natl Acad Sci* [Internet]. 2001 Apr 24 [cited 2021 Jul 6];98(9): 5205–5210. Available from: https://www.pnas.org/content/98/9/5205.
41. Sun Q, Prato FS, Goldhawk DE. Optimizing reporter gene expression for molecular magnetic resonance imaging : Lessons from the Magnetosome. *Bioimaging* [Internet]. 2020 May 26 [cited 2021 Jul 6];201–214. Available from: https://www.taylorfrancis.com/chapters/edit/10.1201/9780429260971-9/optimizing-reporter-gene-expression-molecular-magnetic-resonance-imaging-qin-sun-frank-prato-donna-goldhawk.
42. Allport JR, Weissleder R. In vivo imaging of gene and cell therapies. *Exp Hematol* [Internet]. 2001 Nov 1 [cited 2021 Jul 6];29(11):1237–1246. Available from: http://www.exphem.org/article/S0301472X01007391/fulltext.
43. Enochs WS, Petherick P, Bogdanova A, Mohr U, Weissleder R. Paramagnetic metal scavenging by melanin: MR imaging. [Internet]. 1997 Aug 1 [cited 2021 Jul 6];204(2): 417–423. Availablefrom: https://pubs.rsna.org/doi/abs/10.1148/radiology.204.2.9240529.
44. Paul Winnard, Raman V. Real time non-invasive imaging of receptor—ligand interactions in vivo. *J Cell Biochem* [Internet]. 2003 Oct 15 [cited 2021 Jul 6];90(3):454–563. Available from: https://onlinelibrary.wiley.com/doi/full/10.1002/jcb.10616.
45. Manuel Querol, John W. Chen, Ralph Weissleder, Alexei Bogdanov J. DTPA-bisamide-based MR sensor agents for peroxidase imaging. *Org Lett* [Internet]. 2005 Apr 28 [cited 2021 Jul 6];7(9):1719–1722. Available from: https://pubs.acs.org/doi/abs/10.1021/ol050208v.
46. Kelly JJ, Saee-Marand M, Nyström NN, Evans MM, Chen Y, Martinez FM, et al. Safe harbor-targeted CRISPR-Cas9 homology-independent targeted integration for multimodality reporter gene-based cell tracking. *Sci Adv* [Internet]. 2021 Jan 1 [cited 2021 Jul 6];7(4):eabc3791. Available from: https://advances.sciencemag.org/content/7/4/eabc3791.
47. Gray-Edwards HL, Maguire AS, Salibi N, Ellis LE, Voss TL, Diffie EB, et al. 7T MRI predicts amelioration of neurodegeneration in the Brain after AAV gene therapy. *Mol Ther—Methods Clin Dev*. 2020 Jun 12;17:258–270.
48. Figueroa-Bonaparte S, Llauger J, Segovia S, Belmonte I, Pedrosa I, Montiel E, et al. Quantitative muscle MRI to follow up late onset Pompe patients: A prospective study. *Sci Reports* 2018 81 [Internet]. 2018 Jul 18 [cited 2021 Jul 6];8(1):1–11. Available from: https://www.nature.com/articles/s41598-018-29170-7.
49. Barp A, Carraro E, Albamonte E, Salmin F, Lunetta C, Comi G Pietro, et al. Muscle MRI in two SMA patients on nusinersen treatment: A two years follow-up. *J Neurol Sci*. 2020 Oct 15;417:117067.
50. HI M, X Y. Imaging after vascular gene therapy. *Eur J Radiol* [Internet]. 2005 Nov [cited 2021 Jul 6];56(2):165–170. Available from: https://pubmed.ncbi.nlm.nih.gov/16233890/.

Index

Page locators in **bold** indicate a table Page locators in *italics* indicate a figure

H

I

J

K

L

Printed in the United States
by Baker & Taylor Publisher Services